TRENDS IN THYROID CANCER RESEARCH

HORIZONS IN CANCER RESEARCH
VOLUME 37

HORIZONS IN CANCER RESEARCH

Volume 1: Prostate Cancer
John N. Lucas (Editor)
ISBN 1-59454-100-0
Volume 2: Trends in Ovarian Cancer Research
A. P. Bardos (Editor)
ISBN 1-59454-023-3
Volume 3: Percutaneous Cryotherapy of Renal Cell Carcinoma under an Open MRI System
Junta Harada, Kazuo Miyasaka and Sajio Sumida (Editors)
ISBN 1-59454-169-8
Volume 4: Focus on Colorectal Cancer Research
Julia D. Martinez (Editor)
ISBN 1-59454-101-9
Volume 5: Focus on Leukemia Research
Rafael M. Romero (Editor)
ISBN 1-59454-093-4
Volume 6: Progress in Bladder Cancer Research
A. M. Mallory (Editor)
ISBN 1-59454-129-9
Volume 7: Trends in Prostate Cancer Research
John N. Lucas (Editor)
ISBN 1-59454-265-1
Volume 8: Tumor Budding in Colorectal Cancer Recent Progress in Colorectal Cancer Research
Tadahiko Masaki (Editor)
ISBN 1-59454-189-2
Volume 9: Trends in Breast Cancer Research
Andrew P. Yao (Editor)
ISBN 1-59454-134-5
Volume 10: Trends in Leukemia Research
Rafael M. Romero (Editor)
ISBN 1-59454-311-9
Volume 11: Liver Cancer: New Research
Felix Lee (Editor)
ISBN 1-59454-182-5
Volume 12: Focus on Lung Cancer
Robert L. Carafaro (Editor)
ISBN 1-59454-082-9
Volume 13: Treatment of Ovarian Cancer
A. P. Bardos (Editor)
ISBN 1-59454-022-5
Volume 14: Focus on Kidney Cancer Research
Kelvin R. Nunez (Editor)
ISBN 1-59454-110-8
Volume 15: Focus on Pacreatic Cancer Research
Maxwell A. Loft (Editor)
ISBN 1-59454-270-8
Volume 16: Peritoneal Carinomatosis from Ovarian Cancer
Kostantinos N. Chatzigeorgiou and John N. Bontis (Editors)
ISBN 1-59454-398-4
Volume 17: Trends in Pacreatic Cancer Research
Maxwell A. Loft (Editor)
ISBN 1-59454-524-3
Volume 18: Trends in Kidney Cancer Research
Kelvin R. Nunez (Editor)
ISBN 1-59454-141-8
Volume 19: Ovarian Cancer: New Research
A. P. Bardos (Editor)
ISBN 1-59454-241-4
Volume 20: Gene Therapy in Cancer
Grace W. Redberry (Editor)
ISBN 1-59454-288-0
Volume 21: Lung Cancer New Research
Robert L. Carafaro (Editor)
ISBN 1-59454-
Volume 22: New Developments in Bone Cancer Research
Catherine E. O'Neil (Editor)
ISBN 1-59454-337-2
Volume 23: New Developments in Breast Cancer Research
Andrew P. Yao (Editor)
ISBN 1-59454-809-9
Volume 24: Trends in Bone Cancer Research
E. V. Birch (Editor)
ISBN 1-59454-346-1

Volume 25: Focus on Brain Cancer Research
Andrew V. Yang (Editor)
ISBN 1-59454-973-7

Volume 26: Cancer Vaccine: New Research
(Editor)
ISBN 1-59454-968-0

Volume 27: Brain Cancer Therapy and Surgical Interventions
Andrew V. Yang (Editor)
ISBN 1-59454-974-5

Volume 28: Trends in Brain Cancer Research
Andrew V. Yang (Editor)
ISBN 1-59454-972-9

Volume 29: New Developments in Cancer Research
Lee P. Jeffries (Editor)
ISBN 1-60021-102-X

Volume 30: Progress in Skin Cancer Research
V.L. Heinz (Editor)
ISBN 1-60021-095-3

Volume 31: Skin Cancer: New Research
V.L. Heinz (Editor)
ISBN 1-60021-096-1

Volume32: Trends in Cancer Research
Lee P. Jeffries (Editor)
ISBN 1-60021-100-3

Volume33: Frontiers in Cancer Reseacrh
Lee P. Jeffries (Editor)
ISBN 1-60021-101-1

Volume 34: New Topics in Cancer Research
Fredrick G. Drabell (Editor)
ISBN 1-60021-155-0

Volume 35: Leading Edge Cancer Research
Lee P. Jeffries (Editor)
ISBN 1-60021- 197-6

Volume 36: New Breast Cancer Research
Andrew P. Yao *(Editor)*
ISBN 1-59454-932-X

Volume 37: Trends in Thyroid Cancer
Carl A. Milton (Editor)
ISBN 1-59454-627-4

TRENDS IN THYROID CANCER RESEARCH

HORIZONS IN CANCER RESEARCH
VOLUME 37

CARL A. MILTON
EDITOR

Nova Biomedical Books
New York

Library of Congress Cataloging-in-Publication Data
Available upon request.

ISBN 1-59454-627-4

Published by Nova Science Publishers, Inc. ✦New York

CONTENTS

PREFACE

Thyroid cancer is cancer of the thyroid gland. These may be of many types including papillary, follicular, Hurthle cell (aka oxyphilic or oncocytic), or medullary cancers. Surgery plays an important role in treating these cancers. The thyroid concentrates iodine and so is extremely sensitive to the effects of various radioactive isotopes of iodine produced by nuclear fission. These radioactive isotopes increase the chances of developing cancer, though thyroid cancer can develop even without any exposure to radioactivity. Some evidence suggests that insufficient or excessive dietary iodine may also increase the risk for thyroid cancer. This new book presents the latest research in this field.

According to current data, it seems probable that there is no interruption along the evolution of different follicular thyroid neoplasias. Most likely, transforming events responsible for the transition from a normal to tumoral cell starts with molecular changes that determine the appearance of follicular adenoma. Ulterior changes favor the development of follicular cancer. Probably, the generation of papillary carcinoma follows a different pathway without passing through a previous phase of follicular adenoma. Subsequently, genetic changes render the cell prone to dedifferentiation setting the basis for the development of anaplastic thyroid cancer. Those incidental molecular changes determine a dramatic worsening in the prognosis of thyroid cancer. The investigation of thyroid tumors is likely to be instructive in view of the spectrum they span, from benign adenomas to poorly differentiated carcinomas.

It has been proven that molecular alterations in tumoral thyroid cells are predisposed by genomic instability. Usually, changes of proto-oncogenes represent an early event, whereas mutations of suppressor genes are usually a late phenomenon. The onset of an aggressive behavior may be studied, and perhaps can be predicted in the future, by molecular medicine.

As discussed in chapter one, the clinical application of the growing understanding of gene alterations involved in thyroidal oncogenesis is becoming a reality. Such knowledge might contribute to improve our diagnostic accuracy, by helping us to characterize malignant or benign cells, as well as to predict tumor outcome or to state its origin. Likewise, it might be useful to predict the response to conventional therapies or the future implications of pharmacogenetics.

The impressive advance of molecular medicine over the last few years is providing us an attractive vision of the new possibilities in diagnosis and treatments of thyroid cancer helping us to understand its biological behavior.

In addition, molecular medicine applications ought to be considered in determining the prognosis of spontaneous and familiar carcinomas. Such information can significantly improve our current clinical-pathologic prognostic methods.

In recent years, several alterations involving oncogenes and tumor suppressor genes have been identified in thyroid cancer. However, although some advances have been made to the understanding of the molecular mechanisms that determine thyroid malignancies, the absence of crucial information on the mechanisms underlying increased expansion and survival of thyroid cancer cells does not allow the development of standard and reliable treatments, with the exception of unifocal non-metastatic papillary microcarcinoma. Apoptosis is a key mechanism governing the development of multicellular organisms and maintenance of tissue homeostasis. It is becoming increasingly clear that impaired apoptosis is a critical component of the multi-step tumorigenesis process as discussed in chapter two. Although CD95 is expressed in essentially all the histological variants of thyroid carcinomas, CD95 cross-linking fails to induce cell death in thyroid tumor cells. It has been demonstrated that thyrocytes produce CD95L and are able to kill infiltrating T lymphocytes expressing CD95. Therefore refractoriness to CD95 stimulation in thyroid tumors may be a critical event in tumorigenesis. Indeed, the abundant expression of CD95L in malignant tumors may result in the so called "tumor counterattack", a defence process that helps cancer cells to escape immune surveillance mechanisms by eliminating infiltrating lymphocytes. Traditional antineoplastic therapy is based on the use of chemotherapeutic compounds, which exert a cytotoxic effect on proliferating cells and promote the destruction of sensitive tumors. Therefore, the development of effective anti-apoptotic mechanisms can result in the resistance of malignant cell to chemotherapy. It has been recently investigated the mechanisms responsible for the widespread refractoriness to chemotherapeutic drugs observed in thyroid cancers. It has been found that malignant thyroid carcinoma cells express high levels of Bcl-2 and Bcl-xL. All the histological thyroid cancer variants examined produced interleukin-4 (IL-4) and interleukin-10 (IL-10), which increased FLIP, PED, Bcl-2 and Bcl-xL levels and protected thyroid cells from chemotherapeutic agents and from cell death induced by CD95. Exposure to neutralizing antibodies against IL-4 and IL-10 resulted in down modulation of FLIP, PED, Bcl-2 and Bcl-xL, death of a considerable percentage of thyroid cancer cells and sensitization of the residual tumor population to cytotoxic drugs- and CD95- induced apoptosis. Thus, IL-4 and IL-10 may represent new therapeutic targets for the treatment of epithelial cancer. It is therefore likely that presence of these cytokines in the cancer microenvironment should promote survival activating the ability of cancer cells to up regulate anti-apoptotic genes leading to apoptosis resistance. These studies may provide key molecular bases to the understanding of thyroid cancer pathogenesis and the definition of novel therapeutic strategies.

Papillary cancer and follicular cancer are types of differentiated thyroid cancers. They are considered to share the same developmental origin, the same thyroid follicular epithelial cells and show distinct biological behavior. Although several studies have demonstrated differences in the biological characteristics of these cancers, little is known about the genetic backgrounds that underlie the differences in these cancers. The clarification of the genetic background can lead to the understanding of thyroid carcinogenesis, proper therapeutic strategies, and development of the molecular targeting drugs. Aberrant activation of RAS-RAF-MEK-MAP kinase signaling pathway is frequently found in thyroid cancer. The pathway transmits the mitogenic signal to the nucleus, and constitutive activation of the pathway is thought to promote uncontrolled cell division. In our series, BRAF mutation was detected exclusively in papillary cancer (30-60%), and was exclusively V599E (a single nucleotide change of A-T at nucleotide 1796), but not in follicular cancers or adenomas. RAS mutations are rare in sporadic papillary cancers, but are observed in 20-50% of follicular cancers, being particularly common as NRAS Q61R mutations. In chapter 3, the authors explain the role of RAS-RAF-MEK-MAP kinase pathway in carcinogenesis of the thyroid and its clinical implication based on our study. In addition, we review the current knowledge in this field.

Iodine is the heaviest and richest in electrons among required elements in the animal diet. Inorganic iodides are necessary for all living vegetable and animal cells, but only the vertebrates have the thyroid gland and its iodinated hormones.

Impaired intrathyroidal iodine metabolism represents one of the most peculiar abnormalities present in thyroid neoplastic tissue. The biological activity of peroxidase, although normal in benign cold adenomas, was decreased or absent in thyroid carcinomas, resulting in a low iodine organification. As a consequence, in thyroid cancer tissues, a low intrathyroidal iodine concentration, a low degree of iodination of thyroglobulin and a low rate of thyroid hormones synthesis were observed. The altered iodine intrathyroidal metabolism may confer on tumor cells a proliferative advantage as a result of the loss of the iodine autoregulating process.

Malignant disease of the thyroid gland is a heterogeneous disorder that affects all age groups, but is more serious in the elderly. The relation of iodine deficiency to enlargement of the thyroid gland, or goiter, was first shown by David Marine, who found that hyperplasic changes occurred regularly in the thyroid when the iodine concentration fell below 0.1%. Papillary carcinoma of the thyroid may be more common in areas with iodination of salt or a high-iodine diet. Follicular carcinoma is much more common in iodine-deficient goiterous areas. The high incidence of follicular neoplasia in goiterous area may be related to the prolonged stimulatory effects of thyroid-stimulating hormone (TSH). In animals, the chronic stimulation of the thyroid by TSH is known to produce thyroid neoplasmes.

In chapter four, the authors discuss how the role of iodine nutrition in the pathogenesis of thyroid cancer (TC) is both complex and controversial. Several investigators have reported an association between iodization and subsequent changes in thyroid cancer, an increase for papillary carcinoma and a decline for follicular and anaplastic carcinoma. Improved iodine intake in previously iodine-deficient communities has also been associated with an increased incidence of papillary thyroid cancer (PTC). These so-called "papillarization" is characterized by an increase in the ratio of papillary to follicular thyroid cancers (FTC), a decrease in PTC size, and an attenuation of the malignant phenotype. There is, however, no clear relationship between increased dietary iodine and higher total TC rates. Other factors such as geographic and ethnic variations in the incidence of thyroid cancer are considerable. The relationship between thyroid cancer and iodine status has often been debated without agreement being reached on many aspects, including on a possible causal relationship. Overall, many data have shown that correction of iodine deficiency decreases the risk of, and the morbidity form, thyroid cancer.

Although prognosis of patients with differentiated thyroid cancer is generally favorable, undifferentiated/anaplastic thyroid cancer is one of the most aggressive malignancies. The remarkable difference in prognosis between two types of thyroid cancer indicates that there is a large biological difference between them. The authors of chapter five have been involved in the studies for exploring new biomarkers to evaluate aggressiveness of thyroid cancer. These markers are useful not only for predicting prognosis but also for developing new strategies against aggressive thyroid cancer.

They recently established three different thyroid cancer cell lines, KTC-1, KTC-2 and KTC-3. KTC-1 cells are derived from a patient with poorly differentiated thyroid papillary carcinoma. KTC-2 cells are derived from a patient with anaplastic transformation from papillary thyroid carcinoma. KTC-3 cells are derived from a patient with primary anaplastic thyroid carcinoma.

To test the hypothesis that overexpression of human epidermal growth factor receptor (HER) 1 promotes malignant progression in thyroid cancer, the relationship among expression levels of HER1 and a cognate receptor HER2 and effects of a HER1 tyrosine kinase inhibitor, gefitinib on cell proliferation, cytokine secretion and the expression level of one of thyroid differentiation markers, thyroglobulin were investigated using these three cell lines. Gefitinib inhibited *in vitro* growth of the thyroid cancer cells in dose- and time-dependent manners. No significant correlation was observed between the antitumor effect of gefitinib and expression level of HER1 or HER2. Gefitinib significantly decreased secretion of angiogenic cytokines, vascular endothelial growth factor (VEGF) and interleukin (IL)-8 in KTC-2 cells. In contrast, gefitinib significantly increased secretion of both angiogenic cytokines in KTC-3 cells. Changes in secretion of IL-6 and parathyroid hormone-related protein (PTHrP) induced by gefitinib were also different among thyroid cancer cell lines. Gefitinib did not significantly change the expression level of thyroglobulin in any thyroid cancer cell lines. These findings suggest that gefitinib is effective for the treatment of aggressive thyroid cancer but its influences on cytokine secretion from tumor cells are different among thyroid cancers.

Thrombospondin (TSP)-1 has been identified as an anti-angiogenic factor. The authors recently demonstrated that TSP-1 expression negatively related to extrathyroidal infiltration as well as angiogenesis in patients with papillary thyroid carcinoma. To elucidate the relationship between expression levels of p53 and TSP-1 in thyroid cancer, they studied their expression levels in 75 papillary thyroid carcinomas. There was an inverse correlation between expression levels of TSP-1 and p53. Additionally, the effects of TSP-1 and anti-TSP-1 antibody on invasion were investigated in six thyroid cancer cell lines using the *in vitro* invasion assay. Angiogenesis-related factors, VEGF, VEGF-C, TSP-1 and TSP-1 receptor (CD36) were expressed at various levels in all cell lines. Invasion tended to be inhibited by TSP-1 in five of the six cell lines. These effects inversely related to the expression level of VEGF or VEGF-C. The effects of anti-TSP-1 antibody on invasion differed among cell lines. These findings indicate that TSP-1 plays a certain role in invasion of thyroid cancer cells, and that the effects of TSP-1 and anti-TSP-1 antibody on invasion are different among thyroid cancers.

In chapter six, the authors will review the role of telomerase in carcinogenesis of thyroid and its potential aplication for the diagnosis of carcinomas. Human telomeres are composed of 5,000 to 15,000 base pairs, with a repeat sequence of TTAGGG. Their role is to protect the end of chromosomes. Under unknown circumstances, cells may become immortal by stabilizing the length of telomeres and this almost always occurs through the activation of telomerase. Telomerase is a ribonucleoprotein that adds the telomeric repeats onto the 3′end of chromosomes. It has two major components: the human telomerase RNA (hTR), which is present in all somatic cells as a template on which telomeric repeats are added to the chromosome, and the catalitic subunit called human telomerase reverse transcriptase (hTERT). Activity of Telomerase (TA) plays a major role in maintaining genetic integrity while the cells are in mitotic cycles and it is normally detected in germ cells, stem cells and lymphocytes. Also, TA has been demonstrated in neoplasms, mainly in those with endocrine differentiation, such as neoplasms of the thyroid, breast, prostate, parathyroid and adrenal gland. Theirr experience, in agreement with scientific literature, shows that around 50% of papillary carcinomas and 80% of follicular carcinomas had TA, whereas adenomas and other benign lesions rarely express TA. This result could be achieved in frozen tissue and also in material obtained by Fine Needle Aspirate (FNA) of thyroid. It is widely accepted that thyroid FNA is a useful tool in the screening of nodules for surgery, with sensitivity ranging from 65% to 99%, and specificity from 72% to100%. Nevertheless, 15-20% of FNAs are not diagnostic because the distinction between adenomatous nodules and follicular neoplasms could not be achieved. The authors attempted to determine whether TA could improve the sensitivity of cytology, mainly in this group of lesions with inconclusive cytological diagnosis, for a more accurate selection of patients before thyroidectomy.

Malignant alterations in the thyroid gland, especially carcinoma, can occur in solitary nodules, diffuse enlarged gland or in a gland with multiple nodules, and they are of special interest in the diagnosis and treatment because of uncertain clinical evaluation as well as their frequency and malignant potential as discussed in chapter seven.

Finding of malignances in solitary thyroid gland nodules represent an entity itself in thyroid surgery and endocrinology because of frequency in occurrence and differential diagnosis of thyroid diseases.

Similarities in clinical characteristics and differences in the histological structure and development of the disease, request quick and adequate application of all available diagnostic procedures in evaluation of disease.

After all clinic methods of examination, surgery includes necessary range of extraction of tissue at benign changes while at malignant changes radical intervention of the gland is suggested and if it is necessary on the surrounding structures of the neck.

“Biopsio Ex Tempore” still represents vital method in histological diagnosis and help in making a decision about extensiveness of operative procedure. Because of that, surgery represents both a diagnostic and therapeutic procedure. Data analysis shows the presence of carcinoma in solitary thyroid gland nodules in 15% of all cases.

The aim of this study is to point out validity of diagnostic procedures, frequency of occurrence and types of changes as well as principles in treatment of thyroid gland carcinoma with emphasis on solitary nodules where carcinoma is the most frequent.

Radioiodine-131 is used in differentiated thyroid cancer (DTC) for ablation of post surgical thyroid remnants and destruction of metastasis. As it is commonly accepted that repeated RAI treatments in metastatic DTC with lower doses are less effective, large doses of I-131 are routinely administered to patients for this purpose. The dose limiting toxicity of radioiodine treatment on the bone marrow and the absorbed doses in the subsequent organs (act as platform during iodine excretion) are a great concern in internal dosimetry. The dosimetric calculations to determine the radiation doses in different organs involve many factors; e.g. percent uptake, effective half life, tumor size, turnover of activity etc. An extensive study has been performed on 29 thyroid cancer patients with the following objects: To calculate i) the effective half lives of iodine for different organs, ii) the absorbed doses in major organs act as platform during excretion process, iii) to find a relation between drinking water and bladder dose, iv) to determine the effective dose equivalent due to uptake of iodine in the therapeutic as well as secondary organs (act as platform of iodine uptake during excretion) and v) to find the phase wise absorbed doses to the remnant thyroid-tissue.

In chapter eight, a total of twenty-nine patients (all female, age ranged from 40-60 y, mean 50 y) were treated with I-131 (dose-range 3700-7400 MBq, mean 5550 MBq) for thyroid cancer. The radioiodine uptake was measured at 1cm distance from three organs (previously marked by ultrasonography): thyroid, thigh-muscle and stomach by a calibrated Eberline ESP-2 GM counter under special arrangement of each patient. Urine sample was collected 12 hourly for first 72 h and then 24 hourly for the next 96 h. The individual biologic half-life of excreted urine was calculated using individual effective half-life. Absorbed doses were calculated for an adult female phantom using dynamic bladder model of MIRDOSE 3 program.

The effective half lives were calculated in two phases for the urine sample and it was found (24.81± 0.74) h for the first 72 h and (73.25±0.64) h for the next 96 h. (87±0.9)% of total activity passed through the urinary tract within first 72 h and the amount was (9±0.05)% for the next 96 h. The absorbed doses were calculated in groups of patients at different voiding intervals. The absorbed dose increased around 100% when the voiding interval was changed from 1 h to 2 h. This dose increased by 50% for the next hour and 33% for one more hour consecutively. The effective half lives for thyroid, thigh and stomach were found 39±0.85, 31.50±0.40 and 33.11±0.70 h consecutively. The correlation coefficient (r) among the measured uptakes was found very significant ($p<0.001$) for thyroid-thigh and stomach-urine, fairly significant ($p<0.01$) for thigh-stomach and non-significant for thyroid-stomach and thyroid-urine ($p<0.1$). The effective dose equivalent (EDE) for different target organs (sensitive for fatal occurrences) was calculated separately using MIRDOSE 3 program depending on absorbed doses to three source organs (Thyroid, Stomach and Urine bladder). The doses for stomach are found remarkably highest among the three source organs. The absorbed dose per unit mass (Gy/g) of remnant tissue (calculated using nodule-module protocol of MIRDOSE 3) is found as high as 1.72E+05 Gy and as low as 1.22E+04 Gy.

Extra water drinking in first few days after giving I-131 to the thyroid cancer patients reduces the absorbed doses to bladder. This study indicates that the subsequent uptake of radioiodine in stomach and urine bladder of thyroid cancer patients undertakes some extra burden of probabilistic fatal occurrence than other organs. The long-term post therapeutic follow up of the concerned organs is necessary to reduce the occurrences. The target-absorbed dose strongly depends on the size and mass of the remnant tissue and smaller tissue spot (radius<0.75 cm) shows high uncertainties in dose calculation.

Cancer of thyroid gland is an uncommon tumor that predominantly affects women most often in the third to fifth decade. Thyroid tumors develop when the growth of a single thyroid epithelial cell escapes from the normal mechanisms regulating cell divisions and gains a selective growth advantage. Unregulated cell division can result from mutations in both oncogenes and tumor suppressor genes. An understanding of mutations of the proto-oncogenes and tumor suppressor genes that occur in these tumors should eventually explain the diverse clinical characteristics of thyroid tumors and also direct therapy. These genetic abnormalities usually represent somatic/acquired mutations as opposed to germline/inherited mutations because most thyroid tumors are sporadic and not familial.

Chapter nine will discuss the tumorigenic changes found in thyroid epithelial (non-medullary) cancers.

Papillary thyroid carcinomas (PTC), representing most common malignant tumor of thyroid, are associated with rearrangements of 2 different transmembrane tyrosine kinase genes—RET and NTRK1 resulting in production of chimeric proteins (RET/PTC and TRK) that contribute to the development of malignant phenotype. Expression of wild type RET is detected in half of RET positive tumors and is an independent risk factor for aggressive PTC. Mutation of BRAF gene is present in 30% of PTC. This is isoform of RAF proteins (serine-threoninekinases) that activate RAF/ MEK/ MAPK signaling pathway.

A small number of PTC cases show deletions in the expressed RNA for p21/ Waf1, a cell cycle inhibitor protein. It also shows increased incidence in patients with familial adenomatous polyposis caused by germline mutations of APC gene. Familial predisposition has been linked to chromosomes 19 and 1. Follicular variant of PTC is characterized by a high frequency of ras mutations as compared to classical PTC that shows almost no ras mutations.

Recently PAX8-PPAR rearrangement has been identified in majority of follicular carcinomas (FC). A translocation has been shown in many FCs t(2,3)(q13;p25) that results in fusion of part of PAX8 gene (thyroid transcription factor) and PPAR-gamma-1 gene (transcription factor that stimulates cell differentiation and inhibits cell growth). The fusion product blocks action of PPAR-gamma-1 gene and thus most likely stimulates cell growth and inhibits cell differentiation. Mutations of K-ras, N-ras, and H-ras proto-oncogenes and over-expression of normal c-myc and c-fos genes are also found in FCs and occasionally PTCs. Hypermethylation of RASSF1A, a tumor suppressor gene, is also described in 2/3 of FC and minority of PTC. The frequency of allelic loss (FAL) using a panel of tumor suppressor genes in follicular derived neoplasms correlates with histological aggressiveness of the tumor.

Mutation of p53 tumor suppressor gene leading to production of an inactive p53 protein is seen in most anaplastic carcinomas which are the most aggressive of all thyroid carcinomas. Some cases, in particular those with areas of papillary differentiation, also show mutational activation of BRAF gene.

Immunohistochemically focal CK 19 staining may be seen in benign lesions however diffuse positivity is characteristic of PTC. HBME-1 positivity indicates malignancy but not papillary differentiation. Ret reflects RET/ PTC rearrangement and is seen in majority of classic PTCs. Only rarely all these markers are negative in PTC. Over-expression of cyclin-D1 and under-expression of p27 is also reported to predict lymph node metastasis in PTCs and thus has a role in identifying PTC with metastatic potential.

This chapter reviews and updates in detail, yet in a simplified manner, the tumor markers and genes involved in thyroid cancers.

Thyroid cancer is increasingly being diagnosed at an earlier stage and treatment is now usually associated with a long life expectancy. New information from large retrospective series has helped identify prognostic factors more accurately so that management can be adapted appropriately as discussed in chapter ten.

Results from recent studies show that differentiated carcinoma in the elderly behaves more aggressively and has a less favourable prognosis compared with younger patients. In a series of 111 patients aged 70 years or older at the time of initial diagnosis, 70% of tumours at presentation were pathological stage T3 or over, 44% demonstrated lymphatic spread and 23% had evidence of distant metastases. Cause specific survival was only 50% at 5 years. By contrast, thyroid cancer discovered incidentally at surgery for benign thyroid disease, or presenting in pregnancy has an excellent prognosis.

The use of diagnostic radioiodine scanning is declining both for initial diagnosis in a thyroid nodule and in the detection of recurrence. There is new evidence that it adds little additional information to influence clinical management.

In a retrospective analysis of 153 consecutive patients treated between 1990 and 2000, no patient with a positive diagnostic scan received radioiodine therapy which would not otherwise have been given based on clinical findings and serum thyroglobulin. Thyroglobulin estimation following rhTSH stimulation is rapidly gaining acceptance as the preferred way for detecting persistent or recurrent disease.

As the majority of patients with differentiated carcinoma are young with a good prognosis, the effect of treatment on reproductive function is an important area of concern. In 122 young men treated for differentiated thyroid cancer with a median follow-up of 21 years, no effect was observed on long term fertility even after multiple administrations. Similarly, no case of permanent ovarian failure was seen in 409 young women with a median follow-up of 18 years.

Prognostic factors for medullary thyroid cancer (MTC) have recently been clarified and include age at diagnosis, lymph node involvement and completeness of initial surgical resection. Prognosis for MTC when part of multiple endocrine neoplasia (MEN) 2A is excellent and is mainly accounted for by the earlier stage at which disease is diagnosed, thus emphasizing the need for early detection.

There is now general agreement that management of patients with thyroid cancer should be within a multidisciplinary team, working in specialised units and following evidence-based guidelines.

The aim of the study in chapter eleven was to test some hypothetical risk factors for anaplastic carcinoma, the most lethal type of thyroid cancer. A case-control study comprised 126 histologically or cytologically verified anaplastic thyroid cancer patients and 252 controls individually matched with cases by sex, age and place of residence. In the analysis of data univariate and multivariate logistic regressions analysis were used.

According to the multivariate conditional logistic regression analysis following factors were significantly and independently related to anaplastic thyroid cancer: lower education level (OR=1.42, 95%CI=1.09-1.86), history of goiter (OR=37.55, 95%CI=4.86-290.11), personal history of other non-thyroid malignant tumors (OR=2.42, 95%CI=0.99-5.95), blood group B (OR=2.41, 95%CI=1.03-5.66) and age at menarche after 15 year (OR=4.06, 95%CI=1.76-9.46).

The results obtained are in line with the current knowledge on factors related to thyroid cancer, except for the associations between anaplastic thyroid cancer and blood group B, which has not been reported.

Hurthle cell carcinoma represents about 5% of differentiated thyroid carcinomas [1]. When Hurthle cell population represents more than 75% of cell population, the lesion can be considered a Hurthle cell tumor. Hurthle cell tumor can be classified as malignant when capsular or vascular invasion is reported or if there is a perithyroid infiltration or distant metastases occur. Until now, there is a controversy about its classification; in fact, the World Health Organization (WHO) Committee considers this tumor the oxyphilic variant of follicular thyroid cancer, while for the Armed Forces Institute of Pathology (AFIP) Hurthle cell carcinoma should be separated into a category of thyroid neoplasm, different from true follicular cancer. The prognosis of the malignant variant of the tumor is still under debate as some authors have reported that Hurthle cell adenoma occasionally behaves like Hurthle cell carcinoma.

The purpose of the current study in chapter twelve was to evaluate previously reported data and the authors' own experience on the clinical and pathological features of patients affected by Hurthle cell tumor that can predict disease progression and death. Factors potentially associated with decreased survival for all patients were identified as: age, disease stage, tumor size, extraglandular invasion, lymphnodes disease, distant metastases, extensive surgery, radioiodine therapy and external beam radiation therapy. From 1992 to 2003, the authors identified 28 patients affected by Hurthle cell tumor, 9 patients with Hurthle cell adenomas and 19 patients with Hurthle cell carcinomas. Twenty-two were females and 6 males. Mean age of patients affected by adenoma was 49.7 years (30-72 yrs) versus 49.3 years (15 –72 yrs) of Hurthle cell carcinoma patients. In all patients a total thyroidectomy was performed. At hystology 9 adenomas, 5 "minimally invasive" and 14 invasive carcinomas were found. Average size of primary tumor was: 28.8 mm medium diameter in Hurthle cell adenoma versus 25.8 mm in Hurthle cell carcinoma. None of the patients had lymph nodes metastases. Postoperatively, in Hurthle cell carcinoma patients TNM staging showed 9 patients stage I, 5 stage II, 4 stage III and 1 stage IVa (UICC, 2002). All invasive carcinomas underwent ^{131}I therapy (91-150 mCi). One Hurthle cell carcinoma patient received external beam radiotherapy. The average follow-up period was 62 months (range 6-324). In none of their cases with adenoma a relapse was observed. Only one Hurthle cell carcinoma patient showed distant lung metastases at 60 months of follow up. She was submitted to repeated treatments and she is still in follow-up. In conclusion, several clinical and pathologic prognostic factors were rewieved from literature and from the authors' own series of patients with Hurthle cell adenoma and Hurthle cell carcinoma in order to analyze factors that could be associated with worse prognosis. Hurthle cell carcinoma was not found to have an aggressive behaviour when risk factors, including extent of tumour invasion, were taken into account. None of Hurthle cell adenoma showed a relapse or death caused by the tumor.

Graves' disease (GD) is a complex organ-specific autoimmune pathology that affects thyroid gland. A specific clinical outcome of GD is the presence of autoantibodies, which activate thyroid-stimulating hormone receptor and cause thyroid hyperfunction, or hypertyroidism. Clinical and subclinical hyperthyroidism is widely distributed in humans affecting up to 2% of Caucasians and occurs mostly in women. GD has a strong genetic background, which accounts up to 80% of the predisposition to disease. During the last five years, with the availability of the complete human genome sequence, a significant progress was made in the identification and functional characterization of genes conferring susceptibility to GD.

In chapter thirteen, the authors summarized recent findings in searching the susceptibility loci. To date, strong and consistent evidence for the involvement in GD pathogenesis was shown for HLA class II (chromosome 6p21), CTLA-4 (2q33), thyroglobulin (8q24) and CD40 (20q11) genes. The list of GD susceptibility genes can be extended by including of the VDR (12q12) and PTPN22 (1p13) genes, a role of which in thyroid autoimmunity is rather general, since they are shown to be involve in several autoimmune diseases. These loci are likely to interact, and their interactions could determine disease severity and clinical outcome. The review is also focused on recent advances in the identification of common susceptibility genes responsible for shared genetic background between several autoimmune disorders. In the near future, additional GD-specific and general susceptibility loci will be found that will help to clarify tight pathogenic mechanisms of the induction and progression of this disease as well as to dissect common pathways in the etiology of autoimmune diseases.

In: Trends in Thyroid Cancer Research
Editor: Carl A. Milton, pp. 1-31
ISBN 1-59454-627-4

Chapter I

MOLECULAR BIOLOGY OF FOLLICULAR THYROID CELL CANCER

Juan C Galofré*, Francisca Payeras, Amparo Calleja and Javier Salvador

Departamento de Endocrinología y Nutrición, Clínica Universitaria,
Facultad de Medicina
Universidad de Navarra, Pamplona, Spain.

ABSTRACT

According to current data, it seems probable that there is no interruption along the evolution of different follicular thyroid neoplasias. Most likely, transforming events responsible for the transition from a normal to tumoral cell starts with molecular changes that determine the appearance of follicular adenoma. Ulterior changes favor the development of follicular cancer. Probably, the generation of papillary carcinoma follows a different pathway without passing through a previous phase of follicular adenoma. Subsequently, genetic changes render the cell prone to dedifferentiation setting the basis for the development of anaplastic thyroid cancer. Those incidental molecular changes determine a dramatic worsening in the prognosis of thyroid cancer. The investigation of thyroid tumors is likely to be instructive in view of the spectrum they span, from benign adenomas to poorly differentiated carcinomas.

It has been proven that molecular alterations in tumoral thyroid cells are predisposed by genomic instability. Usually, changes of proto-oncogenes represent an early event, whereas mutations of suppressor genes are usually a late phenomenon. The onset of an aggressive behavior may be studied, and perhaps can be predicted in the future, by molecular medicine.

* Correspondence concerning this article should be addressed to Dr. Juan C Galofré, Departamento de Endocrinología y Nutrición, Clínica Universitaria, Facultad de Medicina Avda Pio XII 36. Universidad de Navarra, 311008 Pamplona, Spain. e-mail: jcgalofre@unav.es

The clinical application of the growing understanding of gene alterations involved in thyroidal oncogenesis is becoming a reality. Such knowledge might contribute to improve our diagnostic accuracy, by helping us to characterize malignant or benign cells, as well as to predict tumor outcome or to state its origin. Likewise, it might be useful to predict the response to conventional therapies or the future implications of pharmacogenetics.
The impressive advance of molecular medicine over the last few years is providing us an attractive vision of the new possibilities in diagnosis and treatments of thyroid cancer helping us to understand its biological behavior.
In addition, molecular medicine applications ought to be considered in determining the prognosis of spontaneous and familiar carcinomas. Such information can significantly improve our current clinical-pathologic prognostic methods.

Keywords: Thyroid Carcinoma, Molecular Markers, Diagnosis, Treatment

Molecular Bases of Thyroid Carcinogenesis

Introduction

According to a recent review, the neoplastic process follows a correlation of events [1]. In the developing of all malignancies at least six essential biological cell functions are altered. First, the cell cannot rule its own growth signals (with a predominant role of proto-oncogenes). Second, there is a lack of sensitivity to cellular growth inhibitory signals (mediated mainly by the tumor suppressor genes). Third, there exists an escape from programmed cell death (apoptosis). Fourth, tumor cells have an unlimited replicative capacity. Fifth, neoplastic cells synthetize several factors in order to elicit a permanent promotion of angiogenesis. And finally, there are alterations in the cellular adhesive capacity that provides the cells with the ability to spread leading to tisular invasion and metastasis development. Each of these alterations may be determined by several mutations and most of them still remain elusive to investigators. These six events normally occur in a cell with some degree of genetic instability. Usually these changes are correlative in time, and do not always take place in the same order. However, some of these alterations are predisposed to others. In addition to these six events, the tumor cells must elude the immune system to make possible the development of malignancy.

Genetic changes that determine alterations in the expression of proteins related with cell replication have special importance in the carcinogenic process. Regarding this subject, the remarkable role of two groups of genes must be stressed: proto-oncogenes and tumor suppressor genes. The former group is responsible for starting replicative signals, while the second group's role has the opposite effects. The expression of both genes is activated by transmembrane receptors and depends on extracellular signals. An oncogen is a mutated proto-oncogen that maintains the ability to mimic the growth or replicative signal, but without a normal control. Ordinarily, tumor suppressor genes drive the cell to a quiescent state (G0) in a postmitotic situation after the differentiation. Usually these mutations are a late event, in the carcinogenic development process and cause the lack of arrest in the replicative cell cycle stimulated by the oncogenes.

Thyroid Cancer Classification. Significance of Molecular Studies

The classical morphological classification of thyroid malignancies, according with their cellular origin (follicular or parafollicular) or with the differentiation degree (papillary, follicular, poor differentiated and undifferentiated) is generally accepted. It may be wise to evaluate whether this classification fits properly with the current knowledge or if nowadays we are in the situation to propose a new molecular classification for thyroid cancer (TC). Progress in this new TC classification might offer other perspectives that allow the increase of the efficacy in the diagnosis and therapy [2,3].

Carcinogenesis is an extensively influenced open process by its own nature. There are constant genetic and epigenetic changes. It is probably that in cell TC subtypes, despite their pathological classification, follow the alternate carcinogenic phenomena summarized by Hanahan and Weinberg [1]. Nevertheless, it has not yet been possible either to determine molecular bases of different TC phenotypes nor the genetic changes that condition the evolution to an undifferentiated pattern. However, the efforts in this direction are outstanding [4,5,6]. Experimental data show firm signals to suspect that the neoplastic shift from differentiated to undifferentiated state happens without interruption, by the accumulation of deleterious mutations.

Current advances are focused in the study by microarrays of TC tissue specimens, in order to look for associations between genetic expression and the TC morphological profiles. In a recent study, the investigators observed an overexpression of 18 genes and underexpression of 40 genes in the metastatic tissue [7]. The altered expressed genes were related with the cell cycle regulation, apoptosis, DNA repair, angiogenesis, adhesion and mobility, and with the immune response. Furthermore, the authors observed a different genetic expression in the primary tumor and in metastatic tissue.

Mutations and Carcinogenesis in Thyroid Cancer

Some TCs are characterized by the existence of genetic instability with a state of hypermutation. The amount of genetic changes in DNA is the origin of the different neoplasias [8,9,10,11]. Likewise, changes in the DNA methylation pattern can be an early event in carcinogenesis, and this circumstance may contribute to genetic instability [8]. Usually hyper-methylation takes place in gene promoters. In a similar way this phenomenon may help to understand the progression from differentiated to undifferentiated carcinoma [12].

In TC, genetic alterations like rearrangements and chromosomic translocations, which exceptionally occur in other epitelial tumors, are specifically involved [13]. Some rearrangements as *ret/PTC* (characteristic of papillary neoplasias), *NTRK* and *Pax-8/PPARγ* have also been described [14]. The latter is typical of follicular thyroid cancer (FC) because it is found in more than 60% of these tumors [15], and rarely is described in papillary tumors. An empirical observation in papillary tumors shows an alteration in the DNA repair mechanism, which motivates the presence of microsatellite instability as another potential mechanism in the cancer development and progression [16]. Furthermore, in poor differentiated carcinomas epigenetic changes like dinucleotides CpG deamination, which are associated with tumor progression and methylation in *p16* genes, even in 33% of the samples have been described [17].

Other alterations that cause defective protein synthesis without the presence of gene mutations also occur in the development of thyroid neoplasias. Alternative splicing has been observed in some suppressor genes, such as *FHIT* (*Fragile histidine triad gene*) and *TSG 101* (*Tumor supresor gene 101*) [18]. These alterations determine a different codon association and consequently intron and exon changes that induce mRNA changes and, therefore, a modified pattern of protein synthesis. However, the consequences of alternative splicing are not precisely established. Current data show neither a relation with the evolution phase nor with the grade of tumor differentiation. The fact that these changes are found in both benign and malignant neoplasias point out that it probably represents an early event in thyroid carcinogenesis.

The current knowledge in genetic changes that determine the evolution from adenoma to carcinoma is scant. Some phenomena like activation, mutation or de novo expression of some oncogenes and growth factors as *ras, ret, TDK, met* and *PTEN* at the beginning of the change from adenoma to carcinoma have been reported in some cases [19]. Mutations in tumor suppressor genes may occur as well [20], but at present, the presence of inactive mutations in TSH receptor (TSH-R) in thyroid neoplastic cells has yet to be shown. However, the expression of GRK-5 (a protein that regulates downstream TSH-R signaling pathway) is significantly reduced in TC. This finding may represent a decreased TSH-R sensitivity with the consequence of a low cell differentiate capacity [21]. Other reasons need to be looked at when the absence of TSH-R expression is found in cancer cells. Recently, TSH-R gene promoter aberrant methylation pattern has been reported in TC, and these changes are not described in benignant adenomas [22]. In addition, a possible role for mutated thyroid hormone receptors in the tumorigenesis of human papillary thyroid carcinoma has been suggested (PC) [23].

As it has been noted before, the development of a neoplasia is the result of a number of mutations in several genes, in both proto-oncogenes and tumor suppressor genes. Any event related with proliferation may be inside the scope of the carcinogenesis. It is well known, for instance, that both TGF-β and Activin A are two of the most potent inhibitors of normal follicular cell proliferation [24]. The tumoral cells show resistance to the action of these substances. In fact, a decrease in the TGF-β receptor in PC thyrocytes has been found [26], and likewise changes in the expression of Activin A receptor have also been described [25].

Somatic mitochondrial ADN mutations have been determined in PC and in Hürthle cell carcinoma. These findings indicate that such changes can be present in the development of this type of neoplasias and may have a promoting effect on tumor progression [27]. However the significance of these findings remains elusive.

A well-known feature of malignant neoplasias is the ability to avoid the immune surveillance system. This particular characteristic is related with the tumoral cell capacity to express Fas-L and, as a consequence, activate the Fas (CD 95) receptor of immunological cells, inducing apoptosis. The presence of this ligand has been observed in both PC and FC cells [28]. On the other hand, in medullary carcinoma cell Fas-L expression is mild or absent.

In addition, a low expression of Fas has been observed in malignant cells as a putative effect to avoid a fratricide action [28].

The membrane protein CD 97 or GR1 is generally expressed by activated lymphocytes and its ligand is CD 55 or DAF. Recently, CD 97 has been designated to act as a marker of cellular differentiation. This molecule is not expressed in the normal thyroid gland but is detected in neoplasias without a clear relation with the tumoral stage [29].

Similarly, a link between type 1 deiodinase activity and cellular differentiation has been established, since its activity is high in healthy thyroid tissue while it is low in differentiated FC and almost undetectable in anaplastic thyroid carcinoma [30].

Proto-Oncogene Mutations: An Early Event

Cell growth regulation and differentiation is mediated by ras proto-oncogen activity. ras mutations have been found in almost all types of thyroid carcinomas [31]. Mutations of ras proto-oncogenes are related with the initial phase of tumoral development [32]. These changes are found in 10-15% of all human carcinomas. Three types of ras proto-oncogenes have been described (H-ras, K-ras and N-ras), and all are involved with punctual mutations in the carcinogenic process. Probably ras activating mutations are an early event in the evolution of thyroid neoplasm and are usually linked with genetic instability. Therefore, these mutations increase the chance of new additional mutations [9,33,34]. It has been shown experimentally that these alterations destabilize the genome in the PCCL3 thyroid cell line. This finding is consistent with the beginning of the carcinogenic process because the biological function of ras proto-oncogen is the phenotypical progression [35]. Any mistake in its proper function favor the predisposition to develop genomic abnormalities on a great scale. In addition, a correlation has been described between the presence of ras mutation and the age of cancer onset. In fact, these mutations are rare in thyroid tumors of young population, whereas their prevalence increases with age [36]. History of previous radiation increases the prevalence of these mutations [34]. The current available information is consistent with the hypothesis of an evolution from benign follicular adenoma, time when ras mutation occur, to any other type of neoplasias, depending on subsequent mutations [10,31,32].

Nearly 5-20% of PC, have these mutations, though a high expression of ras proto-oncogen has been observed. The follicular subtype of PC shows a major predisposition to present ras mutations [37]. Between 24-53% of FC carry ras mutations and its expression can be increased to 53% of the cases. Furthermore, mutations of proto-oncogen ras are more common in FCs with metastasic behavior. Undifferentiated thyroid cancer shows a prevalence of proto-oncogen ras mutation ranging from 20% in some series to a maximum of 60% in other series.

Some authors were not able to establish a clear relationship between the presence of ras mutations and aggressive tumor behavior. In spite of this lack of relationship, others reported a clear correlation between N-ras codon 61 mutation and a different evolution in TC. Of note, this mutation is unusual in medullary thyroid cancer [38].

Many cell responses after ras activation follow its downstream efector Raf. Three Raf isoforms have been described: A-Raf, B-Raf and C-Raf (Raf-1). Once activated, Raf phosphorylizes MAPK kinase (MEK), starting the cascade events of cell growth and inhibiting apoptosis. A common feature in several cancers is braf mutations [39]. It has recently been described that this gene mutation is the most common genetic aberration in PC, reaching 40-45% of the cases, whereas is rare in anaplasic subtype, and almost nonexistent in other thyroid tumors [8,41]. Activated mutations of braf stimulate tumor proliferation and have been considered as a useful prognostic marker in patients with advanced cancer [42]. Other studies show the utility of its early detection in cytological samples in order to program preoperatively the preoperative extension or surgical excision, because braf mutations are associated with a poor prognosis [41]. At the same time, these patients deserve a follow-up.

Very often CCND1, erbB2 and myc proto-oncogenes are found altered in solid neoplasias. All of them have been studied in TC with the result of frequent variable expression [43]. Some authors point out that c-erbB2 is regularly overexpressed in PC subtypes, but mutations are unusual. On the other hand, in FC and anaplasic cancer subtypes the erbB2 expression is poor [44]. In contrast, CCND1 is overexpressed in both malignant and benign neoplasias. Some authors show a relation between the expression, and of these proto-oncogenes tumor aggressiveness [45]. Data on myc expression are conflicting. All together these findings show that in the development of TC CCND1 mutations may have an early role whereas erbB2 changes probably represent a late event [43].

The study of HGF (hepatocyte growth factor) and its receptor HGF-R (or c-met) shed light in understanding some events in the natural history of thyroid neoplasias. This proto-oncogen is overexpressed, but not mutated, in follicular adenoma and PC [46]. Nevertheless, this situation may be the result of preceding mutations because previous reports show RNA accumulation of MET in relation with ras and ret overactivity. In other words, lack of met regulation may be the final result of different molecular senseless pathways with the ability of induction thyroid cell transformation. Cells with met overexpression can synthesize and activate HGF. Interestingly, neither in anaplasic nor in follicular malignancies HGF or c-met expression have been found. This deficiency is related to the loss of chromosome 7q genetic material, which is lacking in follicular adenomas and in PCs with good prognosis. The same finding is found in the equal subtype with poor evolution, especially when the presentation is multicentric [12,47].

The proto-oncogen TRK codifies a membrane tyrosine kinase with Neuronal Growth Factor receptor activity. The overactivity of N-TRK1 (also known as TRKA, located in 1q22) is usual in PC. As in ret proto-oncogen, the gene activation is produced by rearrangements with the implication of at least three genes [48,49,50].

Ret: An Emblematic Thyroid Proto-Oncogen

Biological activity of ret has been related to a follicular variant of PC and medullary thyroid carcinoma development. However the contribution of ret to the onset of these two neoplasias have different methods. In PC, somatic ret rearrangements with a variety of activated genes can be found. The result is an expression of RET/PTC chimerical oncoproteins. In medullary tumors, point mutations usually occur in germinal line with the corresponding constitutional activation of RET tyrosine kinase response.

Probably the most frequent somatic changes found in PC are the rearrangements of ret proto-oncogen (10q11.2) reaching 10-40% of cases [52]. Eighth types of ret rearrangements have been described, identified from RET/PTC1 to RET/PTC8 [53,54,55,56,57,58,59]. Some unsuccessful attempts have been done in order to associate particular RET/PTC mutations with risk factors as radiation exposure, age and even pathological PC subtypes [60]. There is no agreement on the relation between particular mutations with the biological tumor behavior or treatment responses. At present, the putative interactions have no practical implications [61,62,63]. As a consequence of the efforts in correlationing PC prognosis with the presence of RET/PTC rearrangements, it has been observed that half of these tumors also show RET-TK rearrangement (RET with tyrosine kinase domain), of whom, only a small subset can be explained by RET/PTC rearrangement. On the contrary, the wild-type ret has been detected in 45% of the positive RET-TK tumors and its expression seems to be an independent risk factor of PC aggressiveness [63,64]. In the same way, some authors have shown that RET/PTC1 rearrangements are also associated with an increase in aggressive conduct in adult patients [64]. This alteration is more often found in patients with previous external radiation [65], especially in children [66] and some data demonstrate a shift from RET/PTC3 to RET/PTC1 in patients with prolonged radiation [67]. Two new gene fusions with ret implication have been described (ELKS and PCM-1) [68,69] Of note, no RET rearrangements have been described either in anaplasic or in FC, and this finding underlines the low probability of the RET/PTC rearrangements responsibility in the progression from differentiated to undifferentiated cancer [70]. However, RET/PTC activation has been detected in tumors with the oncocytic feature, suggesting that this pattern can also be characteristic of Hürthle cell neoplasias [71].

Peroxisome Proliferator-Activated Receptor Translocations

Peroxisome proliferator-activated receptor (PPAR) is a nuclear receptor involved in such cellular processes as adipogenesis, inflammation, atherosclerosis, cell cycle control, apoptosis, and carcinogenesis. PAX8 is an essential transcription factor for thyroid cell differentiation and thyroid specific gene regulation like peroxidase and thyroglobulin. PAX8-PPAR1 gene rearrangement frequently generates a chromosomal translocation in thyroid FC [72]. Albeit, initially it was proposed that this alteration was detected only in FC, more recent investigations show PAX8-PPARγ1 rearrangements in both follicular adenomas and carcinomas [73,74]. This finding suggests that this oncogen is not a reliable marker to distinguish between the two entities in cytological specimens [73]. Nevertheless this alteration is more frequent in FC than in PC neoplasias. Other investigators have explored the relation of this modification with the grade of malignancy. The results illustrate an increased aggressiveness in tumors with PAX8-PPARγ rearrangements [75]. However this alteration has not yet been found in anaplasic carcinoma [76].

A Late Event: Mutations in p53 Suppressor Gene

The P53 protein has a determinant role in cell proliferation process. P53 is a key factor in DNA organization and in reparation of mistakes when occurring during the cell replication process. It is well understood that any error in this mechanism can determine the neoplastic onset and development.

PC p53 hypermutability has been proven [17]. The percentage of different mutations found suggests that these alterations happen by chance. These mutations seem to be a late event in the neoplastic multistep development, therefore is considered a typical feature of undifferentiated or poor differentiated tumors.

The expression of p53 is elevated in 11%, 14%, 25-41%, 64-71% of PC, FC, poor differentiated or undifferentiated carcinomas, respectively [77,78]. The overexpression does not mean the existence of the respective gene mutation. On the contrary, the overexpression may represent two phenomena. First, the existence of some alterations or mutations of the genes that encode proteins elicit, by diverse mechanisms, an increase of P53 expression. Another explanation may be the existence of an alteration that takes place in the synthesis of any of the varied proteins that participate in this important suppressor gene metabolic pathway. Thus, these changes determine P53 functional impotence and consequently the intracellular high protein concentration.

As has been mentioned before, there is a clear correlation between p53 mutations or changes and tumor aggressiveness. This is consistent with the gene suppressor loss of biological activity. Any cell with a damaged mechanism in detecting DNA mistakes or without the capacity to repair DNA mismatches may increase the chance of new mutations in every replication. The probability is even higher in malignant neoplasias with an increased cell replication cycle. This alteration can also determine the tumor diversification in new clones with specific mutations, from a common clonal origin. Thus, the same tumor can be made with cells of a wide background with different differentiation stage.

Of note, in tall cell PC subtype, with the exception of the classic one, findings report p53 loss of heterozygosity, and this feature is related with the poor prognosis of the former variant [79]. Likewise in 38% of the worst prognostic insular trait PC p53 mutations have been found. Furthermore, it has been proven that more than 75% of anaplasic cancer carries p53 mutations [34,80,81]. Therefore, it seems clear that these mutations have a central role in clinical-pathological behavior of TC [82]. In fact, the reintroduction of p53 gene in a TC cell line elicits growth arrest.

The aftermath of Chernobyl's accident has been studied in the radiated population with TC. The results show that p53 mutations in codons 167 and 183 may have an important role in the pathogenesis of the radiation related to TC [83]. However, other authors are reluctant to accept the relation between radiation and the incidence of p53 mutations [17]. Nevertheless, it has been speculated that in TC patients with p53 mutations I^{131}, therapy may elicit evolutive changes from differentiated to undifferentiated tumors, propitiating the malignant transformation [84]. However, this statement is not universally accepted.

Other Suppressor Gene Mutations

Anaplasic thyroid cancer phenotype is usually recessive. This association is probably related to the suppressor gene failure, whose expression has a recessive nature, rather than to the dominant character of oncogene activation [85].

PTEN is a suppressor gene that encodes a phosphatase. PTEN loss of heterozygosity in the correspondent locus (10q23) is found in 5-21% of PC, 7-30% of FC and 35-59% of anaplasic cancer. These findings are negatively related with PTEN protein expression, which is underexpressed in these neoplasias [86]. However, PTEN mutations are rarely observed [87]. PTEN re-expression inhibits carcinogenesis with cell growth arrest in engineered cell lines. Furthermore, a close relationship between PTEN and kinase cyclin-dependent inhibitor p27-kip1 has been described. Current available data allow the conclusion that PTEN inactivation may have a role in the development of spontaneous TC [87], mainly FC subset, because mutations have been found on 8% of this subtype [86]. Interestingly, this gene has a fundamental role in Cowden disease, where benign thyroid neoplasia coexists with breast neoplasia and multiple hamartomas.

Rb suppressor gene plays an important role in cell growth arrest by several mechanisms. Rb deletions have been found in 55% of malignant thyroid tumors with increased probability in aggressive and metastatic tumors [20,88]. Both, p27 and p21 have a suppressor gene biological activity. Ten percent of TC have mutations in the p21 gene. TC can display normal p27 expression, however protein banishment is found. Normal protein localization used to be in the nucleus but in cancer cells shift to the cytoplasm [89].

The Role of TSH in the Thyrocyte Morphological and Functional Control

The controversy on TSH receptor (TSH-R) contribution to thyroid carcinogenesis is open. Some authors do not find any role in the differentiated cancer outgrowth, while others state that TSH-R and Gs-α point mutations are oncogenic [90,91,92,93,94]. Isolated hyperfunctioning PC with TSH-R mutations has been found [95]. Somatic TSH-R mutation in FC tissue has been described, and this finding can help to explain the rarity of the hyperfunction associated to these tumors [96]. Nevertheless there is agreement in associate TSH-R mutations with the development of hyperfunctioning thyroid adenomas [90,91,97].

Adhesion Molecule Alterations: a Warning Sign of Aggressiveness

Expression of the intercellular adhesion molecule 1(ICAM-1) in the thyrocyte is not normally detected. This expression may be stimulated by a huge variety of factors interacting with the immune system, such as the proinflammatory cytokine interferon-γ (IFN-γ), tumor necrosis factor-α (TNF-α), interleukin-1 (IL-1) and retinoic acid. ICAM-1 is overexpressed in thyroid neoplasias and this feature might contribute to the tumor's ability to elude the immune system [98].

Catenins (-α, -β and -γ) are a group of cytoplasmatic proteins with ubiquitous expression. Their attributed function deals with the crucial cell to cell adhesion system and works through E-cadherin action [99,100]. Catenins make a specific bond between the cytoskeleton and extracellular adhesion system. It is well known that a reduction in E-cadherin expression is associated with a poor TC prognosis, albeit lack of catenin expression properly reflects the neoplastic future evolution [101,102]. Mutations of these molecules occur in more than 60% of TC [103]. Low expression of the three catenin types has been described in TC [104]. Likewise, significant relations between prognostic traits and catenin expression in tumors have been established [104]. A positive correlation between a decrease in α- and β- catenin expression with the age of diagnosis and the TNM stage has also been observed. In addition, tumor size association with reduction in catenin β- and γ- expression has been found. More investigations have found a link between node metastasis and decreased α-catenin expression, whereas distant metastases are more frequent in tumors with reduced expression of the β- and γ- subtypes. Recurrences are associated with a drop in the α-catenin presence, whereas mortality is increased in tumors with a declined β- expression. These findings allow recommending the opportunity of α-catenin expression assessment as a prognostic marker in

TC [104]. Furthermore, it has also been speculated that β-catenin may act as an oncogen in TC. That supposition is supported by the findings of nuclear heterotopic β-catenin expression in neoplasias. The localization of intranuclear β-catenin is restricted to poor differentiated tumors (25%) or undifferentiated (66%), hence, the association of nuclear localization and poor membrane β- expression with poor prognosis, despite the presence of other prognostic factors of tumor differentiation. Analysis of this characteristic may help to put in order TC and predict its evolution [105]. Moreover, as has been mentioned before, β-catenin expression is diminished in 66% and 100% of thyroid adenomas and carcinomas respectively.

E-cadherin is downregulated by dysadherin. Also findings show that the level of dysadherin expression is closely related to prognosis, dedifferentiation, tumor size and local and pulmonary metastasis in TC [106].

Changes that take place in association with alterations in Galectin-3 expressions are of special interest. It is well known that normal thyrocytes do not express either CD44v6, nor Galectin-3 adhesion molecules. However, these molecules are invariably present in thyroid cell proliferation. Therefore, such results allow the speculation that Galectin-3 expression is a specific feature of malignancy [107,108], albeit some authors have found that Galectin-3 is also expressed in inflammatory areas of normal thyroid tissue [109]. Galectin-3 plays an important role in intracellular adhesion and in cell matrix interaction. The usual expression of this molecule in neoplastic cells is cytoplasmatic. The grade of expression is diverse in different tumors. Protein expression can be mildly detected in adenomas in contrast with FC and even more in PC, where Galectin-3 is expressed with high intensity. Furthermore, a direct relationship between expression level and the existence of metastasis has been described in PC [110].

Lack of CD44v6 expression is associated with a worse evolution of TC, especially in the PC subtype. Furthermore, a correlation has been found between the deficit of CD44 expression and several poor prognosis factors like old age (more than 60 years), distant metastasis, advanced TNM stage, tumor recurrence and cancer related mortality. However, this point is controversial because other investigators have found a relation among high CD44 expression and prognosis worsening in thyroid tumors [112].

Antiangiogenic Factors and Growth Factors

Malignant thyrocytes have the capacity to synthesize the angiogenic factor VEGF (Vascular endotelial growth factor), and its expression level is related with aggressive disease patterns [32,113,114]. An association of VEGF expression with tumor dedifferentiation has been proven by some authors [115,116] while others [117] did not find any increase in VEGF expression, neither in nodes nor in pulmonary metastasis, when compared with the primary tumor. Probably, due to its relation with the risk of metastasis development, this marker may predict the evolution of PC. Expression of VEGF is related with TSH stimulus but surprisingly, recombinant human TSH does not increase its expression [118]. Even more, in the follow-up of TC patients, the administration of recombinant TSH can induce a significant VEGF plasma level decrease in absence of thyroid tissue [119]. In immunodeficient mice with induced FC, either transfection of endostatin gene or administration of the recombinant protein shows a therapeutic effect [120].

Another important growth factor is EGF (epidermal growth factor). This growth factor has an important role in thyroid cell proliferation and as such inhibits significant thyroid specific functions, like iodine transport and organification, or characteristic thyroid protein synthesis like thyroglobulin and peroxidase. Therefore, its main biological activity in thyroid cells is to promote the proliferation, but not its differentiation. Hence, it is a characteristic protagonist of tumor growth. Normal EGF function starts with cell membrane receptor interaction followed by the internalization of the complex ligand-receptor to exert a second action in the nucleus. It is known that TGFα (tumor growth factor α) also interacts with EGF receptors (EGF-R) contributing to the proliferative stimulus. Nuclear expression of EGF and EGF-R is a typical trait of both follicular adenoma and carcinoma. This expression has also been found in the thyroid tissue of patients with Graves' disease. Surprisingly, a decrease in nuclear EGF expression has been observed in PC cells, albeit is present in cytoplasm [121].

TC cells, especially in those that are more undifferentiated, synthesize IGF II (insulin growth factor type II) and also overexpress insulin receptors. Therefore, a continuous cell growth promoter feedback is mantained by an autocrine loop [122].

Chromosome Alterations

A relationship between the loss of heterozygosity and prognosis has been found in TC. This association is more frequent in FC than in PC [123]. However, loss of heterozygosity is found in 36% of anaplasic cancer cases and this figure surpasses both former cancer types [12,48]. In addition, anaplastic tumors may display a localized loss in the short arm of chromosome 16. This finding probably indicates the lack of a suppressor gene in this locus [124]. This hypothesis is supported by the observation of frequent loss of 16p in anaplasic thyroid cancer cell lines in contrast with differentiated cancer thyroid cell lines [125].

Changes in the number of DNA copies have been frequently observed in FC, medullar and anaplasic thyroid carcinomas, while this finding is rare in PC. Loss of chromosome 22 is particularly frequent in FC, and is associated with an extensive invasive behavior [126]. A loss in chromosome 7q and 11p has also been found [128].

Immune Reaction

Immune response against TC is both humoral and cellular, and may be important for long-term survival. This hypothesis has been proved by the study of lymphocyte characteristics of the infiltrated tumor areas [129]. Carcinomas with lymphocytic infiltrate are associated with long-term disease-free survival [130].

Experimental TC gene therapy with interleukin-12 and Granulocyte Macrophage Colony Stimulator Factor accomplish a dramatic therapeutic result with 90% of remission and generates an immune response against rechallenge [131,132,133].

Clinical Applications

Introduction

It is not rare in clinical practice to see patients with identical TC pathological subtype diagnosis and equal initial tumor extension whose evolution is quite different. Currently, there is no explanation for this conflicting behavior, and even worse, it is not possible to strictly predict the sense of evolution in every particular case. However, recent data on molecular medicine sheds light on future possibilities. Probably, in the near future, cancer classification and staging will depend not only on morphological data. The concurrent molecular changes are going to be of great help [3], and probably new data will guide new better prognostic classification of cancer patients.

With reference to TC patients, these new findings may render valuable information in order to have an accurate diagnostic and treatment orientation in every individual patient. Today, it is known that some features determine the biological evolution of TC and the dramatic shift in clinical progress that takes place may be explained by the alteration of molecular background. Nevertheless, current available data are partial and limited. Hopefully, the precise classification of several molecular treats will facilitate the knowledge on the probable evolution of a particular neoplasia. In addition, the use of tumoral markers can be useful to find out the metastasis origin in the case of an unknown primary tumor.

Diagnostic Applications of Molecular Biology in Thyroid Cancer

Benign and Malignant Prediction by Cytological Studies

Morphological data of cytological specimen observation from material obtained by Fine Needle Aspiration (FNA) are not always enough to diferentiate between malignant or benign thyroid nodules. This technique is blind to distinguish this circumstance in follicular neoplasias. Therefore, any attempt to improve the diagnostic procedure in order to increase the information on nature and evolution of cells from a thyroid nodule is of special interest. Molecular markers look like the most probable candidates to offer this information.

In addition, as has been mentioned before, molecular analysis provides data on the most likely tumor conduct and aggressiveness. This information can be of paramount importance when therapeutic decisions should be adopted.

The use of microarrays has been experimentally started in TC in order to identify changes in protein expression and to assess the differences between primary tumors, metastasis and normal tissue [3,7].

As stated above, galectin-3 is a protein of the lectin family that has been associated with neoplastic processes in various tissues. Expression of this protein has been described in differentiated FC suggesting that the immunohistochemical study of galectin-3 may be a potential marker of malignancy in thyroid neoplasms. Some authors have shown the utility of measurement galectin-3 or CD44v6 expression in cytological samples from thyroid nodules [134] in order to distinguish adenoma from carcinoma. Authors that have published good results studying galectin-3 show a 99% of sensitivity, a 98% of specificity, a positive predictive value of 92% and a 99% in the diagnostic accuracy. Other findings confirm these results [107,108,135,136]. However, in contrast with previously published data, it has been published that benign lesions also express galectin-3. Thus, the use of galectin-3 immunodetection as a molecular marker for thyroid carcinoma must be interpreted with caution, particularly in the differentiation between FC and follicular adenoma [137,138]. Another approach has been attempted by measuring galectin-3 mRNA, but results of studies done in order to distinguish benign from malignant nodules do not reach statistical significance [138b], and it has even been postulated that the origin of galectin-3 mRNA detected is not the follicular thyroid cell [139]. Galectin-3 is not a universal marker for children and adolescent neoplasias and, of note, has found its expression in tissue of Hashimoto thyroiditis [140].

Ninety five percent of TC expresses CD57 (leu-7) (HNK-1), while only 27% is found in follicular adenomas and 10% of colloid nodules. Normal thyroid tissue does not express this antigen [141].

Follicular Cytology

Overexpression of HGF in cytological thyroid samples may be a useful assistance to the pathologist in the difficult task of differentiating adenoma from carcinoma in the case of a cytological pattern of follicular proliferation, because it is overexpressed in benign tumors whereas it is not in malignant [47]. Nevertheless, this overexpression is not an exclusive feature of adenomas, since they have also been found in PC.

It has been speculated that the study of PAX8-PPARγ fusion may be useful in the cytological classification of follicular proliferation [15]. However, recent data show that this rearrangement is not restricted to malignant lesions. On the other hand, data on telomerase expression are not uniform and offer scanty guidance in the differentiation of adenomas from carcinomas [145], despite its expression in children's thyroid cancer is related with aggressiveness [146].

Papillary Cytology

It is well known that ret (ret/PTC) oncogen rearrangements have specificity for PC. This feature has been used in samples from FNA for cell classification by assessment of RNA by RT-PCR. Specific probes have been used in the localization of ret/PTC-1, 2 and 3. The result was consistent with the final pathological outcome, without false positives. Therefore, this technique can be useful when the result is doubtful or in the case of inadequate samples albeit rarely cytological diagnosis of PC is problematic [142]. The study by immunohistochemistry of Met protein can also help in the diagnosis. However, it is not a specific marker, because a high expression also has been found in thyroid cells from Graves' disease or Hashimoto thyroiditis [143].

Cytokeratin-19 is a sensitive PC marker, particularly when diffuse cytoplasmatic pattern is found in immunohistochemistry observation, while focal expression is more characteristic of normal cells, Hashimoto thyroiditis and some benign tumors [144].

Metastasis

Molecular studies can also help in the diagnosis of primary tumor from metastatic samples. It has been postulated that the use of RT-PCR in the analysis of specific transcripts from TSH receptor or thyroglobulin in cytological node specimen when PC is suspected, in order to improve the diagnostic performance previous to surgery [147].

Differentiation

Transcription factors TTF-1 and Pax-8 expression have been studied both in cytological and surgical TC samples. Results show that the expression of the two factors is correlated with tumor differentiation and, interestingly, with scanty expression in undifferentiated cancer [11].

Thyroid peroxidase is expressed in normal thyroid tissue and benign nodules, but its expression falls in malignancies. Therefore, it may be useful to increase the diagnostic accuracy when cytological samples from FNA are studied. Some authors found good results with the MoAb47 antibody.

Multifocality

PC is multicentric in 20 to 80% of cases and bilateral in 30 to 44% [148]. Molecular biology helps in the assessment of tumor differentiation from single to multiple origins. The fact of discover multifocal tumors who do not share same RET/PTC mutation is in favor of a polyclonal PC origin [149], though this it is not a valid explanation for all the cases. *In vitro* studies show that HGF (Hepatocyte growth factor) increases the motility and invasiveness capacity of tumoral cells and induce synthesis and release of active chemokines with the ability to mobilize dendritic cells. HGF is overexpressed in PC [143]. This tumor condition may explain three particular features of this TC subtype i.e, the typical early node metastasis; second, the important peritumoral inflammatory reaction and finally, the multifocality.

Loss of the Radioiodine Trapping Ability

Remnant ablation with radioiodine after surgery is an essential procedure in current therapy strategies for follicular cell origin TC [150]. This management has the advantage of treating not only thyroid remnant but possible locoregional or distant metastasis as well. However, in some cases follicular thyroid cell loses the iodine trapping competence and therefore the chance of being treated by this method [151].

Sodium-iodide symporter (NIS) expression is necessary for the iodine element to be transported inside the thyroid cell, making possible the radioiodine trapping when it is given with therapeutic purpose [152,153]. Therefore, its need to be unharmed is essential [154,155]. Some modifications have been observed (epigenetic changes: histone methylation or acetylation) of NIS promoter in some PC cell lines that determinate a reduction in its expression [156]. These observations are endorsed by the fact that the treatment of undifferentiated thyroid cancer cell lines with the depsipeptide FR 901228 (a new histone deacetylase inhibitor) restore NIS function [157]. In addition, this treatment increases other specific thyroid protein expressions. Those drugs, histone deacetylation inhibitors, induce transcription and expression of genes that were related with the affected nucleosomes leading to cell differentiation [157]. All this information points to the possibility that epigenetic factors related to the histone acetylation have a role in the TC undifferentiating process. Paradoxical results have been observed by different authors because both NIS up-regulation and down-regulation in TC have been published [151,158]. A reduced symporter expression in tumoral tissue in relation with normal surrounding thyroid tissue in the same subject has been reported [155]. Despite the fact that changes have been observed in NIS expression, no mutations have been found that justify the shift in symporter activity [159]. It has been suggested that primary PC and follicular tumors may predict the future recurrent tumor and metastasis capability in trapping radioiodine and thus the efficacy of a possible treatment [151,160]. In addition, in some TCs, a reduction in CREB (trascriptional activator) sequence that regulates NIS expression has also been noticed and this observation may shed more light on the reason for eventual transporter downregulation in these neoplasias [161].

Gene therapy is a promising weapon against cancer [131]. Transfection of NIS-deficient human FC cell lines restores the iodide accumulation ability in xenografted nude mice tumors and their susceptibility to respond to radioiodine therapy [162].

Pendrin is a protein, abundantly expressed in normal thyroid tissue whose function is related with the chloride and iodine transport. Pendrin underexpression has been observed in thyroid neoplastic cell lines. This finding contributes to the explanation of a decrease in iodine trapping by some neoplasias [163]. Epigenetic changes as aberrant hypermethylation have also been observed in 44% of follicular adenomas, 46% of FC, 71% of PC, 71% of anaplasic carcinomas and 100% of TC cell lines. Probably this alteration is an early phenomenon in the process of thyroid carcinogenesis [22].

Thyroglobulin Underexpression

Cell phenotype is determined by the expression of a particular protein array. The possibility of any specific protein expression in a cell is determined by a number of factors including the integrity of the respective transcription factors. It is well known that Pax-8 and thyroid transcription factor-1 (TTF-1) are critical elements in the thyroglobulin, peroxidase, NIS and thyrotropin receptor expression [11]. The observation of the frequent loss of competence to express thyroglobulin by undifferentiated cancer has been explained by a reduction in transcription factors activity such as TTF-1, TTF-2 or Pax-8, that interact with the thyroglobulin promoter [11,164].

Simultaneous thyroglobulin and ras expression have been investigated in TC, with the result of high thyroglobulin level expression in differentiated neoplasias, whereas the protein expression was almost absent in poor differentiated carcinomas. It has been proposed that N-ras mutations seem restricted to a subset of tumors with low or null thyroglobulin expression, suggesting that this genetic change is prevalent in less differentiated neoplasias [38].

FAMILIAL SYNDROMES

Seven to ten percent of all differentiated TC, excluding medullar subtype, are familial [165,166]. Usually, they are PC tumors and their main characteristics features are an early onset with an aggressive behavior. The finding of a genetic marker to identify these neoplasias has been elusive to date, and the inheritance seems to be heterogeneous [165,167].

However, other syndromes with a well-known genetic origin have thyroid neoplasias within their manifestations. Cowden disease and Gardner syndrome are typical examples of these associations. *APC* gene (5q21) has been identified as responsible for Gardner syndrome (familial hereditary poliposis subtype) [168]. TC association with familial poliposis has been described but, surprisingly, the *APC* mutations found in thyroid tissue are different from the same gene mutations found in colon cells [169]. Mutations of *APC* genes are rarely described in spontaneous TC. Current data show that 1-2% of familial adenomatous poliposis have PC. This neoplasia is more frequent in females (ratio female:male, 17:1) and the age of onset seems to be around 25 years. Therefore, in these patients a systematic screening of thyroid diseases is recommended starting in youth (age suggested: 15 years old) [170]. *APC* mutations are usually in germinal line and the association of these mutations with the ret/PTC1 chimeric gene has been studied in these patients. In a substantial proportion of affected subjects both alterations are found. These data suggest some potential cooperation between the deteriorated *APC* function and *ret* activity [171].

Similarly in Hereditary Hamartomatous Syndrome (Cowden disease) *PTEN* suppressor gene (10q23.3) mutations have been identified [172,173]. A relation between frequency of malignancy and mutations in these patients has not yet been established. On the contrary, current data reveal an association with thyroid benign adenoma [174].

A relationship between breast and thyroid diseases has been extensively observed, particularly with FC and PC in premenopausal women [166]. Likewise, non toxic multinodular goiter is connected with a putative gene located in 14q. However, no etiological or genetic association of this region with differentiated TC has been identified to date [175]. Recently, an area in 19p13.2 that determines familial predisposition to have TC from follicular lineage, has been identified and is also associated with an increase oxyphilic cells presence. Nevertheless, no particular responsible gene in this locus has been recognized [176].

Prognosis

Several circumstances have been associated with prognostic value in the development of thyroid carcinoma. Despite the lack of specific molecular markers, TC progression has been related with several factors as aneuploidy, number of microvessels, CD97 or E-cadherin expression, telomerase activity, etc. However, in order to guide thyroid neoplasia prognosis, the value of classical prognostic scores (AGES, MACIS, AMES, TNM, EORTC etc) remain as a valuable tool. These criteria are assessed according with clinical data and are independent from molecular markers [150]. The fact of having several of these clinical evaluating systems indicates their limitations and the existence of several factors that escape their consideration. Perhaps adding molecular information to these score schemes may help to assess the real prognosis with a practical and operational classification.

Good Prognosis Markers

A paradoxical increase of the proapoptotic molecule BAX expression has been observed in TC tissue in contrast with cancer of other origins, where BAX is usually inactivated [177].

These authors did not find any p53 mutation in the studied group, though a protein augmented expression, mainly cytoplasmatic, was detected. Therefore, it was speculated that both data might be related with the good evolution of thyroid neoplasias. Likewise, Her/neu expression has been correlated with prognosis in TC [178].

Metastasis

Currently, in the explanation of potential metastasis mechanism, the homing theory is surpassing soil and seed theory in order to illustrate the special characteristics of peculiar metastasis localization in different neoplasias. This theory postulates that to achieve the implantation of a neoplastic cell in a distant host tissue not only particular neoplastic cell conditions (according with a number of mutations) are needed, but a special admittance conditions by receptor tissue is also essential. These conditions may be related to chemotactic factors. The attractiveness of this theory is, in addition to other reasons, based on the fact that these factors may open a therapeutic window through blocking these factors [179,180]. In the same direction, the use of emerging microarray analysis probably will be of great help in the near future. As has been mentioned before, some attempts in this direction have been done. Gene analysis using microarray technology shows different expression in primary FC from its own metastasis [7]. Genes related to cell cycle regulation and oncogenes were significantly increased in metastatic tissue expression. On the contrary, the expression of fibronectin, a cell adhesion molecule, was reduced.

Important efforts are directed to elucidate specific gene mutations that determine metastasis development. This aspect is inversely related with adhesion molecule expression. In a similar way, an inverse correlation between expression of nm23-H1 (a metastasis suppressor gene) and the metastatic potential of FC, but not in PC has been observed [181]. However, not all the authors have found the same results, and the role of this gene is controversial [182].

CONCLUSION

A dramatic advance in diagnostic methods for thyroid malignancies workout has been achieved over the last few years. However, even now, in some cases it is neither possible to foresee their clinical evolution, nor indicate the appropriate therapy for every patient. Current diagnostic investigations have no sensitivity to detect whether a particular tumor is going to spread locally or systemic metastasis. Today, cytological studies are blind to this discrimination, and cannot distinguish between benign and malignant in some neoplasias.

The recent progression in molecular biology will bring clinicians new suitable tools to perform a quality diagnostic and therapeutic leap in managing thyroid tumors. Therefore, we can expect to overcome the present limitations in the near future. However, there is still a great way to go, knowing that each new advance may answer a question, but generates many new ones.

References

[1] Hanahan, D; Weinberg, RA. The hallmarks of cancer. *Cell*, 2000 100,57-70.

[2] Learoyd DL, Messina M, Zedenius J, Robinson BG. Molecular genetics of thyroid tumors and surgical decision-making. *World J Surg* 2000; 24:923-933.

[3] He YD, Friend SH. Microarrays-the 21st century divining rod? *Nature Med* 2001; 6:658-659.

[4] Golub TR, Slonim DK, Tamayo P, et al. Molecular classification of cancer: class discovery and class prediction by gene expression monitoring. *Science.* 1999. 286:531-537.

[5] Hedenfalk I, Duggan D, Chen Y, Radmacher M, Bittner M, Simon R, Meltzer P,Gusterson B, Esteller M, Kallioniemi OP, Wilfond B, Borg A, Trent J. Gene-expression profiles in hereditary breast cancer. *N Engl J Med.* 2001; 344:539-548.

[6] Khan J, Wei JS, Ringner M, Saal LH, Ladanyi M, Westermann F, Berthold F, Schwab M, Antonescu CR, Peterson C, Meltzer PS. Classification and diagnostic prediction of cancers using gene expression profiling and artificial neural networks. *Nat Med.* 2001 Jun;7(6):673-9.

[7] Chen KT, Lin JD, Chao TC, Hsueh C, Chang CA, Weng HF, Chan EC. Identifying differentially expressed genes associated with metastasis of follicular thyroid cancer by cDNA expression array. *Thyroid* 2001; 11:41-46.

[8] Fagin JA. Molecular genetics of thyroid follicular cells. In: Braverman LE, Utiger RD, eds. *The thyroid.* Philadelphia: Lippincott-Williams & Wilkins, 2000; 886-898.

[9] Gimm O. Thyroid cancer. *Cancer Lett.* 2001; 163:143-156.

[10] Esapa CT, Johnson SJ, Kendall-Taylor P, Lennard TW, Harris PE. Prevalence of Ras mutations in thyroid neoplasia. *Clin Endocrinol* 1999; 50:529-535.

[11] Ros P, Rossi D, Acebrón A, Santisteban P. Thyroid-specific gene expression in the multi-step process of thyroid carcinogenesis. *Biochimie* 1999; 81:389-396.

[12] Kitamura Y, Shimizu K, Tanaka S, Ito K, Emi M. Allelotyping of anaplastic thyroid carcinoma: frequent allelic losses on 1q, 9p, 11, 17, 19p, and 22q. *Genes Chromosomes Cancer* 2000; 27:244-251.

[13] Santoro M, Thomas GA, Vecchio G, Williams GH, Fusco A, Chiappetta G,Pozcharskaya V, Bogdanova TI, Demidchik EP, Cherstvoy ED, Voscoboinik L, Tronko ND, Carss A, Bunnell H, Tonnachera M, Parma J, Dumont JE, Keller G, Hofler H, Williams ED. Gene rearrangement and Chernobyl related thyroid cancers. *Br J Cancer* 2000; 82:315-322.

[14] Dwight T, Thoppe SR, Foukakis T, Lui WO, Wallin G, Hoog A, Frisk T, Larsson C, Zedenius J. Involvement of the PAX8/peroxisome proliferator-activated receptor gamma rearrangement in follicular thyroid tumors. *J Clin Endocrinol Metab.* 2003;88:4440-4445.

[15] Kroll TG, Sarraf P, Pecciarini L, Chen CJ, Mueller E, Spiegelman BM, PAX8-PPARgamma1 fusion oncogene in human thyroid carcinoma. *Science* 2000; 289:1474.

[16] Dobosz T, Lukienczuk T, Sasiadek M, Kuczynska A, Jankowska E, Microsatellite instability in thyroid papillary carcinoma and multinodularhyperplasia. *N. Blin Oncology* 2000; 58:305-310.

[17] Shahedian B, Shi Y, Zou M, Farid NR. Thyroid carcinoma is characterized by genomic instability: evidence from p53 mutations. *Mol Genet Metab* 2001; 72:155-3.

[18] Zou M, Shi Y, Farid NR, al-Sedairy ST, Paterson MC. FHIT gene abnormalities in both benign and malignant thyroid tumours. *Eur J Cancer* 1999; 35:467-472.

[19] Yeh JJ, Marsh DJ, Zedenius J, Dwight T, Delbridge L, Robinson BG, Eng C. Fine-structure deletion mapping of 10q22-24 identifies regions of loss of heterozygosity and suggests that sporadic follicular thyroid adenomas and follicular thyroid carcinomas develop along distinct neoplastic pathways. *Genes Chromosomes Cancer* 1999; 26:322-328.

[20] Moretti F, Nanni S, Pontecorvi A. Molecular pathogenesis of thyroid nodules and cancer. *Baillieres Best Pract Res Clin Endocrinol Metab* 2000; 14:517-539.

[21] Metaye T, Menet E, Guilhot J, Kraimps JL. Expression and activity of g protein-coupled receptor kinases in differentiated thyroid carcinoma. *J Clin Endocrinol Metab.* 2002;87:3279-3286.

[22] Xing M, Usadel H, Cohen Y, Tokumaru Y, Guo Z, Westra WB, Tong BC, Tallini G, Udelsman R, Califano JA, Ladenson PW, Sidransky D. Methylation of the thyroid-stimulating hormone receptor gene in epithelial thyroid tumors: a marker of malignancy and a cause of gene silencing. *Cancer Res.* 2003;63:2316-2321.

[23] Puzianowska-Kuznicka M, Krystyniak A, Madej A, Cheng SY, Nauman J. Functionally impaired TR mutants are present in thyroid papillary cancer. *J Clin Endocrinol Metab.* 2002; 87:1120-1128.

[24] Luisi S, Florio P, Reis FM, Petraglia F. Expression and secrection of activin A: a possible physiological and clinical implications. *Eur J Endocrinol* 2001; 145:225-236.

[25] Schulte KM, Jonas C, Krebs R, Roher HD. Activin A and activin receptors in thyroid cancer. *Thyroid* 2001; 11:3-14.

[26] Matoba H, Sugano S, Yamaguchi N, Miyachi Y. Expression of transforming growth factor-beta1 and transforming growth factor-beta Type-II receptor mRNA in papillary thyroid carcinoma. *Horm Metab Res* 1998; 30:624-628.

[27] Yeh JJ, Marsh DJ, Zedenius J, Dwight T, Delbridge L, Robinson BG, Eng C. Somatic mitochondrial DNA (mtDNA) mutations in papillary thyroid carcinomas and differential mtDNA sequence variants in cases with thyroid tumours. *Oncogene* 2000; 19:2060-2066.

[28] Mitsiades N, Poulaki V, Mastorakos G, Tseleni-Balafouta ST, Kotoula V, Koutras DA, Tsokos M. Fas ligand expression in thyroid carcinomas: a potential mechanism of immune evasion. *J Clin Endocrinol Metab* 1999; 84:2924-2932.

[29] Hoang-Vu C, Bull K, Schwarz I, Krause G, Schmutzler C, Aust G, Kohrle J, Dralle H. Regulation of CD97 protein in thyroid carcinoma. *J Clin Endocrinol Metab* 1999; 84:1104-1109.

[30] Köhrle J. Local activation and inactivation of thyroid hormones: The deiodinase family. *Mol Cell Endocrinol* 1999; 151:103-119.

[31] Vasko V, Ferrand M, Di Cristofaro J, Carayon P, Henry JF, de Micco C. Specific pattern of RAS oncogene mutations in follicular thyroid tumors. *J Clin Endocrinol Metab.* 2003; 88:2745-2752.

[32] Braga-Basaria M, Ringel MD. Beyond radioiodine: a review of potential new therapeutic approaches for thyroid cancer. *J Clin Endocrinol Metab*. 2003;88:1947-1960.

[33] Specht MC, Barden CB, Fahey TJ 3rd. p44/p42-MAP kinase expression in papillary thyroid carcinomas. *Surgery*. 2001; 130:936-940.

[34] Farid NR, Shi Y, Zou M. Molecular basis of thyroid cancer. *Endocr Rev*. 1994; 15:202-232

[35] Saavedra HI, Knauf JA, Shirokawa JM, Wang J, Ouyang B, Elisei R, Stambrook PJ, Fagin JA. The RAS oncogene induces genomic instability in thyroid PCCL3 cells via the MAPK pathway Oncogene 2000; 19:3948-3954.

[36] Fenton C, Anderson J, Lukes Y, Dinauer CA, Tuttle RM, Francis GL. Ras mutations are uncommon in sporadic thyroid cancer in children and young adults. *J Endocrinol Invest* 1999; 22:781-789.

[37] Zhu Z, Gandhi M, Nikiforova MN, Fischer AH, Nikiforov YE. Molecular profile and clinical-pathologic features of the follicular variant of papillary thyroid carcinoma. An unusually high prevalence of ras mutations. *Am J Clin Pathol*. 2003;120:71-77.

[38] Basolo F, Pisaturo F, Pollina LE, Fontanini G, Elisei R, Molinaro E, Iacconi P, Miccoli P, Pacini F. N-ras mutation in poorly differentiated thyroid carcinomas: correlation with bone metastases and inverse correlation to thyroglobulin expression. *Thyroid* 2000; 10:19-23i.

[39] Davies H, Bignell GR, Cox C, Stephens P, Edkins S, Clegg S, Teague J, Woffendin H, Garnett MJ, Bottomley W, Davis N, Dicks E, Ewing R, Floyd Y, Gray K, Hall S, Hawes R, Hughes J, Kosmidou V, Menzies A, Mould C, Parker A, Stevens C, Watt S, Hooper S, Wilson R, Jayatilake H, Gusterson BA, Cooper C, Shipley J, Hargrave D, Pritchard-Jones K, Maitland N, Chenevix-Trench G, Riggins GJ, Bigner DD, Palmieri G, Cossu A, Flanagan A, Nicholson A, Ho JW, Leung SY, Yuen ST, Weber BL, Seigler HF, Darrow TL, Paterson H, Marais R, Marshall CJ, Wooster R, Stratton MR, Futreal PA. Mutations of the BRAF gene in human cancer. *Nature*. 2002; 417:949-954.

[40] Puxeddu E, Moretti S, Elisei R, Romei C, Pascucci R, Martinelli M, Marino C, Avenia N, Rossi ED, Fadda G, Cavaliere A, Ribacchi R, Falorni A, Pontecorvi A, Pacini F, Pinchera A, Santeusanio F. BRAF(V599E) mutation is the leading genetic event in adult sporadic papillary thyroid carcinomas. *J Clin Endocrinol Metab*. 2004; 89:2414-2420.

[41] Xing M, Tufano RP, Tufaro AP, Basaria S, Ewertz M, Rosenbaum E, Byrne PJ, Wang J, Sidransky D, Ladenson PW. Detection of BRAF mutation on fine needle aspiration biopsy specimens: a new diagnostic tool for papillary thyroid cancer. *J Clin Endocrinol Metab*. 2004 Jun;89(6):2867-72.

[42] Namba H, Nakashima M, Hayashi T, Hayashida N, Maeda S, Rogounovitch TI, Ohtsuru A, Saenko VA, Kanematsu T, Yamashita S. Clinical implication of hot spot BRAF mutation, V599E, in papillary thyroid cancers. *J Clin Endocrinol Metab*. 2003; 88:4393-4397.

[43] Bieche I, Franc B, Vidaud D, Vidaud M, Lidereau R. Analyses of MYC, ERBB2, and CCND1 genes in benign and malignant thyroid follicular cell tumors by real-time polymerase chain reaction. *Thyroid* 2001; 11:147-152.

[44] Sugg SL, Ezzat S, Zheng L, Rosen IB, Freeman JL, Asa SL. Cytoplasmic staining of erbB-2 but not mRNA levels correlates with differentiation in human thyroid neoplasia. *Clin Endocrinol* 1998; 49:629-637.

[45] Wang S, Lloyd RV, Hutzler MJ, Safran MS, Patwardhan NA, Khan A. The role of cell cycle regulatory protein, cyclin D1, in the progression of thyroid cancer. *Mod Pathol.* 2000;13:882-887.

[46] Ramirez R, Hsu D, Patel A, Fenton C, Dinauer C, Tuttle RM, Francis GL. Over-expression of hepatocyte growth factor/scatter factor (HGF/SF) and the HGF/SF receptor (cMET) are associated with a high risk of metastasis and recurrence for children and young adults with papillary thyroid carcinoma. *Clin Endocrinol* 2000; 53:635-644.

[47] Trovato M, Fraggetta F, Villari D, Batolo D, Mackey K, Trimarchi F, Benvenga S. Loss of heterozygosity of the long arm of chromosome 7 in follicular and anaplastic thyroid cancer, but not in papillary thyroid cancer. *J Clin Endocrinol Metab* 1999; 84:3235-3240.

[48] Sozzi G, Bongarzone I, Miozzo M, Cariani CT, Mondellini P Calderone C. Cytogenetic and molecular genetic characterization of papillary thyroid carcinomas. *Genes Chromosomes Cancer* 1992; 5:212-218.

[49] Greco A, Pierotti MA, Bongarzone I, Pagliardini S, Lanzi C, Della Porta G. TRK-T1 is a novel oncogene formed by the fusion of TPR and TRK genes in human papillary thyroid carcinomas. *Oncogene* 1992; 7:237-242.

[50] Greco A, Mariani C, Miranda C, Lupas A, Pagliardini S, Pomati M. The DNA rearrangement that generates the TRK-T3 oncogene involves a novel gene on chromosome 3 whose product has a potential coiled-coil domain. *Mol Cell Biol* 1995; 15:6118-6127.

[51] Jhiang SM. The RET proto-oncogene in human cancers. *Oncogene* 2000 20; 19:5590-5597.

[52] Sugg SL, Ezzat S, Zheng L, Freeman JL, Rosen IB, Asa SL. Oncogene profile of papillary thyroid carcinoma. *Surgery* 1999; 125:46-52.

[53] Grieco M, Santoro M, Berlingieri MT, Melillo RM, Donghi R, Bongarzone I. PTC is a novel rearranged form of the ret proto-oncogene and is frequently detected in vivo in human thyroid papillary carcinomas. *Cell* 1990; 60:557-563.

[54] Sozzi G, Bongarzone I, Miozzo M, Borrello MG, Blutti MG, Pilotti S. A t(10;17) translocation creates the RET/PTC2 chimeric transforming sequence in papillary thyroid carcinoma. *Genes Chromosomes Cancer.* 1994; 9:244-250.

[55] Santoro M, Dathan NA, Berlingieri MT, Bongarzone I, Paulin C, Grieco M. Molecular characterization of RET/PTC3; a novel rearranged version of the RETproto-oncogene in a human thyroid papillary carcinoma. *Oncogene* 1994; 9:509-516.

[56] Fugazzola L, Pierotti MA, Vigano E, Pacini F, Vorontsova TV, Bongarzone I. Molecular and biochemical analysis of RET/PTC4, a novel oncogenic rearrangement between RET and ELE1 genes, in a post-Chernobyl papillary thyroid cancer. *Oncogene* 1996; 13:1093-1097.

[57] Klugbauer S, Demidchik EP, Lengfelder E, Rabes HM. Detection of a novel type of RET rearrangement (PTC5) in thyroid carcinomas after Chernobyl and analysis of the involved RET-fused gene RFG5. *Cancer Res* 1998; 58:198-203.

[58] Klugbauer S, Rabes HM. The transcription coactivator HTIF1 and a related protein are fused to the RET receptor tyrosine kinase in childhood papillary thyroid carcinomas. *Oncogene* 1999; 18:4388-4393.

[59] Salassidis K, Bruch J, Zitzelsberger H, Lengfelder E, Kellerer AM, Bauchinger M. Translocation t(10;14) (q11.2:q22.1) fusing the kinetin to the RET gene creates a novel rearranged form (PTC8) of the RET proto-oncogene in radiation-induced childhood papillary thyroid carcinoma. *Cancer Res* 2000; 68:2786-2789.

[60] Elisei R, Romei C, Vorontsova T, Cosci B, Veremeychik V, Kuchinskaya E, Basolo F, Demidchik EP, Miccoli P, Pinchera A, Pacini F. RET/PTC rearrangements in thyroid nodules: studies in irradiated and not irradiated, malignant and benign thyroid lesions in children and adults. *J Clin Endocrinol Metab* 2001; 86:3211-3216.

[61] Pacini F, Elisei R, Romei C, Pinchera A. RET proto-oncogene mutations in thyroid carcinomas: clinical relevance *J Endocrinol Invest* 2000; 23:328-338.

[62] Basolo F, Molinaro E, Agate L, Pinchera A, Pollina L, Chiappetta G, Monaco C, Santoro M, Fusco A, Miccoli P, Elisei R, Capezzone M, Pacini F. RET protein expression has no prognosis impact on the long-term outcome of papillary thyroid carcinoma. *Eur J Endocrinol* 2001; 145:599-604.

[63] Kjellman P, Learoyd DL, Messina M, Weber G, Hoog A, Wallin G, Larsson C, Robinson BG, Zedenius J. Expression of the RET proto-oncogene in papillary thyroid carcinoma and its correlation with clinical outcome. *J. Br J Surg* 2001; 88:557-563.

[64] Fenton CL, Lukes Y, Nicholson D, Dinauer CA, Francis GL, Tuttle RM. The ret/PTC mutations are common in sporadic papillary thyroid carcinoma of children and young adults. *J Clin Endocrinol Metab* 2000; 85:1170-1175.

[65] Mizuno T, Iwamoto KS, Kyoizumi S, Nagamura H, Shinohara T, Koyama K. Preferential induction of RET/PTC1 rearrangement by X-ray irradiation. *Oncogene* 2000; 19:438-443.

[66] Collins BJ, Chiappetta G, Schneider AB, Santoro M, Pentimalli F, Fogelfeld L, Gierlowski T, Shore-Freedman E, Jaffe G, Fusco A. RET expression in papillary thyroid cancer from patients irradiated in childhood for benign conditions. *J Clin Endocrinol Metab.* 2002; 87:3941-3946.

[67] Smida J, Salassidis K, Hieber L, Zitzelsberger H, Kellerer AM, Demidchik EP. Distinct frequency of ret rearrangements in papillary thyroid carcinomas of children and adults from Belarus. *Int. J. Cancer* 1999; 80:32-38.

[68] Nakata T, Kitamura Y, Shimizu K, Tanaka S, Fujimori M Yokoyama S. Fusion of a novel gene, ELKS, to RET due to translocation t(10;12)(q11;p13) in a papillary thyroid carcinoma. *Genes Chromosomes Cancer* 1999; 25:97-103.

[69] Corvi R, Berger N, Balczon R, Romeo G. RET/PCM-1: a novel fusion gene in papillary thyroid carcinoma. *Oncogene.* 2000; 19:4236-4242.

[70] Santoro M, Papotti M, Chiappetta G, Garcia-Rostan G, Volante M, Johnson C, Camp RL, Pentimalli F, Monaco C, Herrero A, Carcangiu ML, Fusco A, Tallini G. RET

activation and clinicopathologic features in poorly differentiated thyroid tumors. *J Clin Endocrinol Metab.* 2002; 87:370-379.

[71] Chiappetta G, Toti P, Cetta F, Giuliano A, Pentimalli F, Amendola I, Lazzi S, Monaco M, Mazzuchelli L, Tosi P, Santoro M, Fusco A. The RET/PTC oncogene is frequently activated in oncocytic thyroid tumors (Hurthle cell adenomas and carcinomas), but not in oncocytic hyperplastic lesions. *J Clin Endocrinol Metab.* 2002; 87:364-369.

[72] Martelli ML, Iuliano R, Le Pera I, Sama' I, Monaco C, Cammarota S, Kroll T, Chiariotti L, Santoro M, Fusco A. Inhibitory effects of peroxisome poliferator-activated receptor gamma on thyroid carcinoma cell growth. *J Clin Endocrinol Metab.* 2002; 87:4728-4735.

[73] Marques AR, Espadinha C, Catarino AL, Moniz S, Pereira T, Sobrinho LG, Leite V. Expression of PAX8-PPAR gamma 1 rearrangements in both follicular thyroid carcinomas and adenomas. *J Clin Endocrinol Metab.* 2002; 87:3947-3952.

[74] Cheung L, Messina M, Gill A, Clarkson A, Learoyd D, Delbridge L, Wentworth J, Philips J, Clifton-Bligh R, Robinson BG. Detection of the PAX8-PPAR gamma fusion oncogene in both follicular thyroid carcinomas and adenomas. *J Clin Endocrinol Metab.* 2003; 88:354-357.

[75] Nikiforova MN, Lynch RA, Biddinger PW, Alexander EK, Dorn GW 2nd, Tallini G, Kroll TG, Nikiforov YE. RAS point mutations and PAX8-PPAR gamma rearrangement in thyroid tumors: evidence for distinct molecular pathways in thyroid follicular carcinoma. *J Clin Endocrinol Metab.* 2003 May; 88:2318-2326.

[76] Dwight T, Thoppe SR, Foukakis T, Lui WO, Wallin G, Hoog A, Frisk T, Larsson C, Zedenius J. Involvement of the PAX8/peroxisome proliferator-activated receptor gamma rearrangement in follicular thyroid tumors. *J Clin Endocrinol Metab.* 2003; 88:4440-4445.

[77] Dobashi Y, Sakamoto A, Sugimura H, Mernyei M, Mori M, Oyama T. Overexpression of p53 as a possible prognostic factor in human thyroid carcinoma. *Am J Surg Pathol* 1993; 17:375-381.

[78] Donghi R, Longoni A, Pilotti S, Michieli P, Della Porta G, Pierotti MA. Gene p53 mutations are restricted to poorly differentiated and undifferentiated carcinomas of the thyroid gland. *J Clin Invest* 1993; 91:1753-1760.

[79] Filie AC, Chiesa A, Bryant BR, Merino MJ, Sobel ME, Abati A. The Tall cell variant of papillary carcinoma of the thyroid: cytologic features and loss of heterozygosity of metastatic and/or recurrent neoplasms and primary neoplasms. *Cancer* 1999; 87:238-242.

[80] Fagin JA, Matsuo K, Karmakar A, Chen DL, Tang SH Koeffler HP. High prevalence of mutations of the p53 gene in poorly differentiated human thyroid carcinomas. *J Clin Invest* 1993; 91:179-184.

[81] Ito T, Seyama T, Mizuno T, Tsuyama N, Hayashi Y, Dohi K. Genetic alterations in thyroid tumor progression: association with p53 gene mutations. *Jpn. J. Cancer Res* 1993; 84:526-531.

[82] Takeuchi Y, Daa T, Kashima K, Yokoyama S, Nakayama I, Noguchi S. Mutations of p53 in thyroid carcinoma with an insular component. *Thyroid* 1999; 9:377-381.

[83] Pisarchik AV, Ermak G, Kartel NA, Figge J. Molecular alterations involving p53 codons 167 and 183 in papillary thyroid carcinomas from Chernobyl-contaminated regions of Belarus. *Thyroid* 2000; 10:25-30.

[84] Sera N, Ashizawa K, Ando T, Ide A, Abe Y, Usa T, Tominaga T, Ejima E, Hayashi T, Shimokawa I, Eguchi K.. Anaplastic changes associated with p53 gene mutation in differentiated thyroid carcinoma after insufficient radioactive iodine (131I) therapy. *Thyroid* 2000; 10:975-979.

[85] Martelli ML, Miano MG, Battaglia C, Trapasso F, Stella A, Iuliano R. The highly malignant phenotype of anaplastic thyroid carcinoma cell lines is recessive. *Eur J Endocrinol* 2000; 143:515-521.

[86] Gimm O, Perren A, Weng LP, Marsh DJ, Yeh JJ, Ziebold U. Differential nuclear and cytoplasmic expression of PTEN in normal thyroid tissue, and benign and malignant epithelial thyroid tumors. *Am J Pathol* 2000; 156:1693-1700.

[87] Bruni P, Boccia A, Baldassarre G, Trapasso F, Santoro M, Chiappetta G, Fusco A, Viglietto G. PTEN expression is reduced in a subset of sporadic thyroid carcinomas: evidence that PTEN-growth suppressing activity in thyroid cancer cells mediated by p27kip1. *Oncogene* 2000; 19:3146-3155.

[88] Farid NR, Zou M, Shi Y. Genetics of follicular thyroid cancer. *Endocrinol Metab Clin North Am.* 1995; 24:865-883.

[89] Blain SW, Massague J. Breast cancer banishes p27 from nucleus. *Nat Med.* 2002; 8:1076-1078.

[90] Parma J, Duprez L, Van Sande J, Cochaux P, Gervy C, Mockel J, Dumont J, Vassart G. Somatic mutations in the thyrotropin receptor gene cause hyperfunctioning thyroid adenomas. *Nature.* 1993; 365:649-651.

[91] Porcellini A, Ciullo I, Laviola L, Amabile G, Fenzi G, Avvedimento VE. Novel mutations of thyrotropin receptor gene in thyroid hyperfunctioning adenomas. Rapid identification by fine needle aspiration biopsy. *J Clin Endocrinol Metab* 1994; 79:657-661.

[92] Michiels FM, Caillou B, Talbot M, Dessarps-Freichey F, Maunoury MT, Schlumberger M, Mercken L, Monier R, Feunteun J. Oncogenic potential of guanine nucleotide stimulatory factor alpha subunit in thyroid glands of transgenic mice. *Proc Natl Acad Sci U S A* 1994; 91:10488-10492.

[93] Matsuo K, Friedman E, Gejman PV, Fagin JA. The thyrotropin receptor (TSH-R) is not an oncogene for thyroid tumors: structural studies of the TSH-R and the alpha-subunit of Gs in human thyroid neoplasms. *J Clin Endocrinol Metab* 1993; 76:1446-1451.

[94] Cetani F, Tonacchera M, Pinchera A, Barsacchi R, Basolo F, Miccoli P, Pacini. Genetic analysis of the TSH receptor gene in differentiated human thyroid carcinomas. *J Endocrinol Invest* 1999; 22:273-278.

[95] Mircescu H, Parma J, Huot C, Deal C, Oligny LL, Vassart G, Van Vliet G. Hyperfunctioning malignant thyroid nodule in an 11-year-old girl: pathologic and molecular studies. *J Pediatr* 2000; 137:585-587.

[96] Camacho P, Gordon D, Chiefari E, Yong S, DeJong S, Pitale S, Russo D, Filetti S. A Phe 486 thyrotropin receptor mutation in an autonomously functioning follicular carcinoma that was causing hyperthyroidism. *Thyroid* 2000;10:1009-1012.

[97] Corvillain B, Van Sande J, Dumont JE, Vassart G. Somatic and germline mutations of the TSH receptor and thyroid diseases. *Clin Endocrinol* 2001; 55:143-158.

[98] Bassi V, Vitale M, Feliciello A, De Riu S, Rossi G, Fenzi G. Retinoic acid induces intercellular adhesion molecule-1 hyperexpression in human thyroid carcinoma cell lines. *J Clin Endocrinol Metab* 1995; 80:1129-1135.

[99] Pötter E, Bergwitz C, Brabant G. The cadherin-catenin system: implications for growth and differentiation of endocrine tissues. *Endocr Rev* 1999; 20:207-239.

[100] Brabant G, Hoang-Vu C, Cetin Y, Dralle H, Scheumann G, Molne J, Hansson G, Jansson S, Ericson LE, Nilsson M. E-cadherin: a differentiation marker in thyroid malignancies. *Cancer Res* 1993; 53:4987-4993.

[101] von Wasielewwski R, Rhein A, Werner M, et al. Immunohistocehmical detection of E-cadherin in differentiated thyroid carcinomas correlates with clinical outcome. *Cancer Res* 1997. 57:2501-2507.

[102] Ishigaki K, Namba H, Nakashima M, Nakayama T, Mitsutake N, Hayashi T, Maeda S, Ichinose M, Kanematsu T, Yamashita S. Aberrant localization of beta-catenin correlates with overexpression of its target gene in human papillary thyroid cancer. *J Clin Endocrinol Metab.* 2002; 87:3433-3440.

[103] Garcia-Rostan G, Tallini G, Herrero A, D'Aquila TG, Carcangiu ML, Rimm DL Frequent mutation and nuclear localization of beta-catenin in anaplastic thyroid carcinoma. *Cancer Res* 1999; 59:1811-1815.

[104] Bohm J, Niskanen L, Kiraly K, Kellokoski J, Eskelinen M, Hollmen S, Alhava E, Kosma VM. Expression and prognostic value of α-, β-, and γ- Catenins in differentiated thyroid carcinoma. *J Clin Endocrinol Metab* 2000; 85:4806-4811.

[105] Garcia-Rostan G, Camp RL, Herrero A, Carcangiu ML, Rimm DL, Tallini G. beta-Catenin dysregulation in thyroid neoplasms: down-regulation, aberrant nuclear expression, and ctnnb1 exon 3 mutations are markers for aggressive tumor phenotypes and poor prognosis. *Am J Pathol* 2001; 158:987-996.

[106] Sato H, Ino Y, Miura A, Abe Y, Sakai H, Ito K, Hirohashi S. Dysadherin: expression and clinical significance in thyroid carcinoma. *J Clin Endocrinol Metab.* 2003; 88:4407-4412.

[107] Gasbarri A, Martegani MP, Del Prete F, Lucante T, Natali PG, Bartolazzi Galectin-3 and CD44v6 isoforms in the preoperative evaluation of thyroid nodules. *J Clin Oncol* 1999; 17:3494-3502.

[108] Saggiorato E, Cappia S, De Giuli P, Mussa A, Pancani G, Caraci P, Angeli A, Orlandi F. Galectin-3 as a presurgical immunocytodiagnostic marker of minimally invasive follicular thyroid carcinoma. *J Clin Endocrinol Metab* 2001; 86:5152-5158.

[109] Fernandez PL, Merino MJ, Gomez M, Campo E, Medina T, Castronovo V, Sanjuán X, Cardesa A, Liu FT, Sobel ME. Galectin-3 and laminin expression in neoplastic and non-neoplastic thyroid tissue. *J Pathol* 1997; 181:80-86.

[110] Kawachi K, Matsushita Y, Yonezawa S, Nakano S, Shirao K, Natsugoe S, Sueyoshi K, Aikou T, Sato E Galectin-3 expression in various thyroid neoplasms and its possible role in metastasis formation. *Hum Pathol* 2000; 31:428-433.

[111] Bohm JP, Niskanen LK, Pirinen RT, Kiraly K, Kellokoski JK, Moisio KI, Eskelinen MJ, Tulla HE, Hollmen S, Alhava EM, Kosma VM. Reduced CD44 standard

expression is associated with tumour recurrence and unfavourable outcome in differentiated thyroid carcinoma. *J Pathol* 2000; 192:321-327.

[112] Takano T, Sumizaki H, Amino N. Detection of CD44 variants in fine needle aspiration biopsies of thyroid tumor by RT-PCR. *J Exp Clin Cancer Res* 1997; 16:267-271.

[113] Stepien HM, Kolomecki K, Pasieka Z, Komorowski J, Stepien T, Kuzdak K. Angiogenesis of endocrine gland tumours. New molecular targets in diagnostics therapy. *EJE* 2002, 146:143-51.

[114] Klein M, Vignaud JM, Hennequin V, Toussaint B, Bresler L, Plenat F, Leclere J, Duprez A, Weryha G. Increased expression of the vascular endothelial growth factor is a pejorative prognosis marker in papillary thyroid carcinoma. *J Clin Endocrinol Metab* 2001; 86:656-658.

[115] Viglietto G, Maglione D, Rambaldi M, Cerutti J, Romano A, Trapasso F, Fedele M, Ippolito P, Chiappetta G, Botti G. Upregulation of vascular endothelial growth factor (VEGF) and downregulation of placenta growth factor (PlGF) associated with malignancy in human thyroid tumors and cell lines. *Oncogene* 1995; 11:1569-1579

[116] Katoh R, Miyagi E, Kawaoi A, Hemmi A, Komiyama A, Oyama T, Shibuya M. Expression of vascular endothelial growth factor (VEGF) in human thyroid neoplasms. *Hum Pathol* 1999; 30:891-897.

[117] Soh EY, Duh QY, Sobhi SA, Young DM, Epstein HD, Wong MG, Garcia YK, Min YD, Grossman RF, Siperstein AE, Clark OH. Vascular endothelial growth factor expression is higher in differentiated thyroid cancer than in normal or benign thyroid. *J Clin Endocrinol Metab* 1997; 82:3741-3747.

[118] Tuttle RM, Fleisher M, Francis GL, Robbins RJ. Serum vascular endothelial growth factor levels are elevated in metastatic differentiated thyroid cancer but not increased by short-term TSH stimulation. *J Clin Endocrinol Metab*. 2002; 87:1737-1742.

[119] Sorvillo F, Mazziotti G, Carbone A, Piscopo M, Rotondi M, Cioffi M, Musto P, Biondi B, Iorio S, Amato G, Carella C. Recombinant human thyrotropin reduces serum vascular endothelial growth factor levels in patients monitored for thyroid carcinoma even in the absence of thyroid tissue. *J Clin Endocrinol Metab*. 2003; 88:4818-4822.

[120] Ye C, Feng C, Wang S, Liu X, Lin Y, Li M. Antiangiogenic and antitumor effects of endostatin on follicular thyroid carcinoma. *Endocrinology*. 2002; 143:3522-3528.

[121] Marti U, Ruchti C, Kampf J, Thomas GA, Williams ED, Peter HJ, Gerber H, Burgi U. Nuclear localization of epidermal growth factor and epidermal growth factor receptors in human thyroid tissues. *Thyroid* 2001; 11:37-145.

[122] Vella V, Pandini G, Sciacca L, Mineo R, Vigneri R, Pezzino V, Belfiore A. A novel autocrine loop involving IGF-II and the insulin receptor isoform-A stimulates growth of thyroid cancer. *J Clin Endocrinol Metab*. 2002; 87:245-254.

[123] Gillespie JW, Nasir A, Kaiser HE Loss of heterozygosity in papillary and follicular thyroid carcinoma: a mini review. *In Vivo* 2000; 14:139-140.

[124] Kadota M, Tamaki Y, Sakita I, Komoike Y, Miyazaki M, Ooka M, Masuda N, Fujiwara Y, Ohnishi T, Tomita N, Sekimoto M, Ohue M, Ikeda T, Kobayashi T, Horii A, Monden M. Identification of a 7-cM region of frequent allelic loss on chromosome band 16p13.3 that is specifically associated with anaplastic thyroid carcinoma. *Oncol Rep* 2000; 7:529-533.

[125] Komoike Y, Tamaki Y, Sakita I, Tomita N, Ohue M, Sekimoto M, Miyazaki M, Kadota M, Masuda N, Ooka M, Ohnishi T, Nakano Y, Kozaki T, Kobayashi T, Matsuura N, Ikeda T, Horii A, Monden M. Comparative genomic hybridization defines frequent loss on 16p in human anaplastic thyroid carcinoma. *Int J Oncol* 1999; 14:1157-1162.

[126] Hemmer S, Wasenius VM, Knuutila S, Franssila K, Joensuu H. DNA copy number changes in thyroid carcinoma. *Am J Pathol.* 1999; 154:1539-1547.

[127] Kitamura Y, Shimizu K, Ito K, Tanaka S, Emi M. Allelotyping of follicular thyroid carcinoma: frequent allelic losses in chromosome arms 7q, 11p, and 22q. *J Clin Endocrinol Metab.* 2001; 86:4268-4272.

[128] Ouyang B, Knauf JA, Ain K, Nacev B, Fagin JA. Mechanisms of aneuploidy in thyroid cancer cell lines and tissues: evidence for mitotic checkpoint dysfunction without mutations in BUB1 and BUBR1. *Clin Endocrinol.* 2002; 56:341-350.

[129] Modi J, Patel A, Terrell R, Tuttle RM, Francis GL. Papillary thyroid carcinomas from young adults and children contain a mixture of lymphocytes. *J Clin Endocrinol Metab.* 2003; 88:4418-25.

[130] Shah R, Banks K, Patel A, Dogra S, Terrell R, Powers PA, Fenton C, Dinauer CA, Tuttle RM, Francis GL. Intense expression of the b7-2 antigen presentation coactivator is an unfavorable prognostic indicator for differentiated thyroid carcinoma of children and adolescents. *J Clin Endocrinol Metab.* 2002; 87:4391-4397.

[131] DeGroot LJ, Zhang R. Gene therapy for thyroid cancer: where do we stand? *JCEM*; 2001; 86:2923-2928.

[132] Zhang R, DeGroot LJ. Gene therapy of a rat follicular thyroid carcinoma model with adenoviral vectors transducing murine interleukin-12. *Endocrinology.* 2003; 144:1393-1398.

[133] Barzon L, Bonaguro R, Castagliuolo I, Chilosi M, Gnatta E, Parolin C, Boscaro M, Palu G. Transcriptionally targeted retroviral vector for combined suicide and immunomodulating gene therapy of thyroid cancer. *J Clin Endocrinol Metab.* 2002; 87:5304-5311.

[134] Bartolazzi A, Gasbarri A, Papotti M, Bussolati G, Lucante T, Khan A, Inohara H, Application of an immunodiagnostic method for improving preoperative diagnosis of nodular thyroid lesions. *Lancet* 2001; 357:1644-1650.

[135] Inohara H, Honjo Y, Yoshii T. Expression of galectin-3 in fine-needle aspirates as a diagnostic marker differentiating benign from malignant thyroid neoplasms. *Cancer* 1999; 85:2475-2484.

[136] Orlandi F, Saggiorato E, Pivano G et al. Galectin-3 is a presurgical marker of human thyroid carcinoma. *Cancer Res* 1998; 58:3015-3020.

[137] Martins L, Matsuo SE, Ebina KN, Kulcsar MA, Friguglietti CU, Kimura ET. Galectin-3 messenger ribonucleic acid and protein are expressed in benign thyroid tumors. *J Clin Endocrinol Metab.* 2002; 87:4806-4810.

[138] Kovacs RB, Foldes J, Winkler G, Bodo M, Sapi Z. The investigation of galectin-3 in diseases of the thyroid gland. *Eur J Endocrinol.* 2003; 149:449-453.

[138b] Bernet VJ, Anderson J, Vaishnav Y, Solomon B, Adair CF, Saji M, Burman KD, Burch HB, Ringel MD. Determination of galectin-3 messenger ribonucleic Acid

overexpression in papillary thyroid cancer by quantitative reverse transcription-polymerase chain reaction. *J Clin Endocrinol Metab.* 2002; 87:4792-4796.

[139] Feilchenfeldt J, Totsch M, Sheu SY, Robert J, Spiliopoulos A, Frilling A, Schmid KW, Meier CA. Expression of galectin-3 in normal and malignant thyroid tissue by quantitative PCR and immunohistochemistry. *Mod Pathol.* 2003; 16:1117-1123.

[140] Niedziela M, Maceluch J, Korman E. Galectin-3 is not an universal marker of malignancy in thyroid nodular disease in children and adolescents. *J Clin Endocrinol Metab.* 2002; 87:4411-4415.

[141] Khan A, Baker SP, Patwardhan NA, Pullman JM. CD57 (Leu-7) expression is helpful in diagnosis of the follicular variant of papillary thyroid carcinoma. *Virchows Arch.* 1998; 432:427-432.

[142] Cheung CC, Carydis B, Ezzat S, Bedard YC, Asa SL. Analysis of ret/PTC gene rearrangements refines the fine needle aspiration diagnosis of thyroid cancer. *J Clin Endocrinol Metab* 2001; 86:2187-2190.

[143] Ruco LP, Stoppacciaro A, Ballarini F, Prat M, Scarpino S. Met protein and hepatocyte growth factor (HGF) in papillary carcinoma of the thyroid: evidence for a pathogenetic role in tumourigenesis. *J Pathol* 2001; 194:4-8.

[144] Haugen BR, Woodmansee WW, McDermott MT. Towards improving the utility of fine-needle aspiration biopsy for the diagnosis of thyroid tumours. *Clin Endocrinol.* 2002; 56:281-290.

[145] Aogi K, Kitahara K, Urquidi V, Tarin D, Goodison S. Comparison of telomerase and CD44 expression as diagnostic tumor markers in lesions of the thyroid. *Clin Cancer Res.* 1999; 5:2790-2797.

[146] Straight AM, Patel A, Fenton C, Dinauer C, Tuttle RM, Francis GL. Thyroid carcinomas that express telomerase follow a more aggressive clinical course in children and adolescents. *J Endocrinol Invest.* 2002; 25:302-308.

[147] Arturi F, Russo D, Giuffrida D, Ippolito A, Perrotti N, Vigneri R. Early diagnosis by genetic analysis of differentiated thyroid cancer metastases in small lymph nodes. *J Clin Endocrinol Metab* 1997; 82:1638-1641.

[148] Schlumberger M & Pacini F. (1999) *Thyroid tumors.* Paris; Editions Nucléon.

[149] Chua EL, Wu WM, Tran KT, McCarthy SW, Lauer CS, Dubourdieu D, Packham N, O'Brien CJ, Turtle JR, Dong Q. Prevalence and distribution of ret/ptc 1, 2, and 3 in papillary thyroid carcinoma in New Caledonia and Australia. *J Clin Endocrinol Metab* 2000; 85:2733-2739.

[150] Mazzaferri EL, Kloos RT. Current approaches to primary therapy for papillary and follicular thyroid cancer. *J Clin Endocrinol Metab* 2001; 86:1447-1463

[151] Carrasco N. The thyroid sodium-iodide symporter (NIS): cloning and potential clinical applications. *Thyroid today* 1999 XXII:1-11.

[152] Spitzweg C, Harrington KJ, Pinke LA, Vile RG, Morris JC. The sodium iodide symporter and its potential role in cancer therapy. *J Clin Endocrinol Metab.* 2001; 86:3327-3335.

[153] Peter H K Eng, Guemalli R Cardona, Michael C Previti, William W Chin and Lewis E Braverman. Regulation of the sodium iodide symporter by iodide in FRTL-5 cells. pages 139-144.

[154] Dai G, Levy O, Carrasco N. Cloning and characterization of the thyroid iodide transporter. *Nature* 1996; 379:458-460.

[155] Ringel MD, Anderson J, Souza SL, Burch HB, Tambascia M, Shriver CD, Tuttle RM. Expression of the sodium iodide symporter and thyroglobulin genes are reduced in papillary thyroid cancer. *Mod Pathol* 2001; 14:289-296.

[156] Kogai T, Hershman JM, Motomura K, Endo T, Onaya T, Brent GA. Differential regulation of the human sodium/iodide symporter gene promoter in papillary thyroid carcinoma cell lines and normal thyroid cells. *Endocrinology* 2001; 142:3369-3379.

[157] Kitazono M, Robey R, Zhan Z, Sarlis NJ, Skarulis MC, Aikou T, Bates S, Fojo T. Low concentrations of the histone deacetylase inhibitor, depsipeptide (FR901228), increase expression on the Na^{+}/I^{-} symporter and iodine accumulation in poorly differentiated thyroid carcinoma cells. *J Clin Endocrinol Metab* 2001; 86:3430-3435.

[158] Saito T, Endo T, Kawaguchi A, Ikeda M, Katoh R, Kawaoi A, Muramatsu A, Onaya T. Increased expression of the sodium/iodide symporter in papillary thyroid carcinomas. *J Clin Invest* 1998;101:1296-1300.

[159] Russo D, Manole D, Arturi F, Suarez HG, Schlumberger M, Filetti S, Derwahl M. Absence of sodium/iodide symporter gene mutations in differentiated human thyroid carcinomas. *Thyroid* 2001; 11:37-39.

[160] Castro MR, Bergert ER, Goellner JR, Hay ID, Morris JC. Immunohistochemical analysis of sodium iodide symporter expression in metastatic differentiates thyroid cancer: correlation with radioiodine uptake. *J Clin Endocrinol Metab* 2001; 86:5627-5632.

[161] Luciani P, Buci L, Conforti B, Tonacchera M, Agretti P, Elisei R, Vivaldi A, Cioppi F, Biliotti G, Manca G, Vitti P, Serio M, Peri A. Expression of cAMP response element-binding protein and sodium iodide symporter in benign non-functioning and malignant thyroid tumours. *Eur J Endocrinol.* 2003 May;148(5):579-86.

[162] Smit JW, Schroder-van der Elst JP, Karperien M, Que I, Stokkel M, van der Heide D, Romijn JA. Iodide kinetics and experimental (131)I therapy in a xenotransplanted human sodium-iodide symporter-transfected human follicular thyroid carcinoma cell line. *J Clin Endocrinol Metab.* 2002; 87:1247-1253.

[163] Arturi F, Russo D, Bidart JM, Scarpelli D, Schlumberger M, Filetti S. Expression pattern of the pendrin and sodium/iodide symporter genes in human thyroid cell lines and human thyroid tumors. *Eur J Endocrinol* 2001; 145:129-135.

[164] Shimura H, Suzuki H, Miyazaki A, Furuya F, Ohta K, Haraguchi K, Endo T, Onaya T. Transcriptional activation of the thyroglobulin promoter directing suicide gene expression by thyroid transcription factor-1 in thyroid cancer cells. *Cancer Res* 2001; 61:3640-3646.

[165] Links TP, van Tol KM, te Meerman GJ, de Vries GE. Differentiated thyroid carcinoma: a polygenic disease. *Thyroid* 2001; 11:11351140.

[166] Malchoff CD, Malchoff DM. The genetics of hereditary nonmedullary thyroid carcinoma. *J Clin Endocrinol Metab.* 2002; 87:2455-2459.

[167] Bevan S, Pal T, Greenberg CR, Green H, Wixey J, Bignell G, Narod SA, Foulkes WD, Stratton MR, Houlston RS. A comprehensive analysis of MNG1, TCO1, fPTC, PTEN,

TSHR, and TRKA in familial nonmedullary thyroid cancer: confirmation of linkage to TCO1. *J Clin Endocrinol Metab* 2001; 86:3701-3704.

[168] Nishisho I, Nakamura Y, Miyoshi Y, Miki Y, Ando H, Horii A. Mutations of chromosome 5q21 genes in FAP and colorectal cancer patients. *Science* 1991; 253:665-669.

[169] Miyaki M, Iijima T, Ishii R, Hishima T, Mori T, Yoshinaga K, Takami H, Kuroki T, Iwama T. Molecular evidence for multicentric development of thyroid carcinomas in patients with familial adenomatous polyposis. *Am J Pathol* 2000; 157:1825-1827.

[170] Cetta F, Montalto G, Gori M, Curia MC, Cama A, Olschwang S. Germline mutations of the APC gene in patients with familial adenomatous polyposis-associated thyroid carcinoma: results from an European cooperative study. *J Clin Endocrinol Metab* 2000; 85:286-292.

[171] Cetta F, Curia MC, Montalto G, Gori M, Cama A, Battista P, Barbarisi A. Thyroid carcinoma usually occurs in patients with familial adenomatous polyposis in the absence of biallelic inactivation of the adenomatous polyposis coli gene. *J Clin Endocrinol Metab* 2001; 86:427-432.

[172] Liaw D, Marsh DJ, Li J, Dahia PL, Wang SI, Zheng Z. Germline mutations of the PTEN gene in Cowden disease, an inherited breast and thyroid cancer syndrome. *Nat Genet* 1997; 16:64-67.

[173] Sawada T, Hamano N, Satoh H, Okada T, Takeda Y, Mabuchi H. Mutation analysis of the PTEN/MMAC1 gene in Japanese patients with Cowden disease. *Jpn J Cancer Res* 2000; 91:700-705.

[174] Fackenthal JD, Marsh DJ, Richardson AL, Cummings SA, Eng C, Robinson BG, Olopade OI. Male breast cancer in Cowden syndrome patients with germline PTEN mutations. *J Med Genet* 2001; 38:159-164.

[175] Bignell GR, Canzian F, Shayeghi M, Stark M, Shugart YY Biggs P. Familial nontoxic multinodular thyroid goiter locus maps to chromosome 14q but does not account for familial nonmedullary thyroid cancer. *Am J Hum Genet* 1997; 61:1123-1130.

[176] Canzian F, Amati P, Harach HR, Kraimps JL, Lesueur F, Barbier J. A gene predisposing to familial thyroid tumors with cell oxyphilia maps to chromosome 19p13.2. *Am J Hum Genet* 1998; 63:1743-1748.

[177] Hermann S, Sturm I, Mrozek A, Klosterhalfen B, Hauptmann S, Dorken B, Daniel PT. Bax expression in benign and malignant thyroid tumours: Dysregulation of wild-type P53 is associated with a high Bax and P21 expression in thyroid carcinoma. *Int J Cancer* 2001; 92:805-811.

[178] Kremser R, Obrist P, Spizzo G, Erler H, Kendler D, Kemmler G, Mikuz G, Ensinger C. Her2/neu overexpression in differentiated thyroid carcinomas predicts metastatic disease. *Virchows Arch.* 2003; 442:322-328.

[179] Murphy PM. Chemokines and the molecular basis of cancer metastasis. *N Engl J Med* 2001; 345:833-835.

[180] Muller A, Homey B, Soto H, Ge N, Catron D, Buchanan ME, McClanahan T, Murphy E, Yuan W, Wagner SN, Barrera JL, Mohar A, Verastegui E, Zlotnik A. Involvement of chemokine receptors in breast cancer metastasis. *Nature* 2001; 410:50-56.

[181] Zafon C, Obiols G, Castellvi J, Tallada N, Galofre P, Gemar E, Mesa J, Simo R. nm23-H1 immunoreactivity as a prognostic factor in differentiated thyroid carcinoma. *J Clin Endocrinol Metab* 2001; 86:3975-3980.

[182] Shi Y, Zou M, Farid NR. The mystery of nm23H1 in thyroid cancer. *J Endocrinol Invest*. 2002; 25:663-664

In: Trends in Thyroid Cancer Research
Editor: Carl A. Milton, pp. 33-47

ISBN 1-59454-627-4

Chapter II

Role of IL-4 and IL-10 Cytokines in the Pathogenic Mechanism of Thyroid Cancer

Matilde Todaro**, Sebastiano Bonventre, Enzo Mannino and Giorgio Stassi

Department of Surgical and Oncological Sciences, University of Palermo, Italy.

Abstract

In recent years, several alterations involving oncogenes and tumor suppressor genes have been identified in thyroid cancer. However, although some advances have been made to the understanding of the molecular mechanisms that determine thyroid malignancies, the absence of crucial information on the mechanisms underlying increased expansion and survival of thyroid cancer cells does not allow the development of standard and reliable treatments, with the exception of unifocal non-metastatic papillary microcarcinoma. Apoptosis is a key mechanism governing the development of multicellular organisms and maintenance of tissue homeostasis. It is becoming increasingly clear that impaired apoptosis is a critical component of the multi-step tumorigenesis process. Although CD95 is expressed in essentially all the histological variants of thyroid carcinomas, CD95 cross-linking fails to induce cell death in thyroid tumor cells. It has been demonstrated that thyrocytes produce CD95L and are able to kill infiltrating T lymphocytes expressing CD95. Therefore refractoriness to CD95 stimulation in thyroid tumors may be a critical event in tumorigenesis. Indeed, the abundant expression of CD95L in malignant tumors may result in the so called "tumor counterattack", a defence process that helps cancer cells to escape immune surveillance mechanisms by eliminating infiltrating lymphocytes. Traditional antineoplastic therapy is based on the use of chemotherapeutic compounds, which exert a cytotoxic effect on proliferating cells and

* Correspondence concerning this article should be addressed to: Matilde Todaro MD, Department of Surgical and Oncological Sciences, Via Liborio Giuffrè, 5, 90127 Palermo, University of Palermo, Italy, Voice: +39 091 6553211, Fax: +39 091 6553238, e-mail: matilde.todaro@tiscali.it

promote the destruction of sensitive tumors. Therefore, the development of effective anti-apoptotic mechanisms can result in the resistance of malignant cell to chemotherapy. It has been recently investigated the mechanisms responsible for the widespread refractoriness to chemotherapeutic drugs observed in thyroid cancers. It has been found that malignant thyroid carcinoma cells express high levels of Bcl-2 and Bcl-xL. All the histological thyroid cancer variants examined produced interleukin-4 (IL-4) and interleukin-10 (IL-10), which increased FLIP, PED, Bcl-2 and Bcl-xL levels and protected thyroid cells from chemotherapeutic agents and from cell death induced by CD95. Exposure to neutralizing antibodies against IL-4 and IL-10 resulted in down modulation of FLIP, PED, Bcl-2 and Bcl-xL, death of a considerable percentage of thyroid cancer cells and sensitization of the residual tumor population to cytotoxic drugs- and CD95- induced apoptosis. Thus, IL-4 and IL-10 may represent new therapeutic targets for the treatment of epithelial cancer. It is therefore likely that presence of these cytokines in the cancer microenvironment should promote survival activating the ability of cancer cells to up regulate anti-apoptotic genes leading to apoptosis resistance. These studies may provide key molecular bases to the understanding of thyroid cancer pathogenesis and the definition of novel therapeutic strategies.

Keywords: Thyroid cancer, IL-4, IL-10, apoptosis, CD95, chemoresistance.

Introduction

Thyroid carcinoma constitutes over 1% of incident cancer and is considered the most common endocrine malignancy responsible for about 60% of deaths secondary to endocrine cancer [1] [2]. Thyroid malignancies comprise a broad range of neoplasms of the thyroid gland with differing biologic and clinical implications. Usually, most thyroid carcinomas present as an asymptomatic thyroid mass, unintentionally discovered. The first evidence of cancer may be a palpable cervical lymphonode or an incidental finding on a radiological study for some other purpose (as carotid ultrasonography). Immunohistochemistry of a fine–needle aspirate (FNA) or surgical samples may reveal staining for thyroglobulin, a marker for papillary or follicular cancer.

Clinical thyroid cancers are less common in children with a female yearly incidence and prevalence than male.

According to the WHO thyroid cancer are classified in two types: differentiated, such as papillary thyroid carcinomas (PTC) and follicular thyroid carcinomas (FTC), and undifferentiated or anaplatic thyroid carcinoma (UTC). Differentiated carcinomas of thyroid epithelial cells are the most common; while undifferentiated tumors, medullary cancers (MTC) and tumours of the parafollicular (calcitonin-secreting) cells, are quite infrequent.

Papillary Thyroid Carcinoma

PTC is the most common type of thyroid malignancy, constituting about 80% of primary thyroid tumors. It can occur at any age and rarely it has been diagnosed as a congenital tumor [3], the mean age at the time of initial diagnosis being approximately 40 years. Women are affected more than men in ratios of 2:1 to 4:1 [4, 5]. In fact, some studies have suggested the involvement of various hormonal factors in the development of papillary carcinoma (i.e. late of first pregnancy, fertility problems and oral contraceptives). The PTC diagnosis is based on the presence of certain architectural features mainly in form of papillae and characteristic nuclear changes (Fig. 1).

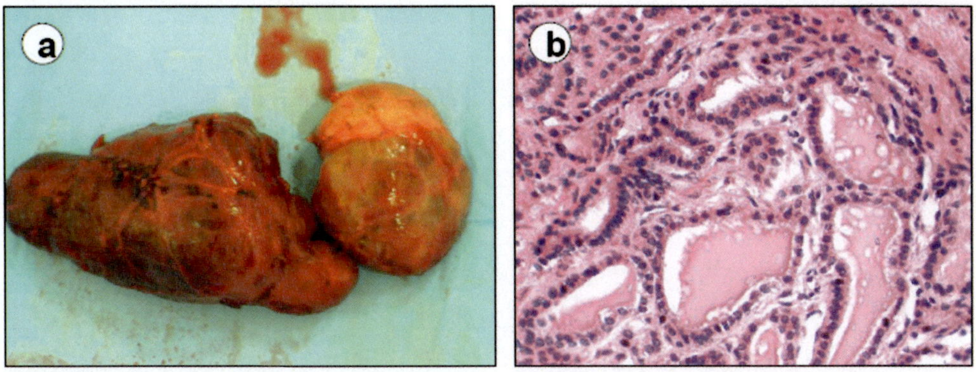

Fig. 1. a - Gross appearance of papillary thyroid carcinoma. b- H&E staining of papillary thyroid carcinoma (40x).

FOLLICULAR THYROID CARCINOMA

FTC comprise about 5% of thyroid cancers [6] whose identification largely depends on the presence of invasion of the capsule, blood vessels or adjacent thyroid. Like PTC, it shares the same predilection for female but older age.

Its histological appearance is extremely variable, ranging from well-formed follicles to predominantly solid growth pattern. In contrast to papillary carcinomas, follicular carcinomas of either subtypes are almost always solitary and practically never occult. It disseminates haematogenously and metastasises to bone, lungs, brain and liver [7,8] (Fig. 2).

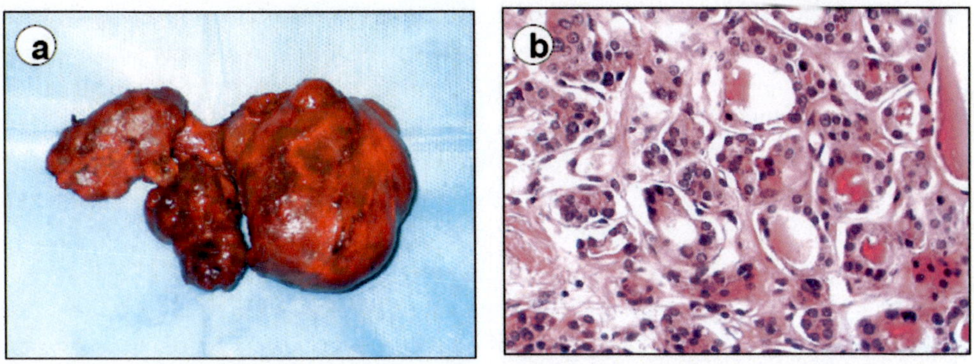

Fig. 2. a - Gross picture of follicular thyroid carcinoma. b - Microscopic examination of follicular thyroid carcinoma (H&E 40x).

Undifferentiated Thyroid Carcinomas

UTC also known as anaplastic or sarcomatoid carcinoma, represents approximately 10% of thyroid malignancies. Anaplastic thyroid carcinoma usually present in older adult women as a rapidly enlarging mass, which often result in dyspnea. They have an extremely poor prognosis, in fact many patients surviving less than 6 months following diagnosis [9]

In contrast, MTC is rare and comprises less than 10% of all thyroid carcinomas. It has been described as solid, non-encapsulated but relatively well-circumscribed tumor. Most lesions are situated in the middle portion or upper half of the thyroid, corresponding to a greater concentration of C-cells. MTC diagnosis is significant for its aggressiveness, its close association with MEN IIa and IIb and a relationship to a C-cell hyperplasia as probable precursor lesion (Fig. 3).

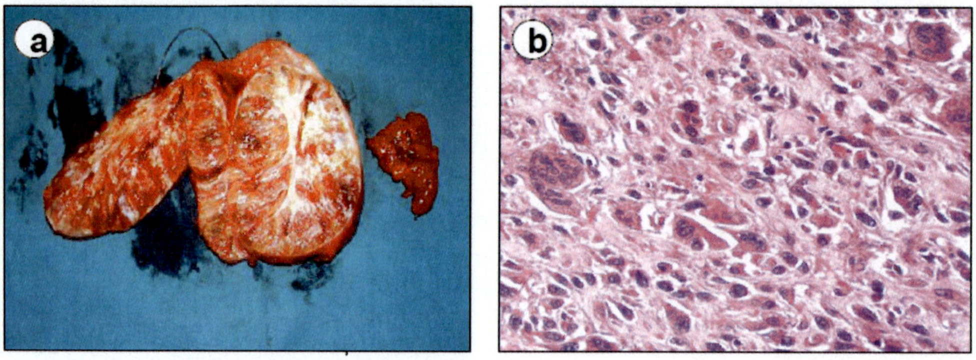

Fig. 3. a - Gross appearance of undifferentiated thyroid carcinoma. b - Undifferentiated thyroid carcinoma (H&E 40x).

Prognosis

Although most patients have a good prognosis, approximately 1200 patients develop progressive metastatic disease and die from thyroid cancer yearly. These progressive cancers either lose or have reduced responsiveness to radioactive iodine rendering them resistant to standard therapeutic approaches. Effective alternative therapies for thyroid cancer have been identified, there is a critical need to develop novel approaches to treat thyroid cancer.

In recent years, several alterations involving oncogenes and tumor suppressor genes have been identified in thyroid cancer. However, although some advances have been made to the understanding of the molecular mechanisms that determine thyroid malignancies, the absence of crucial information on the machinery underlying increased expansion and survival of thyroid cancer cells does not allow the development of standard and reliable. treatments. It is becoming increasingly clear that impaired apoptosis is a critical component of the thyroid cancer pathogenesis.

Apoptosis

Apoptosis is known to play a fundamental role in the development, the maintenance of tissue homeostasis and repair of tissues [10] (Fig. 4). In particular, the apoptosis machinery is essential for the ability to induce suicide of supernumerary, misplaced or damaged cells with high specificity and efficiency [11]. The study of apoptosis has provide a significant contribution to know the physiology of several organ systems and the pathogenesis of many human disease. Dysfunctions in the regulation or execution of cell suicide are concerned in a wide range of developmental abnormalities, autoimmune and neurodegenerative diseases or cancer [12-14].

In fact, improperly excessive cell death leads to parenchymal cell loss consequently impaired organ function, while inadequate cell death contributes to the emergence of hyperplasias and neoplasias.

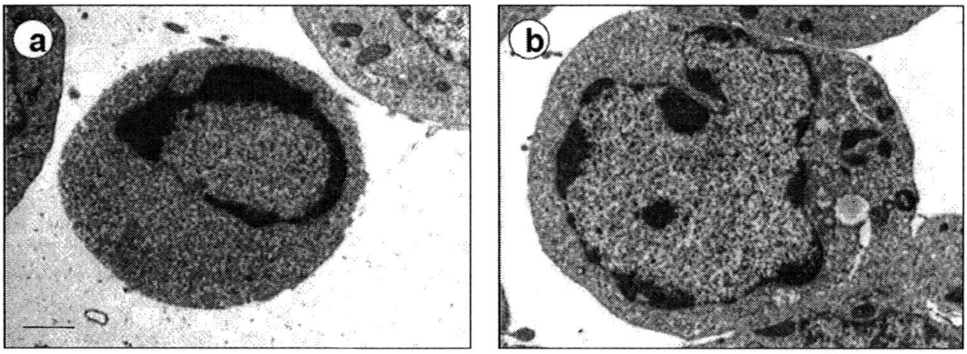

Fig. 4. Morphological features of apoptotic cells. The scale bar represents 1 μm.

The Balance Between Life and Death is Regulated by Pro-Apoptotic and Anti-Apoptotic Factors

The apoptotic process can be divided into three phases: an induction phase, the nature of which depends on the specific death-inducing signals; an effector phases, during which the death executioner machine is activated and the cells becomes committed to die, and a degradation phase, during which cells acquire the biochemical and morphological features of end stage of apoptosis. In this cascade of events, we can identify two "executioner" pathways that activated the "point of no return", a step in which cells becomes irreversibly commitment to the loss of essential cellular functions. In mammalian cells, apoptosis may be triggered through two executioner major pathways: the death-receptor pathway and the mitochondrial pathway [11,15].

The first pathway is triggered by members of Tumor necrosis factor death receptor (TNFR) (such as CD95, TRAIL-R1 and TRAIL-R2) [16-19]. Death receptors are a subgroup of the tumour-necrosis-factor receptor (TNFR) which are characterized by a cytoplasmic death domain that is able to transmit of the apoptotic signal through the activation of caspase, a family of fourteen cysteine protease that cleave selected substrates at aspartic acid residues [20]. Caspases exist in an inactive form in the cytosol of the most cells as a single polypeptide chain that is activated by cleavage to produce the active protease and this cleavage can be mediated by caspases either the same one or others determining proteolytic cleavage of several cellular targets. They can be differentiated into initiator and effector caspases, which are activated in hierarchical manner. One way of starting this cascade is through the activation of membrane bound death receptors.

CD95 (Fas/Apo-1) has a significant role in the immune system; it is a type I transmembrane receptor, but alternative splicing can result in a soluble form. CD95 expression can be increased by cytokines (such as IFNγ and TNF) and in addition by activation of lymphocytes. CD95-mediated apoptosis is activated by its natural ligand, CD95L. TRAIL (Apo2L or tumor necrosis factor-related apoptosis –inducing ligand) receptor 1 (TRAIL-R1 or DR4) and TRAIL-receptor 2 (TRAIL-R2 , DR5, TRICK2 or KILLER) have cytoplasmic death domains and signal for apoptosis and for NF.kB [21]. After binding their specific receptor, TRAIL has been shown to induce apoptosis in various tumor cell lines, while most primary cells seem to be resistant.

The contact of death receptors with their ligands (such as CD95 ligand bond to CD95 or TRAIL to TRAIL-R1 and R2) triggers similar apoptotic pathways in several physiological and pathological cell-death processes. In detail, the death ligand interaction induces receptor clustering and formation of death-inducing signaling complex (DISC) [22,23] assembles at the plasma membrane, within few seconds from receptor engagement. The adaptor FADD (Fas-associated death domain protein, also known as Mort-1) binds via its own death domain in CD95. FADD also carries a so-called death –effector domain (DED) and, again by homologous interaction, recruits the DED-containing procaspase-8, also called FLICE, into the DISC. Next, procaspase-8 is proteolytically activated and active caspase-8 is released from the DISC into cytoplasm in the form of a heterotetramer . Active caspase-8 cleaves various proteins in the cell including pro-caspase-3 that under activated form coordinate DNA fragmentation [24], nuclear condensation [25], and membrane blebbing [26,27] through cleavage of specific substrates, but these are unlikely to fully account for the rapidity of caspase-dependent death once the proteases are activated.

Recapping, apoptosis by death receptors subfamily seems to follow the same basic rules and is initiated by same sequential steps: ligand binding; receptor trimerization and DISC formation; attraction of the adapter molecule FADD into the DISC; association of pro-caspase-8 and autocatalytic cleavage of the procaspase and formation of active caspase-8 that serves as the initiator caspase to active other downstream caspase that cleaves cellular death substrate resulting in apoptosis.

This process can be inhibited by FLICE inhibitor protein (FLIP), also designated as casper, CLARP, FLAME-1, I-FLICE, CASH, MRIT or usurpin [28]. cFLIP exists in two splice forms: cFLIP-long (FLIP-L) comprising two N-terminal DEDs and an enzymatically inactive pseudo caspase domain and cFLIP-short (FLIP-S) containing only the two DEDs.

Both splice forms seem to act as dominant negative molecules in respect to CD95-mediated caspase-8 processing at an intermediate state [29,30].

The second pathway is induced extensively in response to extra and intracellular stimuli such as DNA damage [15] and chemotherapeutic drugs. This particular pathway converges on mitochondria determining activation of pro-apoptotic members of the Bcl-2 family like Bax, Bak, Bim, Bik or Bid. By contrast, some anti-apoptotic members of Bcl-2 family such as Bcl-x_L can block the apoptosis triggered by the mitochondrial pathway [31-33]. In fact, pro- and anti-apoptotic Bcl-2 family members compete to regulate the release of cytochrome c that is a powerful inducer of pro-caspase-e cleavage. Although cytochrome c is not the sole mitochondrial intermembrane protein capable of activating caspases [34], the cytochrome c stimulated pathway of caspase activation is the best characterized. Cytochrome c, in association with Apaf-1(a mammalian homologue of CED-4) and procaspase-9, forms a holoenzyme complex called the apoptosome [33,35] that triggers activation of caspase-9 and executioner caspase responsible for completion of the death program [15,16]. Both pathways, the death-receptor pathway and the mitochondrial pathway, converge at the level of caspase-3 activation that is able to cleave intracellular substrates such as Poly (ADP-ribose) polymerase (PARP) and laminins, leading to the execution phase of apoptosis which results in dismantling and removal of the cell [36]. Bid, a pro-apoptotic member of Bcl-2 family cleaved by caspase-8, integrates the death receptor and the mitochondrial pathways, inducing the cytochrome c release [37,38]. However, under most conditions, the two pathways can operate independently of each other.

Cytokines Role in the Pathogenesis of Thyroid Cancer

CD95/CD95L interaction and the activation of some anti-apoptotic members of the Bcl-2 family or cFlip have been demonstrated playing a central role in the pathogenesis of several autoimmune diseases and cancer [39-47].

Tumor immunology has evolved in parallel with the immunology of infection diseases and has attempted to reproduce the successes obtained in the prevention and cure of infections by directing the immune system to attack tumor antigens. Numerous mechanisms have been hypothesized in an attempt to understand the failure of the immune system to control and/or block tumor growth. The following possibilities may include these mechanisms: a) some tumors could be weakly immunogenic and MHC expression could be down-regulated; b) antitumor immunity could select immune response-resistant tumor cells; c) tumor cells could be tolerigenic either because they do not express costimulatory molecules or because they do not produce cytokines.

With regard to cytokines production profiles, it has been identified that qualitative as well as quantitative alterations in cytokine production can result in complex and severe impairments of immune response. Moreover, cytokines have key effects on carcinogenesis. In fact, they can be involved in the activation of immune effector mechanisms that limit the growth of the tumor, but on the other hand, they may involved in carcinogenesis and malignant trasformation, tumor growth, invasion and metastasis.

Cytokines promote the expression of a variety of genes involved in the survival or death of different target cells [48-51]. Three functionally distinct subsets of T-helper cells have been characterized on the basis of cytokine production [52]. T_H1 cells secrete IFN-γ and other cytokines associated with inflammation and cell-mediated immune responses. In contrast, T_H2 cells promote the humoral response and produce IL-4, IL-5 and IL-10, while T_H3 cells inhibit the immune response through the release of IL-10 and transforming growth factor β-1 [39,52,53]. It was recently demonstrated that cytokines released by T helper lymphocytes control autoimmune thyroid destruction through the modulation of pro- and anti-apoptotic proteins in target cells. IFN-γ contributes to autoimmune thyrocyte destruction through the upregulation of CD95, caspase-3 and caspase-8, whereas IL-4 and IL-10 promote thyrocyte survival during non-destructive autoimmunity through the upregulation of cFLIP [39,54]. Thus type1 and type2 cytokines exercise opposite effects on cells targeted by thyroid autoimmunity, such as Hashimoto's thyroiditis and Grave's disease, through the modulation of pro-apoptotic and anti-apoptotic proteins that promote or inhibit CD95 mediated thyrocyte depletion. Moreover it has been showed that thyroid nodule and thyroid cancer are more frequently implicated in Graves' patients than healthy subjects [55] and these thyroid cancers are more aggressive, metastatic and adverse outcome compared with similar cancers occurring in euthyroid subjects [56]. It has been speculated that the modulation of apoptosis-related proteins by IL-4 and IL-10 cytokines was not restricted to normal thyrocytes, but could be involved in the survival of thyroid cancer cells.

Patients with various malignancies have been report to be immune compromised. About cytokine production profiles, it has been understood that qualitative as well as quantitative alterations in cytokine production can result. Alterations in Th1 and Th2 cytokine levels have been observed to be present in different human tumors. Autocrine production of Type 2 cytokines, in particular IL-4 and/or IL-10 production [57], was reported to be abnormally elevated in human neoplasia including thyroid [58] (Fig. 5), colon cancers, pancreatic and gastric adenocarcinomas [59] or only IL-4 autocrine production in bladder, prostate and breast carcinomas [60]. In contrast, a concomitant reduction in type 1 cytokines has been reported in patients with same tumors. Thus, human neoplastic diseases are frequently associated with dysregulation of the equilibrium between the production of certain type 1 and type 2 cytokines. Recently data proved the presence of IL-4 and IL-10 in the thyroid cancer microenvironment and demonstrated that they were responsible for refractoriness to chemotherapy.

Over the last decades, the treatment of epithelial cancers, including breast, prostate and thyroid cancer has relied primarily on the use of chemotherapeutic drugs that has profound positive effects. However, the effectiveness of chemotherapeutic regimens is hindered by the efficacy of chemotherapy concerning the clinical failure due to the survival and subsequent expansion of apoptosis-resistant malignant cells. Cancer cell resistance to chemotherapy is a major concern in clinical oncology, resulting in increased tumor growth and decreased patient survival. The ability of cancer cells to resist the cytotoxic effects of chemotherapy follows genetic alterations of the mechanisms that control cell-cycle checkpoints and apoptosis. Because cytotoxic drugs act by altering the balance between proapoptotic and antiapoptotic signals, inappropriate activation of antiapoptotic genes may result in the development of drug resistance. It is now widely recognized that chemotherapy resistance is a multistep process originating from the upregulation of key molecules involved in the control of cell proliferation, differentiation and apoptosis. Recent studies have demostrated that, treatment of certain malignant cells with antisense oligonucleotides or with plasmid constructs overexpressing antisense Bcl-2 or Bcl-xL decreased the rates of proliferation and resistance to cytotoxic chemotherapeutic agents [61-64]. Definition of the molecular bases of the mechanisms underlying Bcl-2 and Bcl-xL overexpression, that determine chemoresistance in cancer cells, may allow the development of effective therapeutic strategies.

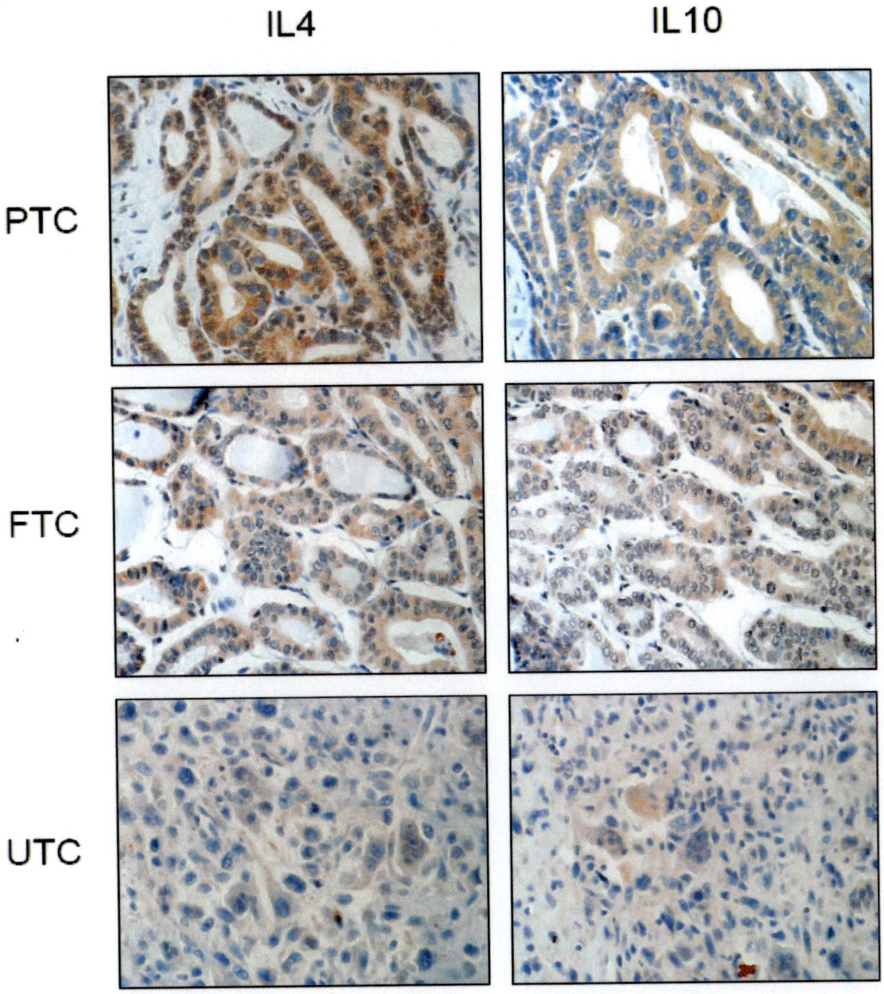

Fig. 5. Immunohistochemical analysis of IL-4 and IL-10 on paraffin-embedded Papillary (PTC), Follicular (FTC) and Undifferentiated (UTC) thyroid carcinoma sections (red staining).

Several cytokines are known to increase Bcl-2 or Bcl-xL expression. For example, IL-3 increases Bcl-xL levels and promotes survival and expansion of myeloid and pro-B cell [65]. Similarly, IL-5 and IL-15 activate Bcl-xL transcription and protect eosinophils and mast cells from apoptosis [66-68], respectively, while IL-10 upregulates Bcl-2 expression and promotes growth and survival of germinal center B cells [69]. Moreover, the increased T_H2 profile of T cells in chronic lymphocytic leukemia results in overproduction of IL-4, which in turn induces Bcl-2 overexpression and increased survival of malignant B cells [70]. This complex network of cytokines and receptors seems particularly relevant in thyroid cancer. Thus, certain cytokines promote cancer cell survival and expansion by stimulating the expression of antiapoptotic genes. Moreover, it has been demonstrated that thyroid carcinoma cells autocrinely produce two antiapoptotic cytokines (IL-4 and IL-10) that alter sensitivity to cytotoxic drugs and to CD95 induced apoptosis. Although loss of FADD expression correlated with tumor development and progression in a transgenic mouse model of thyroid follicular cancer, it was not observed an altered expression of the pro-apoptotic components required for CD95 signaling. Instead, our data clearly indicate that refractoriness to CD95-induced apoptosis in thyroid cancer cells results from high expression of cFLIP and PED/PEA-15, which inhibit the "extrinsic" apoptotic pathway by preventing the interaction between the adaptor molecule FADD and procaspase-8. Thus, as in other tumors, cFLIP and PED/PEA-15 represent two major candidates for cancer cell resistance to death receptor stimulation.

Thyroid cell production of IL-4 and IL-10 is acquired during neoplastic transformation, as in normal thyroid tissue we detect only IL-4 and IL-10 receptors, but neither of the two cytokines. The ability of IL-4 and IL-10 to upregulate cFLIP and PED/PEA-15 in normal thyrocytes, together with the drammatic downregulation of both proteins observed in thyroid cancer cells after exposure to IL-4 and IL-10 neutralizing Abs, clearly indicate that high expression of cFLIP and PED/PEA-15 in thyroid cancer results from autocrine production of IL-4 and IL-10.

All the histological variants of thyroid epithelial cancer are weakly sensitive to chemotherapy and express high levels of Bcl-2 and Bcl-xL. Moreover, exogenous expression of either Bcl-2 or Bcl-xL is sufficient to protect normal thyrocytes from chemotherapeutic drugs, while targeting the increased expression of antiapoptotic proteins sensitized thyroid cancer cells to chemotherapy. The poor cytotoxic effect of chemotherapy on thyroid cancer has directed most of the nonsurgical therapeutic efforts on radioiodine therapy, which exploits the iodide uptake potential of thyroid follicular cells to deliver ^{131}I to well-differentiated thyroid cancer cells. Targeting with radioiodide is far more effective than chemotherapy in the treatment of well-differentiated thyroid cancer. However, the inability to reach complete remission in the absence of surgical treatment restricts the use of radioiodine to a postoperative adjuvant or a second-line treatment.

Importantly, expression of Bcl-2 and Bcl-xL is decreased after treatment with neutralizing Abs against IL-4 and IL-10, which results in the spontaneous death of a considerable percentage of cancer cells, indicating that these cytokines act as survival factors for thyroid tumor cells and may contribute to the progression of cancer. Moreover, neutralization of both IL-4 and IL-10 dramatically increased the effectiveness of antineoplastic drugs of cancer cells [58].

A variety of chemotherapeutic drugs have been investigated for the treatment of thyroid cancer. However, they have shown a very limited efficacy because of the high chemoresistance of thyroid cancer cells that remains a critical obstacle for the treatment of less differentiated tumors unable to uptake radioiodine. We showed that IL-4 and IL-10 neutralization is able to extinguish thyroid cancer cells within two weeks of culture. The possibility to antagonize these cytokines or their receptors could be exploited for therapeutic purposes to induce tumor regression or sensitization to death receptor stimulation or chemotherapeutic drugs. In conclusion, IL-4 and IL-10 can directly act on cancer cells by increasing the expression of antiapoptotic proteins, thus promoting tumor cell progression and resistance to chemotherapy.

REFERENCES

[1] Gimm O: Thyroid cancer. *Cancer Lett* 2001, 163(2):143-156.

[2] Sherman SI: Thyroid carcinoma. Lancet 2003, 361(9356):501-511.

[3] Mills SE, Allen MS, Jr.: Congenital occult papillary carcinoma of the thyroid gland. *Hum Pathol* 1986, 17(11):1179-1181.

[4] Mazzaferri EL, Young RL: Papillary thyroid carcinoma: a 10 year follow-up report of the impact of therapy in 576 patients. *Am J Med* 1981, 70(3):511-518.

[5] Carcangiu ML, Zampi G, Pupi A, Castagnoli A, Rosai J: Papillary carcinoma of the thyroid. A clinicopathologic study of 241 cases treated at the University of Florence, Italy. *Cancer* 1985, 55(4):805-828.

[6] Franssila KO, Ackerman LV, Brown CL, Hedinger CE: Follicular carcinoma. *Semin Diagn Pathol* 1985, 2(2):101-122.

[7] Ruegemer JJ, Hay ID, Bergstralh EJ, Ryan JJ, Offord KP, Gorman CA: Distant metastases in differentiated thyroid carcinoma: a multivariate analysis of prognostic variables. *J Clin Endocrinol Metab* 1988, 67(3):501-508.

[8] Evans HL: Follicular neoplasms of the thyroid. A study of 44 cases followed for a minimum of 10 years, with emphasis on differential diagnosis. *Cancer* 1984, 54(3):535-540.

[9] Carcangiu ML, Steeper T, Zampi G, Rosai J: Anaplastic thyroid carcinoma. A study of 70 cases. *Am J Clin Pathol* 1985, 83(2):135-158.

[10] De Maria R, Testa U, Luchetti L, Zeuner A, Stassi G, Pelosi E, Riccioni R, Felli N, Samoggia P, Peschle C: Apoptotic role of Fas/Fas ligand system in the regulation of erythropoiesis. *Blood* 1999, 93(3):796-803.

[11] Hengartner MO: The biochemistry of apoptosis. *Nature* 2000, 407(6805):770-776.

[12] Tobler A, Maurer R, Hedinger CE: Undifferentiated thyroid tumors of diffuse small cell type. Histological and immunohistochemical evidence for their lymphomatous nature. *Virchows Arch A Pathol Anat Histopathol* 1984, 404(2):117-126.

[13] Harach HR: Solid cell nests of the thyroid. *J Pathol* 1988, 155(3):191-200.

[14] Stanta G, Carcangiu ML, Rosai J: The biochemical and immunohistochemical profile of thyroid neoplasia. *Pathol Annu* 1988, 23 Pt 1:129-157.

[15] Scaffidi C, Fulda S, Srinivasan A, Friesen C, Li F, Tomaselli KJ, Debatin KM, Krammer PH, Peter ME: Two CD95 (APO-1/Fas) signaling pathways. *Embo J* 1998, 17(6):1675-1687.

[16] Krammer PH: CD95's deadly mission in the immune system. *Nature* 2000, 407(6805):789-795.

[17] Klas C, Debatin KM, Jonker RR, Krammer PH: Activation interferes with the APO-1 pathway in mature human T cells. *Int Immunol* 1993, 5(6):625-630.

[18] Leithauser F, Dhein J, Mechtersheimer G, Koretz K, Bruderlein S, Henne C, Schmidt A, Debatin KM, Krammer PH, Moller P: Constitutive and induced expression of APO-1, a new member of the nerve growth factor/tumor necrosis factor receptor superfamily, in normal and neoplastic cells. *Lab Invest* 1993, 69(4):415-429.

[19] Golstein P: Controlling cell death. *Science* 1997, 275(5303):1081-1082.

[20] Nicholson DW, Thornberry NA: Caspases: killer proteases. *Trends Biochem Sci* 1997, 22(8):299-306.

[21] Schneider P, Thome M, Burns K, Bodmer JL, Hofmann K, Kataoka T, Holler N, Tschopp J: TRAIL receptors 1 (DR4) and 2 (DR5) signal FADD-dependent apoptosis and activate NF-kappaB. *Immunity* 1997, 7(6):831-836.

[22] Kischkel FC, Hellbardt S, Behrmann I, Germer M, Pawlita M, Krammer PH, Peter ME: Cytotoxicity-dependent APO-1 (Fas/CD95)-associated proteins form a death-inducing signaling complex (DISC) with the receptor. *Embo J* 1995, 14(22):5579-5588.

[23] Muzio M, Chinnaiyan AM, Kischkel FC, O'Rourke K, Shevchenko A, Ni J, Scaffidi C, Bretz JD, Zhang M, Gentz R et al: FLICE, a novel FADD-homologous ICE/CED-3-like protease, is recruited to the CD95 (Fas/APO-1) death--inducing signaling complex. *Cell* 1996, 85(6):817-827.

[24] Enari M, Sakahira H, Yokoyama H, Okawa K, Iwamatsu A, Nagata S: A caspase-activated DNase that degrades DNA during apoptosis, and its inhibitor ICAD. *Nature* 1998, 391(6662):43-50.

[25] Sahara S, Aoto M, Eguchi Y, Imamoto N, Yoneda Y, Tsujimoto Y: Acinus is a caspase-3-activated protein required for apoptotic chromatin condensation. *Nature* 1999, 401(6749):168-173.

[26] Sebbagh M, Renvoize C, Hamelin J, Riche N, Bertoglio J, Breard J: Caspase-3-mediated cleavage of ROCK I induces MLC phosphorylation and apoptotic membrane blebbing. *Nat Cell Biol* 2001, 3(4):346-352.

[27] Coleman ML, Sahai EA, Yeo M, Bosch M, Dewar A, Olson MF: Membrane blebbing during apoptosis results from caspase-mediated activation of ROCK I. *Nat Cell Biol* 2001, 3(4):339-345.

[28] Thome M, Schneider P, Hofmann K, Fickenscher H, Meinl E, Neipel F, Mattmann C, Burns K, Bodmer JL, Schroter M et al: Viral FLICE-inhibitory proteins (FLIPs) prevent apoptosis induced by death receptors. *Nature* 1997, 386(6624):517-521.

[29] Siegmund D, Mauri D, Peters N, Juo P, Thome M, Reichwein M, Blenis J, Scheurich P, Tschopp J, Wajant H: Fas-associated death domain protein (FADD) and caspase-8 mediate up-regulation of c-Fos by Fas ligand and tumor necrosis factor-related apoptosis-inducing ligand (TRAIL) via a FLICE inhibitory protein (FLIP)-regulated pathway. *J Biol Chem* 2001, 276(35):32585-32590.

[30] Scaffidi C, Schmitz I, Krammer PH, Peter ME: The role of c-FLIP in modulation of CD95-induced apoptosis. *J Biol Chem* 1999, 274(3):1541-1548.

[31] Reed JC: Double identity for proteins of the Bcl-2 family. *Nature* 1997, 387(6635):773-776.

[32] Antonsson B, Martinou JC: The Bcl-2 protein family. *Exp Cell Res* 2000, 256(1):50-57.

[33] Pan G, O'Rourke K, Dixit VM: Caspase-9, Bcl-XL, and Apaf-1 form a ternary complex. *J Biol Chem* 1998, 273(10):5841-5845.

[34] Susin SA, Zamzami N, Castedo M, Daugas E, Wang HG, Geley S, Fassy F, Reed JC, Kroemer G: The central executioner of apoptosis: multiple connections between protease activation and mitochondria in Fas/APO-1/CD95- and ceramide-induced apoptosis. *J Exp Med* 1997, 186(1):25-37.

[35] Hu Y, Benedict MA, Wu D, Inohara N, Nunez G: Bcl-XL interacts with Apaf-1 and inhibits Apaf-1-dependent caspase-9 activation. *Proc Natl Acad Sci U S A* 1998, 95(8):4386-4391.

[36] Pieper AA, Verma A, Zhang J, Snyder SH: Poly (ADP-ribose) polymerase, nitric oxide and cell death. *Trends Pharmacol Sci* 1999, 20(4):171-181.

[37] Li H, Zhu H, Xu CJ, Yuan J: Cleavage of BID by caspase 8 mediates the mitochondrial damage in the Fas pathway of apoptosis. *Cell* 1998, 94(4):491-501.

[38] Gross A, Yin XM, Wang K, Wei MC, Jockel J, Milliman C, Erdjument-Bromage H, Tempst P, Korsmeyer SJ: Caspase cleaved BID targets mitochondria and is required for cytochrome c release, while BCL-XL prevents this release but not tumor necrosis factor-R1/Fas death. *J Biol Chem* 1999, 274(2):1156-1163.

[39] Stassi G, Di Liberto D, Todaro M, Zeuner A, Ricci-Vitiani L, Stoppacciaro A, Ruco L, Farina F, Zummo G, De Maria R: Control of target cell survival in thyroid autoimmunity by T helper cytokines via regulation of apoptotic proteins. *Nat Immunol* 2000, 1(6):483-488.

[40] Stassi G, Todaro M, Bucchieri F, Stoppacciaro A, Farina F, Zummo G, Testi R, De Maria R: Fas/Fas ligand-driven T cell apoptosis as a consequence of ineffective thyroid immunoprivilege in Hashimoto's thyroiditis. *J Immunol* 1999, 162(1):263-267.

[41] Giordano C, Stassi G, De Maria R, Todaro M, Richiusa P, Papoff G, Ruberti G, Bagnasco M, Testi R, Galluzzo A: Potential involvement of Fas and its ligand in the pathogenesis of Hashimoto's thyroiditis. *Science* 1997, 275(5302):960-963.

[42] De Maria R, Testi R: Fas-FasL interactions: a common pathogenetic mechanism in organ-specific autoimmunity. *Immunol Today* 1998, 19(3):121-125.

[43] Arscott PL, Stokes T, Myc A, Giordano TJ, Thompson NW, Baker JR, Jr.: Fas (CD95) expression is up-regulated on papillary thyroid carcinoma. *J Clin Endocrinol Metab* 1999, 84(11):4246-4252.

[44] Hammond LJ, Lowdell MW, Cerrano PG, Goode AW, Bottazzo GF, Mirakian R: Analysis of apoptosis in relation to tissue destruction associated with Hashimoto's autoimmune thyroiditis. *J Pathol* 1997, 182(2):138-144.

[45] Patel VA, Hill DJ, Sheppard MC, Wang F, Logan A, Eggo MC: Apoptosis during goitre involution - the role of Bcl-2. *J Endocrinol* 2000, 164(3):323-330.

[46] Mitsiades N, Poulaki V, Kotoula V, Mastorakos G, Tseleni-Balafouta S, Koutras DA, Tsokos M: Fas/Fas ligand up-regulation and Bcl-2 down-regulation may be significant in the pathogenesis of Hashimoto's thyroiditis. *J Clin Endocrinol Metab* 1998, 83(6):2199-2203.

[47] Basolo F, Pollina L, Fontanini G, Fiore L, Pacini F, Baldanzi A: Apoptosis and proliferation in thyroid carcinoma: correlation with bcl-2 and p53 protein expression. *Br J Cancer* 1997, 75(4):537-541.

[48] Ahn EY, Pan G, Vickers SM, McDonald JM: IFN-gammaupregulates apoptosis-related molecules and enhances Fas-mediated apoptosis in human cholangiocarcinoma. *Int J Cancer* 2002, 100(4):445-451.

[49] Qin JZ, Zhang CL, Kamarashev J, Dummer R, Burg G, Dobbeling U: Interleukin-7 and interleukin-15 regulate the expression of the bcl-2 and c-myb genes in cutaneous T-cell lymphoma cells. *Blood* 2001, 98(9):2778-2783.

[50] Wurster AL, Rodgers VL, White MF, Rothstein TL, Grusby MJ: Interleukin-4-mediated protection of primary B cells from apoptosis through Stat6-dependent up-regulation of Bcl-xL. *J Biol Chem* 2002, 277(30):27169-27175.

[51] Dancescu M, Rubio-Trujillo M, Biron G, Bron D, Delespesse G, Sarfati M: Interleukin 4 protects chronic lymphocytic leukemic B cells from death by apoptosis and upregulates Bcl-2 expression. *J Exp Med* 1992, 176(5):1319-1326.

[52] Abbas AK, Murphy KM, Sher A: Functional diversity of helper T lymphocytes. *Nature* 1996, 383(6603):787-793.

[53] Romagnani S: The Th1/Th2 paradigm. *Immunol Today* 1997, 18(6):263-266.

[54] Stassi G, De Maria R: Autoimmune thyroid disease: new models of cell death in autoimmunity. *Nat Rev Immunol* 2002, 2(3):195-204.

[55] Belfiore A, Russo D, Vigneri R, Filetti S: Graves' disease, thyroid nodules and thyroid cancer. *Clin Endocrinol (Oxf)* 2001, 55(6):711-718.

[56] Vella V, Mineo R, Frasca F, Mazzon E, Pandini G, Vigneri R, Belfiore A: Interleukin-4 stimulates papillary thyroid cancer cell survival: implications in patients with thyroid cancer and concomitant Graves' disease. *J Clin Endocrinol Metab* 2004, 89(6):2880-2889.

[57] Vicari AP, Trinchieri G: Interleukin-10 in viral diseases and cancer: exiting the labyrinth? *Immunol Rev* 2004, 202:223-236.

[58] Stassi G, Todaro M, Zerilli M, Ricci-Vitiani L, Di Liberto D, Patti M, Florena A, Di Gaudio F, Di Gesu G, De Maria R: Thyroid cancer resistance to chemotherapeutic drugs via autocrine production of interleukin-4 and interleukin-10. *Cancer Res* 2003, 63(20):6784-6790.

[59] Fortis C, Foppoli M, Gianotti L, Galli L, Citterio G, Consogno G, Gentilini O, Braga M: Increased interleukin-10 serum levels in patients with solid tumours. *Cancer Lett* 1996, 104(1):1-5.

[60] Conticello C, Pedini F, Zeuner A, Patti M, Zerilli M, Stassi G, Messina A, Peschle C, De Maria R: IL-4 protects tumor cells from anti-CD95 and chemotherapeutic agents via up-regulation of antiapoptotic proteins. *J Immunol* 2004, 172(9):5467-5477.

[61] Jansen B, Schlagbauer-Wadl H, Brown BD, Bryan RN, van Elsas A, Muller M, Wolff K, Eichler HG, Pehamberger H: bcl-2 antisense therapy chemosensitizes human melanoma in SCID mice. *Nat Med* 1998, 4(2):232-234.

[62] Reed JC: Splicing and dicing apoptosis genes. *Nat Biotechnol* 1999, 17(11):1064-1065.

[63] Gautschi O, Tschopp S, Olie RA, Leech SH, Simoes-Wust AP, Ziegler A, Baumann B, Odermatt B, Hall J, Stahel RA et al: Activity of a novel bcl-2/bcl-xL-bispecific antisense oligonucleotide against tumors of diverse histologic origins. *J Natl Cancer Inst* 2001, 93(6):463-471.

[64] Zangemeister-Wittke U, Leech SH, Olie RA, Simoes-Wust AP, Gautschi O, Luedke GH, Natt F, Haner R, Martin P, Hall J et al: A novel bispecific antisense oligonucleotide inhibiting both bcl-2 and bcl-xL expression efficiently induces apoptosis in tumor cells. *Clin Cancer Res* 2000, 6(6):2547-2555.

[65] Kieslinger M, Woldman I, Moriggl R, Hofmann J, Marine JC, Ihle JN, Beug H, Decker T: Antiapoptotic activity of Stat5 required during terminal stages of myeloid differentiation. *Genes Dev* 2000, 14(2):232-244.

[66] Masuda A, Matsuguchi T, Yamaki K, Hayakawa T, Yoshikai Y: Interleukin-15 prevents mouse mast cell apoptosis through STAT6- mediated Bcl-xL expression. *J Biol Chem* 2001, 276(28):26107-26113.

[67] Dibbert B, Daigle I, Braun D, Schranz C, Weber M, Blaser K, Zangemeister-Wittke U, Akbar AN, Simon HU: Role for Bcl-xL in delayed eosinophil apoptosis mediated by granulocyte- macrophage colony-stimulating factor and interleukin-5. *Blood* 1998, 92(3):778-783.

[68] Masuda A, Matsuguchi T, Yamaki K, Hayakawa T, Yoshikai Y: Interleukin-15 prevents mouse mast cell apoptosis through STAT6-mediated Bcl-xL expression. *J Biol Chem* 2001, 276(28):26107-26113.

[69] Levy Y, Brouet JC: Interleukin-10 prevents spontaneous death of germinal center B cells by induction of the bcl-2 protein. *J Clin Invest* 1994, 93(1):424-428.

[70] Dancescu M, Rubio-Trujillo M, Biron G, Bron D, Delespesse G, Sarfati M: Interleukin 4 protects chronic lymphocytic leukemic B cells from death by apoptosis and upregulates Bcl-2 expression. *J Exp Med* 1992, 176(5):1319-1326.

In: Trends in Thyroid Cancer Research
Editor: Carl A. Milton, pp. 49-63
ISBN 1-59454-627-4

Chapter III

GENETIC ALTERATION OF THE RAS-RAF-MAP KINASE PATHWAY IN THYROID CANCER

Toshihiko Fukushima**, Shinichi Suzuki, Koji Sekikawa and Seiichi Takenoshita
Department of Surgery, Fukushima Medical University School of Medicine, 1-Hikarigaoka, Fukushima, 960-1296 Japan.

ABSTRACT

Papillary cancer and follicular cancer are types of differentiated thyroid cancers. They are considered to share the same developmental origin, the same thyroid follicular epithelial cells and show distinct biological behavior. Although several studies have demonstrated differences in the biological characteristics of these cancers, little is known about the genetic backgrounds that underlie the differences in these cancers. The clarification of the genetic background can lead to the understanding of thyroid carcinogenesis, proper therapeutic strategies, and development of the molecular targeting drugs. Aberrant activation of RAS-RAF-MEK-MAP kinase signaling pathway is frequently found in thyroid cancer. The pathway transmits the mitogenic signal to the nucleus, and constitutive activation of the pathway is thought to promote uncontrolled cell division. In our series, BRAF mutation was detected exclusively in papillary cancer (30-60%), and was exclusively V599E (a single nucleotide change of A-T at nucleotide 1796), but not in follicular cancers or adenomas. RAS mutations are rare in sporadic papillary cancers, but are observed in 20-50% of follicular cancers, being particularly common as NRAS Q61R mutations. In this chapter, we explain the role of RAS-RAF-MEK-MAP kinase pathway in carcinogenesis of the thyroid and its clinical implication based on our study. In addition, we review the current knowledge in this field.

* Correspondence concerning this article should be addressed to Dr. Toshihiko Fukushima Department of Surgery, Fukushima Medical University School of Medicine, Hikarigaoka, Fukushima-shi, Fukushima, 960-1296 Japan. Facsimile: +81-24-548-3249; E-mail: fuku@fmu.ac.jp.

Keywords: Thyroid cancer, Braf, Ras, MAP kinase pathway

Introduction

Differentiated thyroid cancers derive from thyroid follicular cells. They account for 95% of all thyroid cancers and are classified into papillary and follicular cancers [1]. Follicular cancers are more common than papillary cancers in iodine-deficient areas, whereas the incidence of papillary cancers is higher in many other areas [2]. In Japan, 80 and 20% of differentiated thyroid cancers are papillary and follicular cancers, respectively. They are known to differ biologically as follows: papillary cancers metastasize frequently to regional lymph nodes but rarely to distant sites [3-5], whereas follicular cancers metastasize rarely to regional lymph nodes but relatively frequently to distant sites such as the lungs and bones [6-8]. However, knowledge on the molecular biological mechanisms in these differences and causing transformation of thyrocytes into papillary or follicular phenotypes is scarce [9].

The RAS gene, a component of the RAS-RAF-MEK-ERK-MAP kinase pathway, which plays important roles in the transduction of cell proliferation signals, has been investigated extensively [10-12]. Activating point mutations in RAS genes have been demonstrated in various cancers, including thyroid cancer, and approximately 5 to 20% of papillary and follicular thyroid cancers are known to harbor specific RAS mutations [13-18]. In 2002, point mutations in BRAF, which encodes a serine/threonine kinase activated by binding to RAS, were reported to occur in 60% of malignant melanomas [19]. BRAF mutations were also observed, though in low frequencies, in 15% of colorectal and 2% of lung cancers, which are known to have RAS point mutations [20, 21]. Thus, BRAF point mutations were also predicted to occur in thyroid cancers, and in 2003, BRAF abnormalities in papillary thyroid cancers were reported with frequencies as high as 30-60%, having a great impact on investigations of thyroid cancers [22-26]. The following chapter discusses RAS and BRAF abnormalities in thyroid cancers, including our data.

Classical MAP Kinase Cascade

Various intracellular signal transduction mechanisms exist to ensure the transmission of extracellular growth stimuli into the cell. Of these, the Mitogen-activated protein (MAP) kinase pathway plays a central role [28]. MAP kinase (MAPK), also known as extracellular signal-regulated kinase (ERK), was discovered as a serine/threonine kinase activated by cell growth factors and other stimuli [29]. Activated MAPK is known to ultimately promote progression of the cell cycle from the G1 to S phase by regulating transcription of immediate early genes such as c-fos, promoting cyclin D1 transcription and activating the cyclin-dependent kinase CDK4/6 [30]. MAPK activation requires the phosphorylation of threonine and tyrosine residues in the kinase domain by MAPK kinases (MAPKK) such as MEK1/2. It also requires the phosphorylation of serine and/or threonie residues in the kinase domain. The serine/threonine kinases responsible for this phosphorylation are designated MAPKK kinase (MAPKKK) [31-33], of which BRAF is one [34]. This kinase cascade has been evolutionally preserved from yeasts to humans, indicating its importance in various intracellular signaling pathways [35-37].

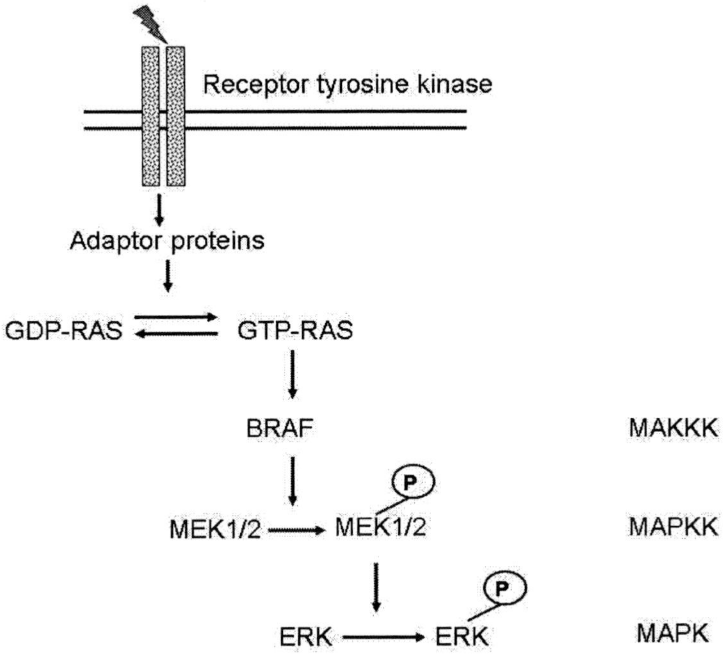

Figure 1. MAP kinase pathway. Growth factor binds to receptor. These signals transduce through the activation of RAS protein, which leads to activation BRAF, and then to activation MAPK kinase. Then MAPKK phosphorylates MAPK. It is this sequential phosphorylation of BRAF, MEK and ERK that is called the MAP kinase cascade.

Ligands such as growth factors bind first to receptors on the cell membrane. These receptors are a receptor-type tyrosine kinase with an intracellular tyrosine kinase domain, which bind to the ligand to form a dimer resulting in phosphorylation of tyrosine residues each other. The self-phosphorylated receptors bind to various adaptor molecules to activate the small G protein RAS by catalyzing replacement of GDP with GTP [38, 29]. When RAS is activated, RAF translocates from the cytosol to the cell membrane. The active GTP-bound RAS binds to the RAS-binding domain of RAF protein, resulting in activation of RAF protein by changing its conformation [40, 41]. In this way, growth stimuli are transmitted from the cell membrane to the cytosol, and this cascade controls cell growth, differentiation and survival.

RAS

Mammals have three kinds of RAS genes, HRAS, KRAS, and NRAS, each of which codes a 21-kD GTP-binding protein (small G protein). RAS is localized in the cell membrane, functioning as a switch protein that controls the transduction of signals from growth factor receptors [42]. Like other G proteins, the small G protein exists as an active

GTP-binding form or inactive GDP-binding form, and has GTPase activity. In normal cells, upstream signals convert RAS from the inactive GDP-binding form to the active GTP-binding form [43]. This reaction is promoted by guanine nucleotide exchange factor (GEF). Binding of GTPase-activating protein (GAP) to active GTP-RAS enhances GTPase activity, and GTP-RAS undergoes hydrolysis to become inactivated [44]. Many of the RAS point mutations found in cancers are miss-sense mutations at codons 12, 13, and 61 [17]. Since these mutations reduce the GTPase activity of RAS, levels of GTP–RAS form becomes predominant, activating the downstream MAPK cascade [45].

BRAF: V-RAF MURINE SARCOMA VIRAL ONCOGENE HOMOLOG B1

The Raf gene was first identified as a murine proto-oncogene [46]. RAF genes are found in various eukaryotes including *Caenorhabditis elegans*, *Drosophila melanogaster*, *Xenopus laevis*, chickens, mice, rats and humans. Its human homologs ARAF, BRAF, and RAF-1 (CRAF) have been cloned. The BRAF gene is located on chromosome 7q34, and has a genomic DNA size of about 190 kb, consisting of 18 exons [47]. These three RAFs contain three conserved regions, CR1, CR2, and CR3 [48, 49]. CR1 contains a GTP-RAS binding domain and cysteine-rich domain that form a zinc finger structure, and is considered important for activation of RAF by RAS binding [50]. CR2 is rich in serine/threonine residues, of which S364 is a regulatory phosphorylation site [51] and CR3 is a kinase domain with the highest homology. S445, D448, T598, and S601 are regulatory phosphorylation sites; the former two correspond to exon 11, and the latter two are present in the region called the activation segment, corresponding to exon 15. The phosphorylation of T598 and S601 plays a central role in the activation of BRAF [52].

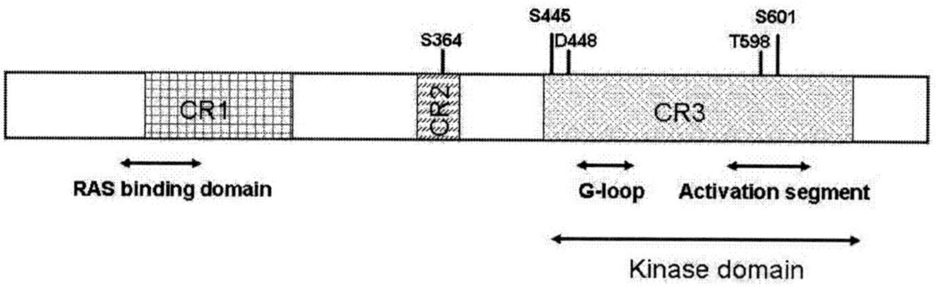

Figure 2. Domain structure of the BRAF. Phosphorylation of S364, S445, D448, T598 and S601 are important for the regulation of activation.

RAS AND BRAF MUTATIONS IN THYROID CANCER

RAS Mutations

The frequencies of RAS mutations in thyroid cancer greatly vary according to reports and have been suggested as being 0-50% in papillary cancers, 14-62% in follicular cancers, 0-60% in undifferentiated cancers, and 0-85% in follicular adenomas. Many studies on the spectrum of mutations have reported that mutations are common in codon 61 of HRAS and NRAS, being rare in other codons [13-15, 53, 54]. PCR-direct sequencing of our series showed mutation rates of 0 in 80 papillary cancers, 4 (50%) in 8 follicular cancers, and 2 (33%) in 6 undifferentiated cancers; all were NRAS Q61R mutations.

The possible causes of the above differences are as follows. The first is the method used for detecting mutations. Earlier studies detected mutations by dot blot hybridization using allele-specific oligonucleotide probes without confirmation by sequencing, suggesting overestimations of mutation frequencies [55, 56]. Direct sequencing is currently considered the most reliable method for detecting mutations. Many recent studies using this method have failed to detect RAS mutations in papillary cancers, in agreement with our results [57, 58]. These studies also reported mutation rates of 20-40% for follicular cancers, with the most common mutation site being Q61R of NRAS (about 60%), which is also in agreement with our results. The frequency of mutations in follicular adenomas was 10%, and the spectra of mutations tended to be the same as those in follicular cancers [57, 58]. The second is the influence of environmental factors such as iodine deficiency, and radiation and chemical exposure. In iodine-deficient regions, RAS mutations were found in 85% of follicular adenomas and in 10% of follicular cancers, with the majority being Q61R mutations of HRAS; no RAS mutations were found in papillary cancers [59]. The effect of radiation on the RAS mutations is controversial. Studies have found KRAS mutations in 60% of radiation-associated follicular cancers but no RAS mutations in childhood thyroid cancers after the Chernobyl nuclear plant accident, or no difference in the RAS mutation rate between radiation-associated and sporadic follicular cancers [60-62]. A previous study reported a high frequency of KRAS G12S mutations in papillary cancers in Thailand, and suggested the influence of environmental chemicals [63]. In summary, the current consensus is that RAS mutations are rare in sporadic papillary cancers, but are observed in 20-50% of follicular cancers, being particularly common as NRAS Q61R mutations.

BRAF Mutations

In 2002, BRAF mutations were reported in 66% of malignant melanomas [19]. Later, BRAF mutations were also confirmed in 1-3% of lung cancers and 5% of colorectal cancers [20, 21, 74]. Eighty-nine percent of the BRAF mutations detected in these cases were present in the activation segment, and 90% were V599E mutations. In addition, V599D, L596V, L596R, and F594L mutations were observed, although at low frequencies [19]. Eleven percent of BRAF mutations are found in glycine residues (G463, G465, and G468) in the G-loop of the N-terminal lobe of the kinase domain; therefore, exons 11 and 15 are hot spots for BRAF mutations.

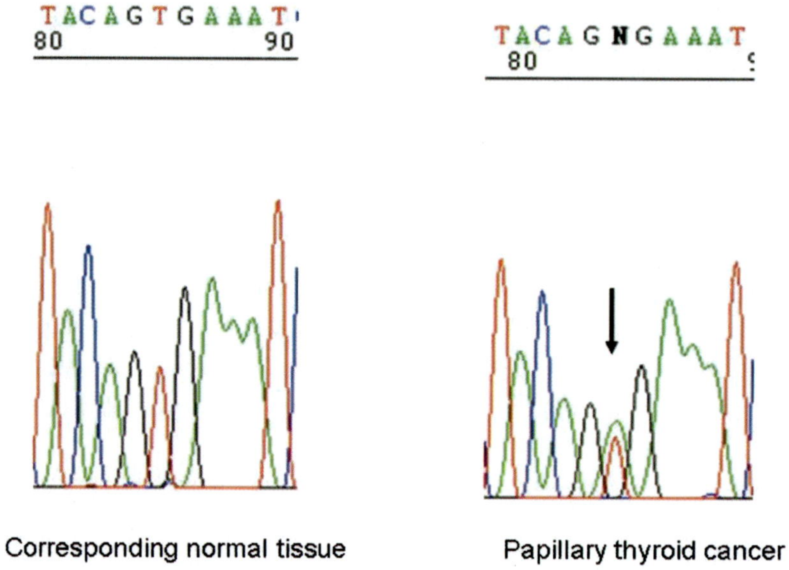

Figure 3. Mutations in the BRAF gene. Sequence electropherogram from tumor DNA shows a heterozygous missense mutation (T1796A/V599E). Nucleotide sequence in the corresponding normal tissue shows a wild type.

Our Study

We analyzed 114 thyroid tumors (80 papillary cancers, 8 follicular cancers, 7 undifferentiated cancers, 9 medullary cancers, and 10 follicular adenomas) for BRAF mutations in exons 11 and 15 using PCR- direct sequencing method. Tumors and corresponding normal tissue samples were obtained from surgical specimens resected at Fukushima Medical University Hospital. All patients gave informed consent. High-molecular-weight DNA was extracted from tumor tissue and corresponding normal tissue separately by treatment with SDS-Proteinase K and phenol-chloroform. DNA from each tumor-normal sample pair was examined by direct sequencing for mutations in hot spots of the BRAF genes (exons 11 and 15), and the NRAS, HRAS, and KRAS genes (exons 1 and 2). The reactions were performed as follows: The 50 μl PCR mixture contained 50 pmol of each primer, 2.5 μM of each dNTP, 500 ng of genomic DNA, and 0.1 units of DNA polymerase (Sigma Co., Ltd.) in 1x reaction buffer supplied by the manufacturer. DNA was amplified by 30 cycles of 30 sec at 94°C, 30 sec at 58°C, and 30 sec at 72°C. The following PCR primers were used to amplify exons 11 and 15 of the BRAF gene, and exons 1 and 2 of the KRAS, NRAS, or HRAS genes: KRAS exon1:F- ATAAGGCCTGCT GAAAATGACTGA, exon 2:R-GAATGGTCCTGCACCAGTAATATGC, exon2:F-CCAGACTGTGTTTCTCCCTTC, exon 2:R- CAGTCCTCATGTACTGGTC, HRAS exon1:F- CAGGAGACCCTGTAGGAGGAC, exon1:R- CTCTATAGTGGGGTCGTATTC, exon2:F- GATTCCTACCGGAAGCAGGTG, exon2:R- CTGTACTGGTGGATGTCCTC, NRAS exon1:F- CTGGTTTCCAACAGGTTCTTG, exon1:R- GATTAGCTGGATTGTCAG TGC, exon 2:F- GTGGTTATAGATGGTGAAACCTG, exon2:R- CAAATACACAGAGGA AGCCTTC, BRAF exon11:F-TCTGTTGGCTTGACTTGACT, exon 11:R-GACTTGTCAC AATGTCACCAC, exon 15:F-GCTTGCTCTGATAGGAAAATGAG, exon15:R-GTAACTC AGCAGCATCTCAGG. PCR products were purified using a QIAGEN PCR purification spin kit (Qiagen). Purified fragments were sequenced using the BigDye Terminator Cycle sequencing FS Ready Reaction Kit (Applied Biosystems) with the ABI PRISM 310 Genetic Analyzer (Applied Biosystems). Sequencing results from tumor samples and corresponding normal samples were compared to identify tumor-specific mutations. Of 80 papillary cancer, 43 (54%) had heterozygous mutations gene at codon 599 (V599E) resulting from a T to A change at nucleotide 1796 (T1796A) (Figure 3). BRAF mutations were not observed in other types of thyroid cancer.

Other Studies

Many studies have reported BRAF mutations in thyroid cancers [22-26]. Other studies have also reported BRAF mutations, exclusively V599E, in 29-69% of papillary cancers, but not in follicular cancers or adenomas (Table 1).

Table 1. Prevalence of BRAF mutation in thyroid cancer.

Ref.	BRAF V599E		
	PTC	FTC	ATC or UTC
22	43/80 (43%)	0/8 (0%)	0/9 (0%)
23	49/170 (28.8%)	0/11 (0%)	2/6 (33.3%)
24	21/56 (38%)	ND	ND
25	24/35 (69%)	0/13 (0%)	ND
26	28/78 (35.8%)	0/14 (0%)	ND

ND: not determined
PTC: Papillary thyroid cancer
FTC: Follicular thyroid cancer
ATC: Anaplastic thyroid cancer
UTC: Undifferentiated thyroid cancer

Significances of BRAF Mutation in Thyroid Cancer

The valine at codon 599 of the *BRAF* gene is located in the evolutionarily conserved activation segment of the kinase domain. An amino acid change from valine to glutamic acid (V599E) is thought to produce a negative charge, which mimics phosphorylation of the regulatory phosphorylation sites T588 and S601, resulting in elevated kinase activity

[19,52,65]. Indeed, the basal kinase activity of the V599E mutant of BRAF has been shown to be elevated in cos cells that can transform NIH3T3 cells [19]. These findings suggest that BRAF V599E mutations activate the MAP kinase cascade, thereby playing an important role in the carcinogenesis of papillary thyroid cancers. In our series and other studies, no cases of simultaneous BRAF and RAS mutations were found. In addition, it has been reported that the microinjection of RAS-neutralizing antibody does not inhibit the proliferation of cells with the V599E *BRAF* mutation [19]. These results suggest that activation of the MAP kinase pathway by BRAF mutations does not depend on RAS mutations.

Thyroid stimulating hormone (TSH) promotes the growth of thyrocytes and differentiated thyroid cancer cells [3]. TSH receptors are G-protein-coupled receptors. Binding of TSH to these receptors elevates intracellular cAMP levels promoting proliferation [66]; this cAMP-dependent pathway is known to activate BRAF [67] (Figure 4). Similar crosstalk is known to exist between melanocyte stimulating hormone and melanocortin receptors [68]. This might account for the higher frequencies of BRAF mutations in papillary thyroid cancer and melanoma than in other cancers such as colorectal and lung cancers, suggesting that BRAF mutations have similar biological effects in the development and progression of papillary thyroid cancer and melanoma.

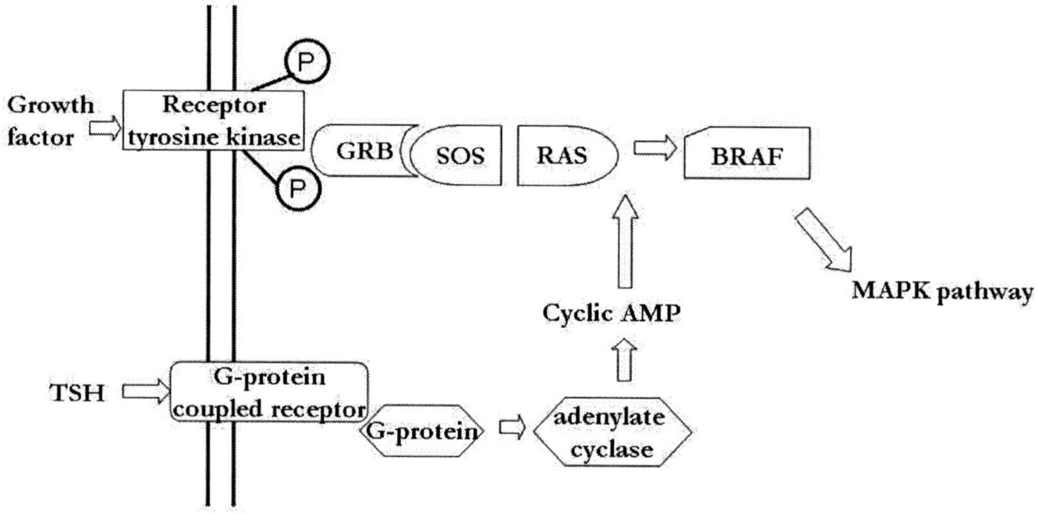

Figure 4. Cross-talk of the MAPK pathway and TSH-cAMP depended pathway. Thyroid stimulating hormone activates adenyl cyclase, and then up-regulates cAMP levels. This cellular response can activate the MAPK pathway.

RET/PTC rearrangement is a genetic abnormality that is known to occur in 5-30% of papillary thyroid cancers [69, 70]. Since there have been no reported cases of simultaneous RET/PTC rearrangement and BRAF mutation, these two genetic abnormalities are considered to be abnormalities with independent pathways [71]. The detection rate of RET/PTC rearrangement was higher (40%) and the prevalence of BRAF mutations was lower (12%) in papillary thyroid cancers after the Chernobyl nuclear plant accident than in sporadic counterparts [72]. A recent study reported that 11% of patients who developed radiation-induced thyroid cancer soon (5-6 years) after radiation, had BRAF rearrangement involving paracentric inversion of chromosome 7q. It has been shown that BRAF rearrangement results from in-frame fusion between exons 1-8 of the A-kinase protein 9 (AKAP9) gene and exons 9-18 of the BRAF gene, and that the fusion protein increases kinase activity [73]. These findings suggest that BRAF is the target of genetic abnormalities in both radiation-induced and sporadic cases, and that activation of the MAPK cascade plays an extremely important role in the carcinogenesis of papillary thyroid cancer.

Some studies have reported that BRAF V599E mutations occur in 20-50% of undifferentiated thyroid cancers, and that similar mutations are found in the coexisting papillary cancer component [74-76]. These results provide an important finding in understanding part of the mechanism involved in development of undifferentiated cancer from the dedifferentiation of differentiated cancer. Undifferentiated cancers with no BRAF mutations might have transformed from follicular cancers, or developed *de novo* from follicular thyroid cells.

Clinical Application

It has been reported that BRAF mutations are often associated with older age, extrathyroidal extension, and advanced TNM stage, and are useful as prognostic predictors [76]. Another report showed that BRAF mutations are correlated significantly with distant metastasis and TNM stage, but have no relation with age or extrathyroidal extension [23]. Large-scale research is necessary to explain this relevance.

BRAF mutations are found at high frequency in papillary thyroid cancers, and appear to be involved in carcinogenesis; therefore, BRAF is a promising target for molecular targeted drugs. Bis-aryl urea has been confirmed to inhibit Raf activity *in vitro* and in mouse xenografts, and clinical trials using melanomas are in progress [77, 78]. Triarylimidazole has also been confirmed to inhibit Raf activity in hematopoietic cell lines [79]. The therapeutic effects of these compounds on papillary thyroid cancer are awaited with interest.

Conclusions

The discovery of BRAF mutations in papillary thyroid cancers has resulted in significant advances in elucidation of the mechanism involved in development of thyroid cancer. However, how BRAF mutations induce changes in downstream signal transduction and expression of target genes, and how these changes are ultimately involved in carcinogenesis remain unknown. Similarly, the mechanism by which papillary cancers develop without BRAF mutations requires clarification. Clues to the answers to these questions might be found in the profile provided by mutational analysis of other factors involved in the MAPK cascade and by comprehensive analysis of the transcriptome and proteotome; however, the details need clarified in further studies.

REFERENCES

[1] Hundahl, SA; Fleming, ID; Fremgen, AM; Menck, HR. A National Cancer Data Base report on 53,856 cases of thyroid carcinoma treated in the US, 1985-1995. *Cancer*, 1998, 83(12), 2638-48.

[2] Franceschi, S; Boyle, P; Maisonneuve, P; La Vecchia, C; Burt, AD; Kerr, DJ; MacFarlane, GJ. The epidemiology of thyroid carcinoma. *Crit Rev Oncog*, 1993, 4(1), 25-52.

[3] Pierotti, MA; Bongarzone, I; Borello, MG; Greco, A; Pilotti, S; Sozzi, G. Cytogenetics and molecular genetics of carcinomas arising from thyroid epithelial follicular cells. *Genes Chromosomes Cancer*, 1996, 16(1), 1-14.

[4] Hay, ID. Papillary thyroid carcinoma. *Endocrinol Metab Clin North Am*, 1990, 19(3), 545-76.

[5] Grebe, SK; Hay, ID. Follicular cell-derived thyroid carcinomas. *Cancer Treat Res*, 1997, 89, 91-140.

[6] Shaha, AR; Shah, JP; Loree, TR. Patterns of nodal and distant metastasis based on histologic varieties in differentiated carcinoma of the thyroid. *Am J Surg*, 1996, 172(6), 692-4.

[7] Shaha, AR; Shah, JP; Loree, TR. Differentiated thyroid cancer presenting initially with distant metastasis. *Am J Surg*, 1997, 174(5), 474-6.

[8] Mazzaferri, EL; Jhiang, SM. Long-term impact of initial surgical and medical therapy on papillary and follicular thyroid cancer. Am J Med., 1994, 97(5), 418-28. *Erratum in: Am J Med*, 1995, 98(2), 215.

[9] Vecchio, G; Santoro, M. Oncogenes and thyroid cancer. *Clin Chem Lab Med*, 2000, 38(2), 113-6.

[10] Lowy, DR; Willumsen, BM. Function and regulation of ras. *Annu Rev Biochem*, 1993, 62, 851-91.

[11] Shih, TY; Weeks, MO. Oncogenes and cancer: the p21 ras genes. *Cancer Invest*, 1984, 2(2), 109-23.

[12] Barbacid, M. Ras genes. *Annu Rev Biochem*, 1987, 56, 779-827.

[13] Suarez, HG; du Villard, JA; Severino, M; Caillou, B; Schlumberger, M; Tubiana, M; Parmentier, C; Monier, R. Presence of mutations in all three ras genes in human thyroid tumors. *Oncogene*, 1990, 5(4), 565-70.

[14] Suarez, HG; du Villard, JA; Caillou, B; Schlumberger, M; Tubiana, M; Parmentier, C; Monier, R. Detection of activated ras oncogenes in human thyroid carcinomas. *Oncogene*, 1988, 2(4), 403-6.

[15] Lemoine, NR; Mayall, ES; Wyllie, FS; Williams, ED; Goyns, M; Stringer, B; Wynford-Thomas, D. High frequency of ras oncogene activation in all stages of human thyroid tumorigenesis. *Oncogene*, 1989, 4(2), 159-64.

[16] Smit, VT; Boot, AJ; Smits, AM; Fleuren, GJ; Cornelisse, CJ; Bos, JL. KRAS codon 12 mutations occur very frequently in pancreatic adenocarcinomas. *Nucleic Acids Res*, 1988, 16(16), 7773-82.

[17] Bos, JL. Ras oncogenes in human cancer: a review. *Cancer Res*, 1989, 49(17), 4682-9 (Review). Erratum in: Cancer Res, 1990, 50(4), 1352.

[18] Rodenhuis, S; van de Wetering, ML; Mooi, WJ; Evers, SG; van Zandwijk, N; Bos, JL. Mutational activation of the K-ras oncogene. A possible pathogenetic factor in adenocarcinoma of the lung. *N Engl J Med*, 1987, 317(15), 929-35.

[19] Davies, H; Bignell, GR; Cox, C; Stephens, P; Edkins, S; Clegg, S; Teague, J; Woffendin, H; Garnett, MJ; Bottomley, W; Davis, N; Dicks, E; Ewing, R; Floyd, Y; Gray, K; Hall, S; Hawes, R; Hughes, J; Kosmidou, V; Menzies, A; Mould, C; Parker, A; Stevens, C; Watt, S; Hooper, S; Wilson, R; Jayatilake, H; Gusterson, BA; Cooper, C; Shipley, J; Hargrave, D; Pritchard-Jones, K; Maitland, N; Chenevix-Trench, G; Riggins, GJ; Bigner, DD; Palmieri, G; Cossu, A; Flanagan, A; Nicholson, A; Ho, JW; Leung, SY; Yuen, ST; Weber, BL; Seigler, HF; Darrow, TL; Paterson, H; Marais, R; Marshall, CJ; Wooster, R; Stratton, MR; Futreal, PA. Mutations of the BRAF gene in human cancer. *Nature*, 2002, 417(6892), 949-54.

[20] Brose, MS; Volpe, P; Feldman, M; Kumar, M; Rishi, I; Gerrero, R; Einhorn, E;Herlyn, M; Minna, J; Nicholson, A; Roth, JA; Albelda, SM; Davies, H; Cox, C; Brignell, G; Stephens, P; Futreal, PA; Wooster, R; Stratton, MR; Weber, BL. BRAF and RAS mutations in human lung cancer and melanoma. *Cancer Res*, 2002, 62(23), 6997-7000.

[21] Yuen, ST; Davies, H; Chan, TL; Ho, JW; Bignell, GR; Cox, C; Stephens, P; Edkins, S; Tsui, WW; Chan, AS; Futreal, PA; Stratton, MR; Wooster, R; Leung, SY. Similarity of the phenotypic patterns associated with BRAF and KRAS mutations in colorectal neoplasia. *Cancer Res*, 2002, 62(22), 6451-5.

[22] Fukushima, T; Suzuki, S; Mashiko, M; Ohtake, T; Endo, Y; Takebayashi, Y; Sekikawa, K; Hagiwara, K; Takenoshita, S. BRAF mutations in papillary carcinomas of the thyroid. *Oncogene*, 2003, 22(41), 6455-7.

[23] Namba, H; Nakashima, M; Hayashi, T; Hayashida, N; Maeda, S; Rogounovitch, TI; Ohtsuru, A; Saenko, VA; Kanematsu, T; Yamashita, S. Clinical implication of hot spot BRAF mutation, V599E, in papillary thyroid cancers. *J Clin Endocrinol Metab*, 2003, 88(9), 4393-7.

[24] Xu, X; Quiros, RM; Gattuso, P; Ain, KB; Prinz, RA. High prevalence of BRAF gene mutation in papillary thyroid carcinomas and thyroid tumor cell lines. *Cancer Res*, 2003, 63(15), 4561-7.

[25] Cohen, Y, Xing, M; Mambo, E; Guo, Z; Wu, G; Trink, B; Beller, U; Westra, WH; Ladenson, PW; Sidransky, D. BRAF mutation in papillary thyroid carcinoma. *J Natl Cancer Inst*, 2003, 95(8), 625-7

[26] Kimura, ET; Nikiforova, MN; Zhu, Z; Knauf, JA; Nikiforov, YE; Fagin, JA. High prevalence of BRAF mutations in thyroid cancer: genetic evidence for constitutive activation of the RET/PTC-RAS-BRAF signaling pathway in papillary thyroid carcinoma. *Cancer Res*, 2003, 63(7), 1454-7.

[27] Davis, RJ. The mitogen-activated protein kinase signal transduction pathway. *J Biol Chem*, 1993, 268(20), 14553-6.

[28] Nishida, E; Gotoh, Y. The MAP kinase cascade is essential for diverse signal transduction pathways. *Trends Biochem Sci*, 1993, 18(4), 128-31.

[29] Robinson, MJ; Cobb, MH. Mitogen-activated protein kinase pathways. *Curr Opin Cell Biol*, 1997, 9(2), 180-6.

[30] Roovers, K; Assoian, RK. Integrating the MAP kinase signal into the G1 phase cell cycle machinery. *Bioessays*, 2000, 22(9), 818-26.

[31] Gotoh, Y; Nishida, E. Activation mechanism and function of the MAP kinase cascade. *Mol Reprod Dev*, 1995, 42(4), 486-92.

[32] Treisman, R. Regulation of transcription by MAP kinase cascades. *Curr Opin Cell Biol*, 1996, 8(2), 205-15.

[33] Matsuda, S; Gotoh, Y; Nishida, E. Signaling pathways mediated by the mitogen-activated protein (MAP) kinase kinase/MAP kinase cascade. *J Leukoc Biol*, 1994, 56(5), 548-53.

[34] Tanoue, T; Nishida, E. Molecular recognitions in the MAP kinase cascades. *Cell Signal*, 2003, 15(5), 455-62.

[35] Tsuda, L; Inoue, YH; Yoo, MA; Mizuno, M; Hata, M; Lim, YM; Adachi-Yamada, T; Ryo, H; Masamune, Y; Nishida, Y. A protein kinase similar to MAP kinase activator acts downstream of the raf kinase in Drosophila. *Cell*, 1993, 72(3), 407-14.

[36] Kosako, H; Nishida, E; Gotoh, Y. cDNA cloning of MAP kinase kinase reveals kinase cascade pathways in yeasts to vertebrates. *EMBO J*, 1993, 12, 787-794

[37] Gotoh, Y; Nishida, E. The MAP kinase cascade: its role in Xenopus oocytes, eggs and embryos. *Prog Cell Cycle Res*, 1995, 1, 287-97.

[38] Marshall, CJ. Specificity of receptor tyrosine kinase signaling: transient versus sustained extracellular signal-regulated kinase activation. *Cell*, 1995, 80(2), 179-85.

[39] Schlessinger, J. How receptor tyrosine kinases activate Ras. *Trends Biochem Sci*, 1993, 18(8), 273-5.

[40] Marais, R; Light, Y; Paterson, HF; Marshall, CJ. Ras recruits Raf-1 to the plasma membrane for activation by tyrosine phosphorylation. *EMBO J*, 1995, 14(13), 3136-45.

[41] Marshall, M. Interactions between Ras and Raf: key regulatory proteins in cellular transformation. *Mol Reprod Dev*, 1995, 42(4), 493-9.

[42] Satoh, T; Nakafuku, M; Kaziro, Y. Function of Ras as a molecular switch in signal transduction. *J Biol Chem*, 1992, 267(34), 24149-52.

[43] Chardin, P. Small GTP-binding proteins of the ras family: a conserved functional mechanism? *Cancer Cells*, 1991, 3(4), 117-26.

[44] Boguski, MS; McCormick, F. Proteins regulating Ras and its relatives. *Nature*, 1993, 366(6456), 643-54.

[45] Grunicke, HH; Maly, K. Role of GTPases and GTPase regulatory proteins in oncogenesis. *Crit Rev Oncog*, 1993, 4(4), 389-402.

[46] Rapp, UR; Goldsborough, MD; Mark, GE; Bonner, TI; Groffen, J; Reynolds, FH Jr; Stephenson, JR. Structure and biological activity of v-raf, a unique oncogene transduced by a retrovirus. *Proc Natl Acad Sci USA*, 1983, 80(14), 4218-22.

[47] Sithanandam, G; Druck, T; Cannizzaro, LA; Leuzzi, G; Huebner, K; Rapp, UR. B-raf and a B-raf pseudogene are located on 7q in man. *Oncogene*, 1992, 7(4), 795-9.

[48] Sithanandam, G; Kolch, W; Duh, FM; Rapp, UR. Complete coding sequence of a human B-raf cDNA and detection of B-raf protein kinase with isozyme specific antibodies. *Oncogene*, 1990, 5(12) , 1775-80.

[49] Stephens, RM; Sithanandam, G; Copeland, TD; Kaplan, DR; Rapp, UR; Morrison, DK. 95-kilodalton B-Raf serine/threonine kinase: identification of the protein and its major autophosphorylation site. *Mol Cell Bio,*. 1992, 12(9), 3733-42.

[50] Kolch, W. Meaningful relationships: the regulation of the Ras/Raf/MEK/ERK pathway by protein interactions. *Biochem J,* 2000, 351 Pt 2, 289-305.

[51] Sendoh, H; Hu, CD; Wu, D; Song, C; Yamawaki-Kataoka, Y; Kotani, J; Okada, T; Shima, F; Kariya, K; Kataoka, T. Role of Raf-1 conserved region 2 in regulation of Ras-dependent Raf-1 activation. *Biochem Biophys Res Commun*, 2000, 271(3), 596-602.

[52] Zhang, BH; Guan, KL. Activation of B-Raf kinase requires phosphorylation of the conserved residues Thr598 and Ser601. *EMBO J,* 2000 19(20), 5429-39.

[53] Learoyd, DL, Messina, M; Zedenius, J; Robinson, BG. Molecular genetics of thyroid tumors and surgical decision-making. *World J Surg*, 2000, 24, 923-33.

[54] Lazzereschi, D; Mincione, G; Coppa, A; Ranieri, A; Turco, A; Baccheschi, G; Pelicano, S; Colletta, G. Oncogenes and antioncogenes involved in human thyroid carcinogenesis. *J Exp Clin Cancer Res*, 1997, 16, 325-332.

[55] Alves, AM; Carr, FJ. Dot blot detection of point mutations with adjacently hybridising synthetic oligonucleotide probes. *Nucleic Acids Res*, 1988, 16(17), 8723.

[56] Vasko, V; Ferrand, M; di Cristofaro, J; Carayon, P; Henry, JF; de Micco, C. Specific pattern of RAS oncogene mutations in follicular thyroid tumors. *J Clin Endocrinol Metab*, 2003, 88(6), 2745-52.

[57] Liu, RT; Hou, CY; You, HL; Huang, CC; Hock-Liew, Chou, FF; Wang, PW; Cheng, JT. Selective occurrence of ras mutations in benign and malignant thyroid follicular neoplasms in Taiwan. *Thyroid*, 2004, 14(8), 616-21.

[58] Zhu, Z; Gandhi, M; Nikiforova, MN; Fischer, AH; Nikiforov, YE. Molecular profile and clinical-pathologic features of the follicular variant of papillary thyroid carcinoma. An unusually high prevalence of ras mutations. *Am J Clin Pathol*, 2003 120(1), 71-7.

[59] Shi, YF; Zou, MJ; Schmidt, H; Juhasz, F; Stensky, V; Robb, D; Farid, NR. High rates of ras codon 61 mutation in thyroid tumors in an iodide-deficient area. *Cancer Res*, 1991, 51(10), 2690-3.

[60] Wright, PA; Williams, ED; Lemoine, NR; Wynford-Thomas, D. Radiation-associated and 'spontaneous' human thyroid carcinomas show a different pattern of ras oncogene mutation. *Oncogene*, 1991, 6(3), 471-3.

[61] Nikiforov, YE; Nikiforova, MN; Gnepp, DR; Fagin, JA. Prevalence of mutations of ras and p53 in benign and malignant thyroid tumors from children exposed to radiation after the Chernobyl nuclear accident. *Oncogene*, 1996, 13(4), 687-93.

[62] Challeton, C; Bounacer, A; du Villard, JA; Caillou, B; de Vathaire, F; Monier, R; Schlumberger, M; Suarez, HG. Pattern of ras and gsp oncogene mutations in radiation-associated human thyroid tumors. *Oncogene*, 1995, 11(3), 601-3.

[63] Naito, H; Pairojkul, C; Kitahori, Y; Yane, K; Miyahara, H; Konishi, N; Matsunaga, T; Hiasa, Y. Different ras gene mutational frequencies in thyroid papillary carcinomas in Japan and Thailand. *Cancer Lett*, 1998, 131(2), 171-5.

[64] Naoki, K; Chen, TH; Richards, WG; Sugarbaker, DJ; Meyerson, M. Missense mutations of the BRAF gene in human lung adenocarcinoma. *Cancer Res*, 2002, 62(23), 7001-3.

[65] Marais, R; Light, Y; Paterson, HF; Mason, CS; Marshall, CJ. Differential regulation of Raf-1, A-Raf, and B-Raf by oncogenic ras and tyrosine kinases. *J Biol Chem*, 1997, 272(7), 4378-83.

[66] Ledent, C; Parmentier, M; Maenhaut, C; Taton, M; Pirson, I; Lamy, F; Roger, P; Dumont, JE. The TSH cyclic AMP cascade in the control of thyroid cell proliferation: the story of a concept. *Thyroidology*, 1991, 3, 97-101.

[67] Busca, R; Abbe, P; Mantoux, F; Aberdam, E; Peyssonnaux, C; Eychene, A; Ortonne, JP; Ballotti, R. Ras mediates the cAMP-dependent activation of extracellular signal-regulated kinases (ERKs) in melanocytes. *EMBO J*, 2000, 19, 2900-2910.

[68] Halaban, R. The regulation of normal melanocyte proliferation. *Pigment Cell Res*, 2000, 13, 4-14.

[69] Nikiforov, YE. RET/PTC rearrangement in thyroid tumors. *Endocr Pathol*, 2002, 13(1), 3-16.

[70] Viglietto, G; Chiappetta, G; Martinez-Tello, FJ; Fukunaga, FH; Tallini, G; Rigopoulou, D; Visconti, R; Mastro, A; Santoro, M; Fusco, A. RET/PTC oncogene activation is an early event in thyroid carcinogenesis. *Oncogene*, 1995, 11(6), 1207-10.

[71] Soares, P; Trovisco, V; Rocha, AS; Lima, J; Castro, P; Preto, A; Maximo, V; Botelho, T; Seruca, R; Sobrinho-Simoes, M. BRAF mutations and RET/PTC rearrangements are alternative events in the etiopathogenesis of PTC. *Oncogene*, 2003, 22(29), 4578-80.

[72] Lima, J; Trovisco, V; Soares, P; Maximo, V; Magalhaes, J; Salvatore, G; Santoro, M; Bogdanova, T; Tronko, M; Abrosimov, A; Jeremiah, S; Thomas, G; Williams, D; Sobrinho-Simoes, M. BRAF mutations are not a major event in post-Chernobyl childhood thyroid carcinomas. *J Clin Endocrinol Metab*, 2004, 89(9), 4267-71.

[73] Ciampi, R; Knauf, JA; Kerler, R; Gandhi, M; Zhu, Z; Nikiforova, MN; Rabes, HM; Fagin JA; Nikiforov YE. Oncogenic AKAP9-BRAF fusion is a novel mechanism of MAPK pathway activation in thyroid cancer. *J Clin Invest*, 2005, 115(1), 94-101.

[74] Begum, S; Rosenbaum, E;, Henrique, R; Cohen, Y; Sidransky, D; Westra, WH. BRAF mutations in anaplastic thyroid carcinoma: implications for tumor origin, diagnosis and treatment. *Mod Pathol*, 2004, 17(11), 1359-63.

[75] Xing, M; Vasko, V; Tallini, G; Larin, A; Wu, G; Udelsman, R; Ringel, MD;, Ladenson, PW; Sidransky, D. BRAF T1796A transversion mutation in various thyroid neoplasms. *J Clin Endocrinol Metab,* 2004, 89(3), 1365-8.

[76] Nikiforova, MN; Kimura, ET; Gandhi, M; Biddinger, PW; Knauf, JA; Basolo, F; Zhu, Z; Giannini, R; Salvatore, G; Fusco, A; Santoro, M; Fagin, JA; Nikiforov, YE. BRAF mutations in thyroid tumors are restricted to papillary carcinomas and anaplastic or poorly differentiated carcinomas arising from papillary carcinomas. *J Clin Endocrinol Metab*, 2003, 88(11), 5399-404.

[77] Bollag, G; Freeman, S; Lyons, JF; Post, LE. Raf pathway inhibitors in oncology. *Curr Opin Investig Drugs*, 2003, 4(12), 1436-41.

[78] Lyons, JF; Wilhelm, S; Hibner, B; Bollag, G. Discovery of a novel Raf kinase inhibitor. *Endocr Relat Cancer*, 2001, 8(3), 219-25.

[79] Shelton, JG; Moye, PW; Steelman, LS; Blalock, WL; Lee, JT; Franklin, RA; McMahon, M; McCubrey, JA. Differential effects of kinase cascade inhibitors on neoplastic and cytokine-mediated cell proliferation. *Leukemia.* 2003, 17(9), 1765-82.

In: Trends in Thyroid Cancer Research
Editor: Carl A. Milton, pp. 65-88
ISBN 1-59454-627-4

Chapter IV

RELATIONSHIP BETWEEN INCIDENCE OF THYROID CANCER IN IODINE RICH AND IODINE DEFICIENT AREAS: THE ROLE OF IODINE IN THYROID CANCER

Bagher Larijani [*] ***and Vahid Haghpanah***
Endocrinology and Metabolism Research Center (EMRC),
Tehran University of Medical Sciences (TUMS), Tehran, Iran

ABSTRACT

Iodine is the heaviest and richest in electrons among required elements in the animal diet. Inorganic iodides are necessary for all living vegetable and animal cells, but only the vertebrates have the thyroid gland and its iodinated hormones.

Impaired intrathyroidal iodine metabolism represents one of the most peculiar abnormalities present in thyroid neoplastic tissue. The biological activity of peroxidase, although normal in benign cold adenomas, was decreased or absent in thyroid carcinomas, resulting in a low iodine organification. As a consequence, in thyroid cancer tissues, a low intrathyroidal iodine concentration, a low degree of iodination of thyroglobulin and a low rate of thyroid hormones synthesis were observed. The altered iodine intrathyroidal metabolism may confer on tumor cells a proliferative advantage as a result of the loss of the iodine autoregulating process.

Malignant disease of the thyroid gland is a heterogeneous disorder that affects all age groups, but is more serious in the elderly. The relation of iodine deficiency to enlargement of the thyroid gland, or goiter, was first shown by David Marine, who found that hyperplasic changes occurred regularly in the thyroid when the iodine concentration fell below 0.1%. Papillary carcinoma of the thyroid may be more common in areas with

[*] Corresponding Author: B. Larijani, MD, Endocrinology and Metabolism Research Center (EMRC) 5th Floor, Shariati Hospital, North Kargar Ave. Tehran 14114, Iran. Tel: 0098 21 88026902-3. Fax: 0098 21 88029399. Email: emrc@sina.tums.ac.ir

iodination of salt or a high-iodine diet. Follicular carcinoma is much more common in iodine-deficient goiterous areas. The high incidence of follicular neoplasia in goiterous area may be related to the prolonged stimulatory effects of thyroid-stimulating hormone (TSH). In animals, the chronic stimulation of the thyroid by TSH is known to produce thyroid neoplasmes.
The role of iodine nutrition in the pathogenesis of thyroid cancer (TC) is both complex and controversial. Several investigators have reported an association between iodization and subsequent changes in thyroid cancer, an increase for papillary carcinoma and a decline for follicular and anaplastic carcinoma. Improved iodine intake in previously iodine-deficient communities has also been associated with an increased incidence of papillary thyroid cancer (PTC). These so-called "papillarization" is characterized by an increase in the ratio of papillary to follicular thyroid cancers (FTC), a decrease in PTC size, and an attenuation of the malignant phenotype. There is, however, no clear relationship between increased dietary iodine and higher total TC rates. Other factors such as geographic and ethnic variations in the incidence of thyroid cancer are considerable. The relationship between thyroid cancer and iodine status has often been debated without agreement being reached on many aspects, including on a possible causal relationship. Overall, many data have shown that correction of iodine deficiency decreases the risk of, and the morbidity form, thyroid cancer.

Keywords: Thyroid Cancer, Incidence, Iodine intake, Iodine Supplementation

INTRODUCTION

Iodine (Molecular, Physiologic and Biochemical Aspects):

Iodine is an essential constituent of the thyroid hormones thyroxin 3,5,3′,5′ tetraiodithyronine (T_4) and 3,5,3′ triiodithyronine (T_3). The major role of iodine in nutrition arises from the importance of thyroid hormones to growth and development [1].

Iodine is the heaviest and richest in electrons among required elements in the animal diet. Inorganic iodides are necessary for all living vegetable and animal cells, but only the vertebrates have the thyroid gland and its iodinated hormones. In humans, the total amount of iodine is about 30-50 mg and less than 30% is present in thyroid gland and in its hormones. Approximately 60%-80% of total iodine is non-hormonal and it is concentrated in extrathyroidal tissues, but its biological role is still unknown. In these cells, iodide acts as an electron donor in the presence of H_20_2 and peroxidase, the remaining iodine readily iodinates the tyrosine and more slowly the histidine or some specific lipid and so, neutralizes its own high oxidant power. Recently Sebastiano Venturi et al reported interesting antioxidant biochemical cooperation (not for thyroid hormonogenesis) in some iodolipids among iodides and omega-6 and omega-3 fatty acids [2].

More than 3 billion years ago, blue-green algae (Cyanobacteria), which are the most primitive oxygenic photosynthetic organisms, ancestors of multicellular eukaryotic algae that contain the highest amount of iodine, were the first living cells to produce oxygen, which was toxic at that time, in the terrestrial atmosphere. So, algal cells required a protective antioxidant action in which Iodides might have had this specific role. In fact iodides are greatly present and available in sea water, where algal phytoplankton acts as a biological accumulator of iodides and selenium [2]. Since approximately 700 million years ago thyroxine (T_4) has been present in fibrous exoskeletal scleroproteins of the lowest Invertebrates (Porifera and Anthozoa), without showing any hormonal action. When some primitive marine vertebrates started to emerge from the iodine-rich sea and transferred to iodine-deficient fresh water, and finally land, their diet became iodine deficient and also harboured vegetable iodide-competitors such as nitrates, nitrites, thiocyanates, and some glycosides. Hence, these animals needed an efficient thyroid gland as reservoir of iodine. Therefore, during progressive slow adaptation to terrestrial life, the primitive chordates started to use the primitive, but not antagonized, T_4 in order to transport antioxidant iodide into the cells. So, the remaining triiodothyronine (T_3), the real active hormone that stimulates the cellular oxidations, became active in the metamorphosis and thermogenesis for a better adaptation of the organisms to terrestrial environment (fresh water, atmosphere, gravity, temperature, and diet) [2].

There are chronologically differentiated on the basis of the phylogenesis and embryogenesis three ways of action of iodine:

1. An ancient and direct action on endodermal foregut and stomach and on ectodermal epidermis, where inorganic iodides probably act as antioxidants.
2. A recent and direct action on fetal prehormonal thyroid and on salivary and mammary glands, thymus, ovary, and on nervous, arterial and skeletal systems, where inorganic iodides are active.
3. A recent and indirect action of the thyroid and its iodinated hormones, on all vertebrate cells, which makes use of specific organic iodine-compounds: T_4 and T_3, which act in very small quantities and utilize T_3-receptors. Indeed thyroid hormones contain less than 1 mg of iodine and less than 1/30-1/50 of total iodine amount [2].

Role of Iodine in Thyroid Physiology and Pathophysiology:

Iodine in thyroid physiology

Iodine represents an essential element in thyroid physiology, being a critical component of thyroxine and tri-iodothyronine molecules, and a key regulator of thyroid gland function. Thus dietary iodide supply influences the functional activity of the thyroid gland, iodine deficiency being the main cause of endemic goiter. Furthermore, iodine directly modulates thyroid sensitivity to thyroid-stimulating hormone (TSH), and intrathyroidal iodine has a generally inhibitory effect on thyroid function, independently of the TSH concentration. This autoregulatory effect of iodine encompasses many aspects of thyroid function, including iodide transport mechanism, iodide organification, thyroid hormone synthesis and secretion, and thyroid intermediary metabolism. The first step of iodine thyroid metabolism is represented by the thyroid trappingand concentration of iodide from the blood, which is achieved by an active, energydependent transport process across the basolateral plasma membrane of the thyrocytes (Figure 1).

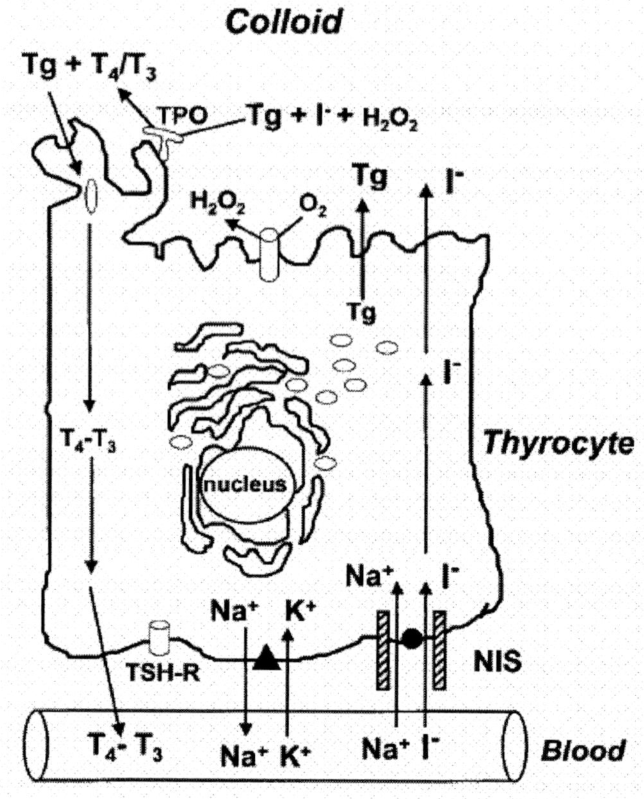

Figure 1: Schematic representation of the iodide uptake and biosynthetic pathway of thyroid hormones in thyrocytes. I[1] is actively accumulated across the basolateral plasma membrane of the thyrocyte in a process catalyzed by the NIS. This transport is driven by the Naþ gradient generated under ATP hydrolysis by Naþ/Kþ-ATPase. The iodide is passively translocated across the apical membrane of the thyrocyte into the colloid, where it is used to iodinate the thyroglobulin (Tg). This reaction, called 'I[1] organification', is catalyzed by TPO and requires H2O2. The iodinated Tg, containing thyroid hormones, is stored in the colloid. Thyroid hormones, thyroxine (T4) and tri-iodothyronine (T3) are released from Tg and secreted in the blood. All steps in the thyroid hormone biosynthetic pathway are stimulated by TSH [4].

The new hormonal action of T_3 was made possible by the formation of T3-receptors in the cells of vertebrates. First, about 600-500 million years ago, in primitive Chordata, the o T3-receptors with a metamorphosing action appeared and then, about 250-350 million years ago, in the birds and Mammalia, the alpha-T3-receptors with metabolic and thermogenetic actions appeared. In water, the iodine concentration decreases step by step from sea water (about 50-60 ~g/L to estuary and source of rivers (less than 0.26 ~g/L in some Triassic mountain regions of northern Italy), and in parallel, salt-water fish (herring) contain about 520 μg of iodine per kilogram compared to freshwater trout about 20 ug/kg (I). So, in iodine-deficient fresh water some trout and other salmonids (anadromous migratory fishes) may suffer thyroid hypertrophy or related metabolic disorders, as do some sharks in captivity. In some anadromous migratory fishes (sea lamprey and salmonids), thyroid hormones play a role in initiation of metamorphosis. After metamorphosis, when these adult marine fish (in-explicably) die in fresh water after reproducing, they release their iodides and selenium in the environment, bringing back upstream from the sea to iodine-deficient areas a considerable quantity of iodine that would normally be flowing downstream in the sea because of gravity and its high atomic weight. During human embryogenesis o T3-receptor genes are expressed before the ~ T3-receptors. Gastric iodide-pump, phylogenetically more primitive than the thyroidal one, has lower affinity for iodide and does not respond to more recent thyrotropin (TSH). In fact, in a pregnant mouse, fetal gastric mucosa shows iodine-concentrating ability earlier than fetal thyroid. On the other hand, from a biochemical point of view, as inhibitors of lipid peroxidation, by 5'-monodeiodinase activity (a seleno-enzyme), T_4 and reverse-T_3 (but not T_3) became and were found to be more effective in this antioxidant activity than vitamin E, glutathione and ascorbic acid . In fact maternal T_4, and not T_3, plays a crucial role in protecting fetal brain from damage caused by hypothyroidism [2]. The antioxidant action of iodides has also been described in isolated rabbit eyes. Rieger et al, Winkler et al , and Buchberger et al reported a beneficial and antioxidant action of iodides in many chronic diseases and in eye cataractogenesis.

Researchers reported the cooperation between antioxidant selenium and iodine. In fact, selenium is also present in some cellular peroxidases and deiodinases, which are able to oxidate iodides and the latter enzymes produce iodides from iodothyronines. Thyroid peroxidase is an important selenium-glutathione-enzyme that utilizes iodides in order to transfer electrons to the oxygen of hydrogen peroxide. The thyroid gland and marine fish have the highest concentration of selenium and iodine. Furthermore, there is an interesting chemical gradient of electronegativity, according to Pauling scale units, among oxygen (3.44), iodine (2.66), selenium (2.55), and hydrogen (2.20). This gradient might clear up the possible roles of iodides in electron transfer. The family of peroxidase enzymes includes mammal, microorganism, plant, algal, and fungal peroxidases. Some of these peroxidases, known as haloperoxidases (io), use halide ions (iodide, bromide, and chloride) as natural electron donors, and also have an antioxidant function in Cyanobacteria. Furthermore, in marine algae, haloperoxidases are able to catalyze iodide incorporation into two-carbon metabolites producing iodomethane gas (CH_3I) in terrestrial atmosphere. Recently, Taurog reported that the relation between animal and nonanimal peroxidases probably represents an example of convergent evolution to a common enzymatic mechanism [2, 3].

Thyroid cells phylogenetically derived from primitive iodide-concentrating gastroenteric cells that, during evolution migrated and specialized in uptake of iodides and storage and elaboration of iodine compounds, in order to adapt to iodine-deficient terrestrial life. The thyroid gland, with a progressively more developed morphology, is a modem organ and its function started and was improved from primitive Chordata to more recent marine and freshwater fishes, Amphibia, reptiles, birds, and finally mammals in which the thyroidectomy and hypothyroidism might be considered like a sort of phylogenetical and metabolical regression to a former stage of reptilian life [2].

Iodine in thyroid pathophysiology:

The recent cloning of the gene encoding the protein responsible for this process, the sodium/iodide symporter (NIS), enabled better characterization of the molecular mechanisms underlying the iodide transport, thus opening the way to clarify its role in thyroid diseases. The evidence that iodine transport is present in thyroid neoplastic tissues has been the basis for the use of radioiodine in the diagnosis and treatment of patients with thyroid cancer [4]. NIS up regulation by TSH has also been described *in vivo*. In hypophysectomized rats with markedly low TSH concentrations, NIS protein expression is low, but increases promptly after a single injection of TSH. Accordingly, in rats maintained on an I–deficient diet or treated with propylthiouracil, increased TSH circulating concentrations paralleled increased NIS protein expression [3, 4, 5].

This suggests that an increase in iodide, probably through its intracellular concentration, may downregulate expression of the *NIS* gene. Factors other than TSH and iodide may participate in the regulation of *NIS* expression. Retinoic acid was found to upregulate iodide transport in human follicular thyroid carcinoma cell lines, whereas a downregulation was observed in non-transfected FRTL-5 cells (differentiated rat thyroid cells that possess specific markers of thyroid function) [4]. Although papillary and follicular thyroid carcinomas retain the majority of biological properties of normal thyroid cells, a variety of biochemical defects has been demonstrated. Indeed, impaired intrathyroidal iodine metabolism represents one of the most peculiar abnormalities present in thyroid neoplastic tissue. The biological activity of peroxidase, although normal in benign cold adenomas, was decreased or absent in thyroid carcinomas, resulting in a low iodine organification. As a consequence, in thyroid cancer tissues, a low intrathyroidal iodine concentration, a low degree of iodination of thyroglobulin and a low rate of thyroid hormones synthesis were observed. The altered iodine intrathyroidal metabolism may confer on tumor cells a proliferative advantage as a result of the loss of the iodine autoregulating process [4].

Proto-oncogene activation, over-expression, or both, have a role in thyroid tumorigenesis and determine a loss of differentiation of thyroid function. PC Cl 3 and FRTL-5 are differentiated rat thyroid cells that possess specific markers of thyroid function – namely, thyroglobulin synthesis and secretion, the ability to trap iodide and TSH-dependent growth. Moreover, the oncogene-transformed cell lines display different degrees of malignancy and differentiation. They exhibit a TSH-independent growth, even if some clones require thyrotropin hormone for optimal proliferation when cultured in conditions of low serum concentration. However, all transformed thyroid cells, exhibiting either a high or a low degree of malignancy, display a loss of iodide uptake function. Moreover, whereas all thyroid specific differentiation markers are lost in highly malignant rat thyroid cell lines (that is, they are transformed by KiMSV, Kirsten murine sarcoma virus), the de-differentiation process appears to be restricted to the loss of iodide uptake in transformed thyroid cells of low malignancy; this suggests that, *in vitro*, the loss of ability to concentrate iodide is an early effect of oncogenic rat thyroid cell transformation. Likewise, the phenotype of transformed thyroid cells may make it possible to define, at the molecular level, the mechanisms whereby oncogene-transformed rat thyroid cells lose the ability to trap iodide. The possibility exists that activation of a specific oncogenic pathway may alter the iodide-trapping ability of transformed cells, through an alteration in *NIS* gene expression [4]. The presence of a transcriptional or post-transcriptional event, or both, responsible for the complete loss of iodide uptake function [4]. Having already been detected in cold follicular adenomas, the low expression of NIS may represent an early abnormality in the thyroid cell transformation pathway, and not be a consequence of cancer progression. Conversely, *Tg* gene expression appears to be well conserved in cancer cells, being absent only in undifferentiated cancer tissue [4]. Immunohistochemistry using anti-NIS antibodies confirmed the much lower expression of the NIS protein in thyroid cancer tissues, and also demonstrated that its expression was heterogeneous, being detected in only a few malignant papillary or follicular thyroid cells [4]. Available data demonstrate that a decrease, loss, or both, of *NIS* gene expression may have a central role in the defective concentration of iodine by neoplastic thyroid carcinomas, in both primary and metastatic tissues. Although the molecular mechanisms of this loss are unclear, the possibility exists that alterations in the iodide symporter may represent a primary defect; thus, in an originally heterogeneous population, a small number of cancer cells carrying this defect may overgrow over time and determine the appearance of an NIS-negative cell population [4]. At the present time, the low expression of *NIS* and of peroxidase genes in thyroid cancer tissues is largely unexplained, although promoter-specific protein: protein or protein: DNA interactions are likely to be involved. Studies of transcription factors and of abnormal methylation of genes are, indeed, being performed [4].

Figure 2 summarizes the possible targets of alterations in the tumorigenic process that are responsible for the loss of iodide uptake in thyrocytes [4].

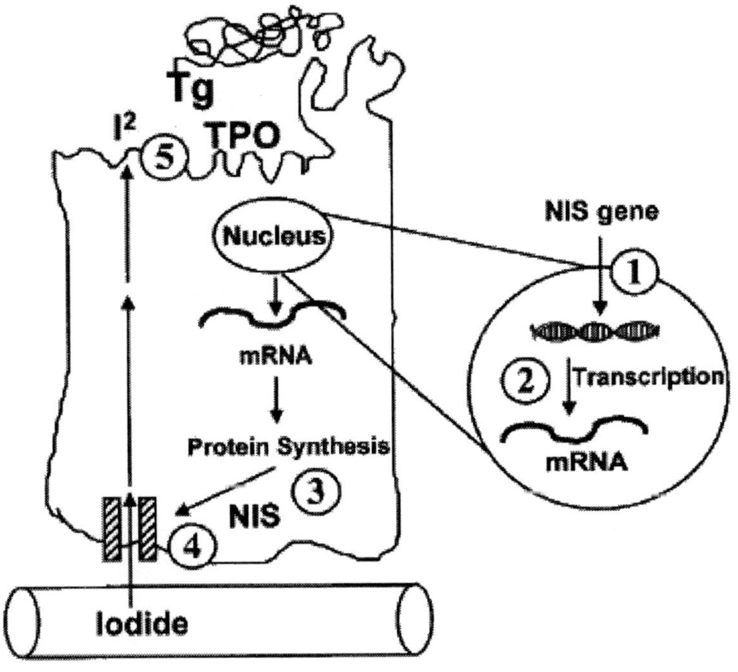

Figure 2: The possible targets of the alterations occurring in the tumorigenic process responsible for the loss of iodide uptake in thyrocytes. 1, Alterations in NIS structural gene; 2, alterations in regulation of NIS transcript expression; 3, alterations in NIS protein synthesis; 4, alterations in NIS transport to the plasma membrane; 5, alterations in iodide organification [4].

In Italy gastric cancer, thyroid cancer and goitre are statistically correlated and more frequent in iodine deficient areas, such as in Alpine and Appennines valleys, and in regions of northern and central Italy compared to southern Italy where the majority of the population lives in seaside areas [6]. an excess of dietary iodine (more than 2 mg) impairs the iodide-pump and the functions of some permanently-concentrating tissues (thyroid, stomach and salivary glands) causing, in the case of greater and prolonged quantities, degenerative, necrotic and also neoplastic lesions, which are well-known in thyroid gland [6]. Several researchers reported also a general anti-tumor activity of iodine-rich edible marine algae (in moderate amount) and a favourable activity in human chemoprevention of oral cancer, not due to the action of retinol or beta-carotene. Noda et al. showed that per-iodate oxidation is necessary to the anti-tumor activity of algae. Recently an inhibition of vacuolation toxin activity of Helicobacter pylori by iodine was also reported. The high iodide-concentration of thymus explains the important role of iodine in immune system. We, also, reported that iodine deficiency impairs immunity and so might reduces defence against tumor cells [6].

Quite recently it has been shown that selenium deficiency may have profound effects on thyroid hormone metabolism and possibly also on the thyroid gland itself. In this situation the function of type I deiodinase (a selenoprotein) is impaired. Type I deiodinase plays a major role in T4 deiodination in peripheral tissues. It has been shown that when, in an area of combined iodine and selenium deficiency, only selenium is supplemented, serum T4 decreases. This effect is explained by restoration of type I deiodinase activity leading to normalization of T4 deiodination while T4 synthesis remains impaired because of continued iodine deficiency. Selenium deficiency also leads to a reduction of the selenium containing enzyme glutathione peroxidase. Glutathione peroxidase detoxifies H_2O_2 which is abundantly present in the thyroid gland as a substrate for the thyroperoxidase that catalyzes iodide oxidation and binding to thyroglobulin, and the oxidative coupling of iodotyrosines into iodothyronines. Reduced detoxification of H_2O_2 may lead to thyroid cell death. Elevated H_2O_2 levels in thyrocytes may be more toxic under situations of increased TSH stimulation such as is present in areas with severe iodine deficiency. Last, but not least, decreased availability of glutathione peroxidase impairs thyroid hormone synthesis in the thyroid gland, a fact that could also contribute to decreased T4 synthesis [7].

Thyroid Cancer (Histopathologic and Clinical features):

The name thyroid comes from the Greek word for shield. The gland was named by Wharton in 1646 either because of its shield like shape or because it shielded the larynx. Malignant disease of the thyroid gland is a heterogeneous disorder that affects all age groups, but is more serious in the elderly. Thyroid cancers exhibit the full range of malignant behavior from the relatively indolent occult differentiated thyroid cancer to the uniformly aggressive and lethal undifferentiated thyroid cancers [8]. Because some thyroid cancers are potentially lethal, a definitive diagnosis of all lesions of the thyroid gland is indicated, which will suggest appropriate therapy.

Malignant thyroid tumors account for only 1% of all human cancers. They are however, the most common endocrine malignancy, accounting for 90% of all endocrine cancers [9, 10, 11, 12, 13, 14, 15]. Malignant epithelial tumors of the thyroid have classically been categorized under the subgroups of follicular, papillary, medullary, and undifferentiated or anaplastic carcinomas [16]. More recently, a classification based on tumor prognosis has been suggested, which included a group with intermediate differentiation (Table 1) [17].

Table 1: Prognostic Classification of Malignant Thyroid Tumors (Li Volsi VA, 1999) [17]

Well differentiated (low-grade malignancy)
Usual papillary carcinoma
Usual follicular carcinoma
Variants of papillary carcinoma
Encapsulated
Cystic
Microcarcinoma
Intermediate differentiation
Tall cell papillary carcinoma
Columnar cell carcinoma
Diffuse sclerosing variant of papillary carcinoma
Solid papillary carcinoma
Hurthle cell (oxyphillic) carcinoma
Insular carcinoma
Medullary carcinoma
Poorly differentiated (high-grade malignancy)
Anaplastic (undifferentiated) carcinoma

The majority of cases occur between 25 and 65 years of age, but thyroid cancer can occur in the very young and the elderly [9]. Globally, age standardized incidence rates have increased by up to 5-fold during the past 60 yr. This increase has largely resulted from a rise in the incidence of differentiated carcinoma, particularly, PTC. The rise in incidence of TC has been observed across regions of disparate geography and ethnicity [10, 11, 18]. The cause remains unclear. Increased exposure to ionizing radiation, changes in iodine nutrition, and greater recognition of prevalent, yet clinically irrelevant, thyroid neoplasia have all been postulated as contributory. Studies documenting the spectrum of TC in iodine-deficient communities commencing iodine prophylaxis have noted a rise in incidence of PTC relative to the other tumor types. Although some authors have reported a rise in the overall incidence of TC after correction of iodine deficiency (ID), the increment in TC is, in general, similar to that occurring contemporaneously in populations with stable iodine nutrition. Additional studies are required to clarify the relationship between iodine nutrition and thyroid tumorigenesis. In particular, longitudinal data spanning transition from iodine sufficiency to deficiency should establish the contributions of improved diagnostic practice, environmental carcinogens, and iodine nutrition, to the observed changes in the spectrum of TC. It is not possible to exclude subtle changes in clinical practice, such as increased use of ultrasonography and fine needle biopsy, as contributory to the rise in PTC incidence. However, based on available anecdotal information, it seems that this unlikely to fully account for the observed increase in PTC. By way of example, despite a rise during recent years of multinodular goiter occurring in association with PTC, the majority of patients with combined PTC and multinodular goiter had evidence of clinically relevant TC [18].

Map of the World's Iodine Nutrition (ICCIDD, 2003) [21]

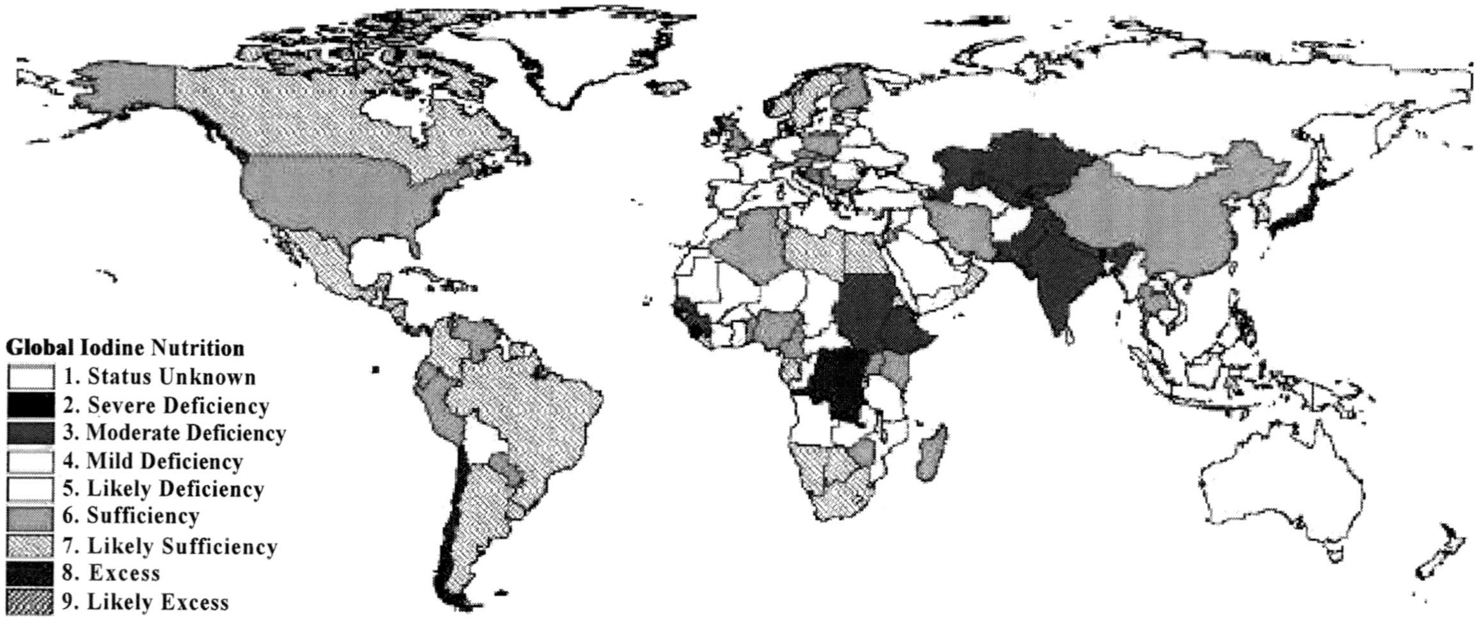

Summary of the World's Iodine Nutrition (ICCIDD, 2003) [21]

	Afr (SS)	Amer	As/Pac	E Eur/CA	China/FE	Mid E/ N Afr	SE Asia	W/C Eur	Total
Population (millions)	633	835	662	287	1,309	514	1,269	580	6,089
Number of Countries	44	25	14	15	3	19	7	32	159
Iodine Nutrition									
By population (millions)									
Deficient	262	49	467	284	25	304	1267	376	3034
Sufficient	311	757	68	3	1284	210	2	204	2839
Excess	54	29	127	0	0	0	0	0	210
Unknown	6	0	0	0	0	0	0	0	6
By population, distribution (%)									
Deficient	41	6	71	99	2	59	99	65	50
Sufficient	49	91	10	1	98	41	1	35	47
Excess	9	3	19	0	0	0	0		3
Unknown	1	0	0	0	0	0	0		0

Summary of the World's Iodine Nutrition (ICCIDD, 2003) [21]

	Afr (SS)	Amer	As/Pac	E Eur/CA	China/FE	Mid E/ N Afr	SE Asia	W/C Eur	Total	
By number of countries										%
Deficient	25	6	9	14	2	9	6	13	84	53
Sufficient	18	18	4	1	1	10	1	19	72	45
Excess	1	1	1	0	0	0	0	0	3	2

Figure 3: Map and summary of the World's Iodine Nutrition (ICCIDD, 2003)

Iodine Deficient (IDA) and Iodine Sufficient Areas (ISA):

The relation of iodine deficiency to enlargement of the thyroid gland, or goiter, was first shown by David Marine, who found that hyperplasic changes occurred regularly in the thyroid when the iodine concentration fell below 0.1% [1].

The recommended daily intake (RDI) of iodine is 100 μg daily for the general population and 150-200 μg daily for women who are pregnant or breastfeeding (iodine demand increases during pregnancy because of increased renal clearance and fetal iodine transfer). Approximately 90% of iodine is excreted in the urine, and iodine status is usually assessed by measuring urinary iodine concentration. The accepted minimum adequate level of urinary iodine (UI) is 100 μg/L, and levels above this are considered normal. Urinary iodine concentrations below 25 μg/L are classified as severe deficiency, and are associated with an increased risk of cretinism; 26-50 μg/L is classified as moderate deficiency, and 51-100 μg/L is regarded as mild iodine deficiency. The World Health Organization (WHO) recommends that the median urinary iodine concentration for populations as a whole should be more than 100 μg/L, that less than 20% of the population should have a urinary iodine concentration below 50 μg/L, and that no cretinism occurs [19].

According to the WHO, the median UI concentration in iodine-sufficient populations should be greater than 10 mg/dl, and no more than 20% of the population should have UI concentrations below 5 mg/dl. A UI concentration adjusted for creatinine concentration (I/Cr) of less than 50 mg iodine/g creatinine also indicates possible iodine deficiency [20]. Figure 3: Map and summary of the World's Iodine Nutrition (ICCIDD, 2003) [21].

History of iodine fortification:

Seaweed has been used to prevent goiter in China for centuries but it is only in the years 1910 to 1920 that systematic programs of salt fortification with iodine were introduced as a strategy for the elimination of IDD (Iodine Deficiency Disorders) almost simultaneously in the United States and in Switzerland. Starting in the early 1950's with pioneering studies in New Guinea, supplementation with iodized oil was introduced in severely affected populations in Asia, Africa and Latin America. Initially, iodized oil was administered intramuscularly, more recently by the oral route [7, 22].

Following the World Summit for Children of 1990 and thanks to the joint efforts and action of the 130 countries with IDD and their governments, with the financial, technical and scientific supports of major agencies of the United Nations, namely UNICEF , WHO, the World Bank ; international NGOs (Non-Governmental Organizations) such as ICCIDD (The International Council for the Control of Iodine Deficiency Disorders) and bilateral ; private partnership for example Kiwanis International and the salt industry, tremendous progress has been achieved during the last decade in insuring access to iodized salt for iodine deficient populations [7, 23, 24, 25, 26, 27].

The social process for successful implementation a national IDD control program includes the following components: situation assessment; communication of results to health professionals, political authorities and the public; development of an action plan; implementation of the plan; and finally, evaluation of its impact at population level. This last phase, monitoring, is often neglected not only because it is the last phase in the process but because it may be over shadowed by other components of the program such as implementation, which is considered as the main or occasionally even the single component to be considered. In addition, many countries affected by IDD belong to the group of countries with low income that therefore do not have the financial or technical resources for the laboratory facilities necessary to proper monitoring of salt quality and iodine status. And yet, monitoring is crucial because IDD is a disease and its prevention and therapy require trained professionals to prescribe the therapy and verify its effects. This absolute ethical duty applies equally to a single individual and to a global population [7].

Technology of Iodine Supplementation

1. Iodized salt

Iodized salt is considered as the most appropriate measure for iodine supplementation. There are two forms of iodine which can be used to iodize salt: "iodide" and "iodate" usually as the potassium salt. Iodate is less soluble and more stable than iodide and is therefore preferred for tropical moist conditions. Both are generally referred to as "iodized" salt. The daily requirement of iodine is 150 ug per person for adults. Levels in the range of 3-6 g per day are being recommended in Western countries [7, 28].

2. Iodized oil

Iodized oil ("lipiodol") was first used for the correction of iodine deficiency in Papua New Guinea. In a controlled trial in the Boana area of the Huon Peninsula of New Guinea, McCullagh carried out a double blind follow-up over 3 years which revealed successful prevention of goiter. Refrigeration is not required, which is a great advantage. Iodized oil is certainly an effective means for the correction of iodine deficiency and has opened up the possibility of elimination of IDD as a public health problem in the next decade. The possibility of linking up an iodized oil program with other preventative programs including the Child Immunization Program (IP) has been considered [7, 29, 30, 31].

3. Other methods

Iodized bread and milk: Iodized bread was used in Tasmania in preference to both iodized salt and iodide tablets distributed through the schools, and shown to be effective. Its use was discontinued because of the availability of other sources of iodine, notably from milk consequent to the use of iodophors in the dairy industry. It is for this reason that milk has become a major adventitious source of iodine in many Western countries such as the USA, the United Kingdom, and in Northern Europe [7, 32].

Iodized water: Water has some of the advantages of salt as a vehicle for iodine fortification. Both are daily necessities and thus their iodization will reach the most vulnerable groups – the poor, the isolated. Water fortified at a regular rate with iodine provides the thyroid with a steadily daily ration, which is physiologically desirable.

Side effects of iodine supplementation

Iodine deficiency is associated with the development of thyroid function abnormalities. Similarly, iodine excess, including following overcorrection of a previous state of iodine deficiency, can also impair thyroid function. The effect of iodine on the thyroid gland is complex with a U shaped relation between iodine intake and risk of thyroid diseases as both low and high iodine intake are associated with an increased risk. It is stated that normal adults can tolerate up to about 1000 μg iodine/day without any side effects. However this upper limit of normal is much lower in a population which was exposed to iodine deficiency in the past. The optimal level of iodine intake to prevent any thyroid disease may be a relatively narrow range around the recommended daily intake at 150 μg [7].

The possible side effects of iodine excess are as follows:

a) Iodide goiter and iodine-induced hypothyroidism.
b) Iodine-induced hyperthyroidism, IIH.
c) Iodine-induced thyroiditis.
d) Thyroid cancer.

In any case, the benefits of iodization programs far outweigh the risks, provided they are implemented and monitored carefully.

Iodine Deficient v/s Iodine Sufficient Areas and Thyroid Cancer:

The relationship between iodine nutrition and thyroid carcinoma pathogenesis is complex. Comparison of incidence rates between iodine-deficient and iodine-sufficient communities yields conflicting results [10, 11, 18, 33]. Some findings argue against the suggested cause-and-effect relationship between iodine and TC. The pattern of distribution of histologic types in some study conforms to that seen in iodine-sufficient areas rather than the pattern observed in iodine-deficient areas [10, 11].

Relative to iodine-sufficient populations, high rates of TC have been found in a number of iodine-deficient communities. Conversely, the populations of Hawaii and Iceland both have high rates of TC, as well as diets rich in iodine. High dietary iodine intake is also typical in Japan, yet similarly high rates for TC to those occurring in Hawaii and Iceland are not observed in this population. Ethnic Japanese living in Hawaii, however, have incidence rates for thyroid cancer up to 2-fold higher than those occurring in Japan. Factors other than iodine nutrition have been proposed to explain these inconsistencies. For example, it has been proposed that the high levels of TC in Hawaii and Iceland relate to volcanic activity rather than iodine nutrition. Case control studies have also produced contradictory findings, iodine-rich diets having been associated with both a heightened and an attenuated risk of TC. Despite these conflicting results, a relatively consistent association has been the link between iodine nutrition and tumor histology. The incidence of FTC and ATC (Anaplastic Thyroid Cancer) is greatest in iodine-deficient populations, whereas the converse is true in regions of iodine sufficiency. Consistent with this observation, iodine prophylaxis is associated with a rise in the proportion of differentiated TC; so called "papillarization" of TC. This is evidenced by a rise in the proportion PTC relative to FTC. The observed increase in PTC incidence in Tasmania has occurred despite the recurrence of mild ID. A complex interaction between iodine nutrition and thyroid tumorigenesis may account for our findings. A study by Galanti *et al.* indicated a possible differential effect for iodine prophylaxis on the spectrum of TC, depending on an individual's age at the time of iodine exposure. The increasing incidence and predominance of PTC despite the fall in contemporary iodine nutrition may reflect either a dose threshold for iodine nutrition and modulation of tumorigenesis, or latency between changes in iodine intake or the clinical expression of neoplastic disease [18].

Whereas total incidence of thyroid cancer is not different between IDA and ISA, increase in iodine supply changes the histologic type of thyroid cancer. The change in iodine supply over the last 40 years in Austria also led to a change in histologic type in thyroid cancer. Whereas the ratio from papillary to follicular thyroid cancer was 0:2 before 1963, it has change to 4:0 after 1990 (Table 2). This underlines observations in other countries that sufficient iodine supply leads to thyroid cancer types with much better prognosis. Follicular thyroid cancer, dedifferentiated follicular thyroid cancer, and anaplastic thyroid cancer have become less frequent in Austria [22].

Table 2: Ratio of Papillary to Follicular Thyroid Cancer in Austria from 1952 to 1995 [22]

Period	Iodine Supply	% Pap DTC	% Foll DTC	Ratio Pap/Foll
1952-1959	IDA	17	83	0.2:1
1970-1975	rIDA	54	46	1.1:1
1984-1989	rIDA	72	28	2.6:1
1990-1995	ISA	80	20	4.0:1

IDA, iodine deficient area; rIDA, relative iodine deficient area; ISA, iodine sufficient area; DTC, differentiated thyroid cancer; Pap, papillary; Foll, follicular

The possible association between iodine intake and occurrence of the various types of thyroid cancer is controversial. Some authors have found an excess of anaplastic and follicular cancers in iodine-deficient areas, whereas papillary cancer seems to dominate in areas with a high natural iodine level [34]. Although the highest follicular carcinoma incidence rates occur in Iceland and Hawaii, both iodine-rich volcanic areas, papillary cancer is still the most common type in these islands. An association between an increase in the iodine supply and a subsequent rise in the incidence of papillary cancer has been reported in several investigations, but it remains unclear whether this reflects a causal relation [35, 36, 37, 38, 39, 40, 41, 42]. Pettersson Bo et al showed in the iodine-deficient area, there was a significant increase of 22% every 5 years among females and 7% (non-significant) among males. The corresponding increase in the iodine-sufficient area was about 20% every 5 years for both sexes. Males in the iodine deficient region had a 2-fold higher risk compared to males in the iodine-sufficient area, but for females, this difference was only 17%. The relative risk of developing follicular thyroid cancer for females compared to males was 1.8 in the iodine deficient area and 3.1 in the iodine-sufficient area [43].

Several investigators have reported an association between iodinization and subsequent changes in thyroid cancer, an increase for papillary carcinoma and a decline for follicular and anaplastic carcinoma, but the theoretical grounds for associating iodine with carcinogenesis in the thyroid appear weak. The introduction of iodinization of the food supply might be expected to produce a period effect if all age groups were affected similarly or a cohort effect if the effect were limited to a critical age. Iodinization would also be expected, over time, to reduce the original differences in incidence patterns between the iodine-deficient and other regions. Pettersson Bo et al showed that papillary cancer is more common in iodine-rich areas, whereas follicular cancer is more common in iodine-depleted areas, confirms previous reports; but overall thyroid cancer incidence was lower in iodine-deficient areas between both sexes, which contrast with earlier findings of a positive association between endemic goiter and thyroid cancer. In Switzerland, Argentina and Paraguay, iodinization of the food supply in areas of endemic goiter was followed by a rise in the incidence of papillary carcinoma and a reduction in follicular and anaplastic carcinoma within 20 years. In Sweden, the prevalence of goiter fell as expected following iodine supplementation (Johnsson, 1965; Sjoberg, 1972), but the subsequent trends in thyroid cancer were more complex. The incidence of papillary cancer rose steeply among successive birth cohorts born after iodine supplementation of the national food supply began, while the relative risk for follicular cancer fell in Sweden. There was no significant difference in the trends of papillary cancer incidence between iodine-deficient and iodine-rich areas, however. This suggests that the increase in papillary cancer was unrelated to iodine supplementation. Introduction of effective (goiter-preventive) iodine supplementation of the national food supply was associated with a greater increase in the incidence of follicular cancer in previously iodine-deficient areas than in iodine-rich areas. Pathological classification of follicular cancer is notoriously difficult, and this is of particular concern when studying time trends. A real increase in follicular carcinoma remains probable, however, since the effect of misclassification should have decreased over time. The usual misdiagnoses of follicular carcinoma arise from benign/atypical adenoma (excluded from this study), from goiter and from the fact that diagnostic criteria for follicular carcinoma have changed; about one-third of follicular carcinomas diagnosed before 1974 would now be assigned to papillary carcinoma (Hedinger and Sobin, 1974). The contribution to follicular carcinoma from misdiagnosed inflammatory goiter would also have vanished after the mid-1960s, and the true trend of follicular cancer is therefore likely to have been an even greater increase in iodine-deficient areas than was actually observed. Anaplastic carcinoma decreased more markedly in the iodine-deficient region, where it was previously higher. Exclusion of less malignant conditions such as inflammatory goiter and small-cell lymphoma, some of which were previously misdiagnosed as anaplastic carcinoma, might have contributed to the decreasing incidence rates since the relative survival from anaplastic carcinoma has actually decreased over time. The incidence of papillary cancer was higher in urban than in rural areas, whereas that of follicular cancer in females and anaplastic cancer in both sexes was higher in rural areas. However, in comparison to the strong effects of age and sex and to the differences between areas defined by iodine status, the effect of urban/rural status was relatively small. It is equally possible, however, that iodine deficiency is not, in fact, a risk factor for thyroid cancer at all, rather than that the increased prevalence of goiter caused by iodine deficiency simply increases the likelihood of thyroid cancer detection because of more frequent thyroid surgery [43].

In iodine deficient area, as long as endemic goiter is a frequent feature in a population, patients are not worried about goiter growth until serious symptoms occur. By that time, initially well-differentiated TC may have change to anaplastic cancer. This phenomenon of late dedifferentiation has been shown in isolated cell lines of papillary TC, in animal studies, and in humans [44].

Environmental factors have an important influence on the development of thyroid cancer, that these factors act at a later stage in the carcinogenic process, and that these factors are changeable within a population. Nutritionally related factors are prime candidates for such exposures. Iodine is a trace element that is essential in the synthesis of thyroid hormones. Both chronic iodine deficiency and chronically high iodine intake have been associated with the development of goiter (*i.e.*, hypertrophy and hyperplasia of the thyroid cells) and attributed to excessive secretion of TSH3 by the pituitary. In turn, goiter has been associated with thyroid cancer risk, particularly in women. In general, chronic iodine deficiency and residence in an endemic goiter area are associated with an increased risk of the follicular histological type of thyroid cancer, whereas chronically high iodine intake may increase the risk of the more common papillary histological type of thyroid cancer. In most epidemiological studies, fish/shellfish consumption has been used as a proxy measure of iodine exposure. For the majority of women, sufficient levels of dietary iodine are associated with either no alteration in risk or reduced risk of papillary thyroid cancer, possibly because of the effects of chronically "sufficient" iodine levels in maintaining normal thyroid levels of thyroxine and TSH [45].

The variations of the histotype rate observed may be consequence of the silent increase of daily iodine intake throughout the subsequent years, while elevations of diagnostic standards (e.g., spread of thyroid scintigraphy, ultrasound, and fine-needle biopsy) available and increased experience of the medical staff have probably increased the number on thyroid ablations performed [46].

Role of other factors in thyroid cancer:

Geographic and ethnic variations in the incidence of thyroid cancer are considerable. Regions of high incidence include Hawaii, Iceland, Kuwait and New Zealand, and there are large differences between ethnic groups in some of these areas. Even in the Nordic countries, where standards of medical care, diagnostic practice, cancer registration and industrialization are closely similar, there is a 10-fold range in incidence of thyroid cancer. The highest overall rates are found in Iceland, with intermediate rates in Finland, Norway and Sweden, while the lowest rates are seen in Denmark. Denmark has one of the lowest thyroid cancer incidence rates in the world [43, 47]. Pronounced differences have been found for individuals who differ in ethnical origin. When interpreting these differences in thyroid rate, socioeconomic factors, differences in food intake, and local environmental influences must be accounted for [48].

Thyroid cancer in female and male (hormonal and reproductive factors):

Numerous investigations have shown that thyroid cancer in 2-4 times more frequent in females than in males. The incidence of thyroid cancer is approximately the same for males and females before puberty and after the female menopause. This suggests an effect of estrogen and/or other factors associated with pregnancy. Several investigations have thus shown a positive correlation between parity and incidence of thyroid cancer, the relative effect increasing with the number of pregnancies. The increase in risk is pronounced in childbearing in the latter half of the reproductive life. The risk is also increased after artificial menopause. The use of oral contraceptives or other exogenous estrogens dose not appears to increase the risk for thyroid cancer [48].

Genetic aspects:

Activating mutations of ras, loss of DNA from the Rb locus and over-expression of both c-met and bFGF are of no pathgenetic relevance in driving thyroid tumorigenesis of iodine-deficient areas [49]. Iodide deficiency predisposes DR1 individuals to thyroid cancer and that this risk is negated by iodide sufficiency unless some other risk factor supervenes [48, 50, 51].

Approximately 3%-5% of patients with thyroid cancer report a family history of the same disease. There are several rare familial syndromes that are associated with a high prevalence of thyroid cancer, in several cases associated with familial adenomatous polyposis.

Influence of body size:

Height, weight, and weight gain appear to be moderately associated with thyroid cancer [48].

Effect of lifestyle, occupation and environmental factors:

Dietary habits may affect the risk for thyroid cancer, which is increased in individuals with high consumption of starchy food, butter and cheese, or high fish consumption, fish-liver oil, and fish sandwich spread. This increase is not related to consumption of vegetables and fruit may have a protective effect. Recently, several reports have appeared indicating a protective effect of cigarette smoking. This effect which is most pronounced in current smokers and that appears to be dose-response related may be caused by the effect of smoking on estrogen metabolism or other factors.

Occupational exposure to low-level radiation such as found in working with diagnostic x-ray equipment constitutes an increased risk for thyroid cancer. Among other occupations associated with increased risk can be wood processing, pulp, and paper making, and work with probable exposure to silica.

The other risk factors for thyroid carcinoma development include exposure to environmental ionization radiation and history of preexisting benign thyroid disease [48, 52, 53].

CONCLUSION

Iodine is an essential constituent of the thyroid hormones thyroxin 3,5,3′,5′ tetraiodithyronine (T_4) and 3,5,3′ triiodithyronine (T_3). The major role of iodine in nutrition arises from the importance of thyroid hormones to growth and development.

Several features cause development of thyroid cancer, although the exact mechanism has not been elucidating until now. The increased prevalence of thyroid cancer associated with iodination programs has caused some concern. It should be realized, that although thyroid cancer is slightly less common in iodine-deficient areas, the cancers are less differentiated and more aggressive. It is, however, apparently important to supervise iodination programs, so that the population dose not receive excess iodine, which could cause an unnecessary increase in thyroid cancer.

The incidence of thyroid cancer is subject to ethnic and geographical variation. The highest incidence rates are reported in areas of high iodine intake; however, there is no general consensus on these findings. In fact, the overall incidence of differentiated thyroid carcinoma is not considered to be influenced by iodine intake in a population, whereas the distribution of the types of thyroid carcinoma seems to be related to the intake of iodine, with fewer of the more aggressive follicular and anaplastic carcinomas and more PTC being observed in iodine-rich areas. This could mean a poorer prognosis for thyroid carcinoma in regions with endemic goiter. Against expectation for an iodine-deficient area, where FTC is more common, some study findings did not reflect this and the distribution of tumors in that study was closer to what seen in iodine rich areas. This can be an argument against a possible association between iodine deficiency and increased risk of follicular carcinomas. It was interesting that during the years that some areas was an iodine deficient area the histologic distribution of thyroid cancer was more similar to iodine rich areas.

Epidemiologic studies show that other factors can affect the incidence of thyroid cancer to a small extent, but with largely unknown mechanisms. Individuals with disease known to be associated with thyroid cancer should be checked regularly.

REFERENCES

[1] Graeme A. Clugston, Basil S. Hetzel. Modern nutrition in health and disease: *Iodine.* 1994 (Eighth ed.) Lea & Febiger. p:252-263

[2] Venturi S. et al. Environmental Iodine Deficiency: A Challenge to the Evolution of Terrestrial Life? *Thyroid 2000.* Volume 10, Number 8 Page 727-729

[3] J. E. Dumont, F. Lamy, P. Roger, and C. Maenhaut. Physiological and Pathological Regulation of Thyroid Cell Proliferation and Differentiation by Thyrotropin and Other Factors. *Physiological Reviews 1992*, vol. 72, No. 3, page: 668-697

[4] Sebastiano Filetti, Jean-Michel Bidart, Franco Arturi, Bernard Caillou, Diego Russo and Martin Schlumberger. Sodium/iodide symporter: a key transport system in thyroid cancer cell metabolism. *European Journal of Endocrinology* 1999. 141**,** 443–457

[5] Fang, W., Qao, B., Wang, J. Iodine deficiency induces thyroid cancer in rats and mice. *Chinese Journal of Oncology 1994.* Volume 16, Issue 5, Pages 341-344

[6] S.Venturi, F.M. Donati, M.Venturi, A.Venturi, L.Grossi and A. Guidi. Role of Iodine in Evolution and Carcinogenesis of Thyroid, Breast and Stomach. *Advances in Clinical Pathology, 2000*, 4, 1 :11-17

[7] R. Francois Delange, MD and Basil Hetzel, MD. The Iodine Deficiency Disorders, Chapter 20. *Thyroid Disease Manager.* http://www.thyroidmanager.org/Chapter20/ 20-frame.htm

[8] Electron Kebebew, Orlo H. Clark. Differentiated Thyroid Cancer: "Complete" Rational Approach. *Word J. Surg. 2000.* 24, 942-951

[9] Mohagheghi M, Moosavi JA, Shariat TS, et al: Annual report of Tehran University of Medical Sciences District Cancer Registry at 1997.

[10] Bagher Larijani, Shahriar Aghakhani, Hossein Khajeh-Dini and Reza Baradar-Jalili: Clinico-pathological features of thyroid cancer as observed in 5 referral hospitals in Iran (review of 1177 cases). *Acta Oncologica 2003.* Vol. 42, No. 4, pp. 334-337

[11] Larijani B., Shirzad M., Mohagheghi MA., Haghpanah V., Moosavi J. AR., Tavangar SM., et al. Epidemiologic Analysis of the Tehran Cancer Institute data system registry (TCIDSR): Focus on Thyroid Cancer. *Asian Pacific J Cancer Prev,* 2004. 5, 36-39

[12] Mishra, A., Mishra, S.K., Agarwal, A. , Das, B.K. , Agarwal, G. , Gambhir, S. Metastatic differentiated thyroid carcinoma: Clinicopathological profile and outcome in an iodine deficient area. *World Journal of Surgery 2002.* Volume 26, Issue 2, Pages 153-157

[13] C Passler, C Scheuba, G Prager, K Kaczirek, K Kaserer, G Zettinig and B Niederle Prognostic factors of papillary and follicular thyroid cancer: differences in an iodine replete endemic goiter region. *Endocrine-Related Cancer 2004.* 11 131-139

[14] Mete Duren, Nihat Yavuz, Yusuf Bukey, etal. Impact of Initial Surgical Treatment on Survival of Patients with Differentiated Thyroid Cancer: Experience of an Endocrine Surgery Center in an Iodine-deficient Region. *World J. Surg. 24,* 1290–1294, 2000

[15] Fabio Levi, Lalao Randimbison, Van-Cong Te, and Carlo La Vecchia. Thyroid cancer in Vaud, Switzerland: An Update. *Thyroid 2002* vol. 12, No. 2 page 163-168

[16] John R. Burgess. Temporal Trends for Thyroid Carcinoma in Australia: An Increasing Incidence of Papillary Thyroid Carcinoma (1982-1997). *Thyroid 2002.* Vol. 12, Number 2 page 141-148

[17] Mark Sywak, Janicel L. Pasieka, Travis Ogilvie. A Review of Thyroid Cancer with Intermediate Differentiation. *Journal of Surgical Oncology 2004*; 86: 44-54

[18] John R. Burgess, Terrence Dwyer, Kathryn Mcardle, Paul Tucker, and Dace Shugg. The Changing Incidence and Spectrum of Thyroid Carcinoma in Tasmania (1978–1998) during a Transition from Iodine Sufficiency to Iodine Deficiency. *The Journal of Clinical Endocrinology & Metabolism 2000,* vol. 85 No 4 Page: 1513-1517

[19] Jenny E Gunton, Graham Hams, Marcelle Fiegert and Aidan McElduff. Iodine deficiency in ambulatory participants at a Sydney teaching hospital: is Australia truly iodine replete? *MJA* 1999; 171: 467-470

[20] Joseph G. Hollowell Norman W. Staehling, W. Harry Hannon, Dana W. Flanders, Elaine W. Gunter, Glen F. Maberly, Lewis E. Braverman, Sam Pino, Dayton T. Miller, Paul L. Garbe, David M. Delozier, and Richard J. Jackson. Iodine Nutrition in the United States. Trends and Public Health Implications: Iodine Excretion Data from National Health and Nutrition Examination Surveys I and III (1971–1974 and 1988–1994). *Journal of Clinical Endocrinology and Metabolism 1998.* vol. 83 No 10

[21] Venturi S, Grossi L, Marra GA, Venturi A, Venturi M. Iodine, Helicobacter Pylori, Stomach Cancer & Evolution. *European Epi-Marker. April 2003.* vol. 7, No. 2, page. 1-7

[22] P. Lind, G. Kumnig, M. Heinisch, et al. Iodine Supplementation in Austria: Methods and Results. *Thyroid 2002.* Vol. 12, No. 10, Page 903-907

[23] Azizi F. Salt iodization, monitoring and evaluation (SIME): an effective replacement for universal salt iodization (USI*). Int J Endocrinol Metab 2003*; 2: 46-47

[24] Parvin Mirmiran, Rambod Hajipour and Fereidoun Azizi. Iodized salt consumption maintains euthyroidism in iodine-deficient hypothyroid subjects. *Int. J Vitam Nutr. Res, 73* (3). 2003, 187-191

[25] Nahid Salarkia, Mehdi Hedayati, Parvin Miramira, Masood Kimiagar and Fereidoun Azizi. Evaluation of the impact of an iodine supplementation programme on severely iodine-deficient schoolchildren with hypothyroidism. *Public Health Nutrition: 2003* 6(6), 529-533

[26] Kimiagar M, Azizi F, Navai L, et al: Survey of iodine deficiency in a rural area near Tehran: association of food intake and endemic goiter. *Eur-J- Clin-Nutr. 1990*; 44(1): 17-22

[27] Azizi F, Kimiagar M, Nafarabadi M, et al: Current status of iodine deficiency in Islamic Republic of Iran. *Emr Health Survey*. 1990; 8: 23-27

[28] Weissel, M. Legal augmentation of iodine content in table salt from 10 to 20 mg Kl/kg: Documented effects a decade later. *Experimental and Clinical Endocrinology and Diabetes 2003.*Volume 111, Issue 4, June, Pages 187-190

[29] Mirmiran P , Hedayati M , Noohi S , Azizi F. The effect of iodized oil administration on the impaired hearing of iodine deficient schoolchildren. *Int J Endocrinol Metab 2003*; 2:61-66

[30] F. Azizi, M. Kimiagar, A.A. Ghazi, and M. Nafarbandi. The effects of iodized oil injection in eu-and hypothyroid iodine deficient girls. *J. Endocrinol. Invest. 1997*, 20: 18-23

[31] F. Azizi, M. Kimiagar, A. Ghazi, M. Nafarabadi, J. Behjati, F. Esfahanian. Treatment of goitrous hypothyroidism with iodized oil supplementation in an area of iodine deficiency. *Exp. Clin. Endocrinol. Diabetes 1996*. 104, 387-391

[32] N Bader, U. Moller, M. Leiterer et al. Pilot study: tendency of increasing iodine content in human milk and cow's milk. *Exp Clin Endocrinol Diabetes 2005*; 113: 8-12

[33] Szpak, S., Zeman, M., Handkiewicz-Junak, D., Kochańska-Dziurowicz, A. etal. Geographic differences in iodine supply in the Silesia terrain in relation to thyroid cancer risk. *Wiadomosci Lekarskie 2001*. Volume 54 Suppl 1, Pages 169-175

[34] Shefali Agrawal, Raja S. Rao, Deepak M. Parikh, et al. Histologic Trends in Thyroid Cancer 1969-1993: A Clinico-pathologic Analysis of the Relative Proportion of Anaplastic Carcinoma of the Thyroid. *J. Surgical Oncology 1996*. 63:251-255

[35] Harach HR, Escalante DA, Day ES. Thyroid cancer and thyroiditis in Salta, Argentina: a 40-yr study in relation to iodine prophylaxis. *Endocr Pathol. 2002* Fall;13(3):175-81

[36] Guan H, Teng W, Yang S. [Comparative epidemiological study on thyroid cancer in areas with different iodine intakes]. Zhonghua Yi Xue Za Zhi. 2001, 25;81(8):457-8

[37] Rolon PA. [Cancer of the thyroid in an area of endemic goiter. "Papillarization" with prophylactic iodization]. *Ann Pathol. 1986*;6(3):170-5

[38] Williams, E.D., Doniach, I., Bjarnason, O., Michie, W. Thyroid cancer in an iodide rich area. A histopathological study. *Cancer 1997*. Volume 39, Issue 1, Pages 215-222

[39] Kristensen, H.L., Vadstrup, S., Knudsen, N., Siersbaek-Nielsen, K. Development of hyperthyroidism in nodular goiter and thyroid malignancies in an area of relatively low iodine intake. *Journal of Endocrinological Investigation1995*. Volume 18, Issue 1, , Pages 41-43

[40] Franceschi, S. Iodine intake and thyroid carcinoma: A potential risk factor. *Experimental and Clinical Endocrinology and Diabetes 1998*. Volume 106, Issue SUPPL. 3, S38-S44

[41] Lind, P., Langsteger, W., Molnar, M., Gallowitsch, H.J., Mikosch, P., Gomez, I. Epidemiology of thyroid diseases in iodine sufficiency. *Thyroid 1998*. Volume 8, Issue 12, Pages 1179-1183

[42] Koutras, D.A. Control of efficiency and results, and adverse effects of excess iodine administration on thyroid function. *Annales d'Endocrinologie 1996*. Volume 57, Issue 6,Pages 463-469

[43] Bo Pettersson, Michel P. Coleman, Elaine Ron and Hans-Olov Adami. Iodine Supplementation in Sweden and Regional Trends in Thyroid Cancer Incidence by Histopathologic Type. *Int. J. Cancer 1996*.65, 13-19

[44] C. Bacher-stier, G. Riccabona, M. Totsch, et al. Incidence and clinical characteristics of thyroid carcinoma after iodine prophylaxis in an endemic goiter country. *Thyroid 1997*. vol. 7, No.5, page: 733-741

[45] Pamela L. Horn-Ross,2 J. Steven Morris, Marion Lee, Dee W. West, Alice S. Whittemore, I. Ross McDougall, Kent Nowels, Susan L. Stewart, Vickie L. Spate, Amy C. Shiau, and Melissa R. Krone. Iodine and Thyroid Cancer Risk among Women in a Multiethnic Population: The Bay Area Thyroid Cancer Study. *Cancer Epidemiology, Biomarkers & Prevention. September 2001*.Vol. 10, 979–985

[46] M. Deandrea, G. Gallone, M. Veglio, et al. Thyroid cancer histotype changes as observed in a major general hospital in a 21-year period. *J. Endocrino. Invest. 1997*. 20: 52 -58

[47] Tmirah Haselkorn, Susan L. Stewart, and Pamela L. Horn-Ross. Why are thyroid cancer rates so high in southeast asian women living in US? The Bay Area Thyroid Cancer Study. *Cancer Epidemiology, Biomarkers & Prevention 2003*. vol. 12, 144-150

[48] Shigenobu Nagataki and Ernst Nystrom. Epidemiology and primary prevention of thyroid cancer. *Thyroid 2002*. vol. 12, No. 10 page: 889-896

[49] L. Bartolone, F Vermiglio, M.D. Finocchiaro. et al. Thyroid follicular oncogenesis in iodine-deficient and iodine-sufficient areas: Search for alterations of the ras, met and bFGF oncogenes and of the rb anti-oncogene. *J Endocrinol Invest. 1998* Nov;21(10):680-7

[50] Larsen B, Thompson C, Kwan A, Farid NR. Lack of association of HLA with thyroid cancer. An effect of iodine sufficiency and safe environment? *Tissue Antigens. 1986* Nov; 28(5):298-300

[51] MR Galanti, A Ekbom, L Grimelius and J Yuen. Parental cancer and risk of papillary and follicular thyroid carcinoma. *British Journal of Cancer 1997*, 75(3), 451-456

[52] Nikiforov, Y.E., Fagin, J.A. Risk factors for thyroid cancer. *Trends in Endocrinology and Metabolism. January 1997*. vol. 8, Issue 1, Pages 20-25

[53] Galanti MR, Hansson L, Bergstrom R, Wolk A, Hjartaker A, Lund E, Grimelius L, Ekbom A. Diet and the risk of papillary and follicular thyroid carcinoma: a population-based case-control study in Sweden and Norway. *Cancer Causes Control 1997*. 8(2),:205-14

In: Trends in Thyroid Cancer Research
Editor: Carl A. Milton, pp. 89-116

ISBN 1-59454-627-4

Chapter V

HUMAN EPIDERMAL GROWTH FACTOR RECEPTOR 1 AND THROMBOSPONDIN-1 IN THYROID CANCER

Junichi Kurebayashi, Katsuhiro Tanaka, Yutaka Yamamoto, Sumiko Okubo and Hiroshi Sonoo

Department of Breast & Thyroid Surgery, Kawasaki Medical School, Japan.

ABSTRACT

Although prognosis of patients with differentiated thyroid cancer is generally favorable, undifferentiated/anaplastic thyroid cancer is one of the most aggressive malignancies. The remarkable difference in prognosis between two types of thyroid cancer indicates that there is a large biological difference between them. We have been involved in the studies for exploring new biomarkers to evaluate aggressiveness of thyroid cancer. These markers are useful not only for predicting prognosis but also for developing new strategies against aggressive thyroid cancer.

We recently established three different thyroid cancer cell lines, KTC-1, KTC-2 and KTC-3. KTC-1 cells are derived from a patient with poorly differentiated thyroid papillary carcinoma. KTC-2 cells are derived from a patient with anaplastic transformation from papillary thyroid carcinoma. KTC-3 cells are derived from a patient with primary anaplastic thyroid carcinoma.

To test the hypothesis that overexpression of human epidermal growth factor receptor (HER) 1 promotes malignant progression in thyroid cancer, the relationship among expression levels of HER1 and a cognate receptor HER2 and effects of a HER1 tyrosine kinase inhibitor, gefitinib on cell proliferation, cytokine secretion and the expression level of one of thyroid differentiation markers, thyroglobulin were investigated using these three cell lines. Gefitinib inhibited *in vitro* growth of the thyroid cancer cells in dose- and time-dependent manners. No significant correlation was observed between the antitumor effect of gefitinib and expression level of HER1 or HER2. Gefitinib significantly decreased secretion of angiogenic cytokines, vascular endothelial growth factor (VEGF) and interleukin (IL)-8 in KTC-2 cells. In contrast, gefitinib significantly increased secretion of both angiogenic cytokines in KTC-3 cells. Changes in secretion of

IL-6 and parathyroid hormone-related protein (PTHrP) induced by gefitinib were also different among thyroid cancer cell lines. Gefitinib did not significantly change the expression level of thyroglobulin in any thyroid cancer cell lines. These findings suggest that gefitinib is effective for the treatment of aggressive thyroid cancer but its influences on cytokine secretion from tumor cells are different among thyroid cancers.
Thrombospondin (TSP)-1 has been identified as an anti-angiogenic factor. We recently demonstrated that TSP-1 expression negatively related to extrathyroidal infiltration as well as angiogenesis in patients with papillary thyroid carcinoma. To elucidate the relationship between expression levels of p53 and TSP-1 in thyroid cancer, we studied their expression levels in 75 papillary thyroid carcinomas. There was an inverse correlation between expression levels of TSP-1 and p53. Additionally, the effects of TSP-1 and anti-TSP-1 antibody on invasion were investigated in six thyroid cancer cell lines using the *in vitro* invasion assay. Angiogenesis-related factors, VEGF, VEGF-C, TSP-1 and TSP-1 receptor (CD36) were expressed at various levels in all cell lines. Invasion tended to be inhibited by TSP-1 in five of the six cell lines. These effects inversely related to the expression level of VEGF or VEGF-C. The effects of anti-TSP-1 antibody on invasion differed among cell lines. These findings indicate that TSP-1 plays a certain role in invasion of thyroid cancer cells, and that the effects of TSP-1 and anti-TSP-1 antibody on invasion are different among thyroid cancers.

Part 1: Epidermal Growth Factor Receptor (EGFR)/HER1 in Thyroid Cancer

Introduction

Epidermal growth factor receptor (EGFR)/HER1 is a member of the human EGFR (HER) family of transmembrane tyrosine kinases. Binding of specific ligands, such as EGF, transforming growth factor-α, heparin binding EGF-like growth factor or betacellulin, to the extracellular domain of HER1 results in homodimerization or heterodimerization with another member of the HER family, such as HER2, HER3 or HER4. This dimerization induces autophosphorylation of tyrosine residues of the intracellular domain of HER1, which activates intracellular signaling cascades, such as the mitogen-activated protein kinase (MAPK), phosphatidylinositol-3-OH-kinase (PI3K), MAPK-independent S6 kinase and phospholipase C-γ signaling pathways. These interactions modulate essential cellular functions, such as cell proliferation, survival, apoptosis, differentiation and migration [1].

Aberrant HER1 signaling, such as overexpression or constitutive activation of HER1, is associated with enhanced tumor cell proliferation, high metastatic potential and poor prognosis in patients with solid malignancies [2]. Preclinical and clinical studies have indicated that overexpression of HER1 relates to aggressive biological characteristics of thyroid cancer, such as high proliferation rate and high invasive potential, and poor clinical outcome in patients with thyroid cancer [3-9].

Recently, molecular targeting agents, such as gefitinib, which targets HER1 signaling pathway, and imatinib, which targets BCR-ABL, c-KIT or platelet-derived growth factor receptor signaling pathway, have been introduced into clinics for the treatment of various malignancies, such as non-small cell lung cancer [10], chromic myeloid leukemia [11] and gastro-intestinal stromal tumors [12]. These agents are safer than conventional anticancer agents and very potent in a part of patients in whom various conventional anticancer agents are ineffective.

Prognosis of patients with well-differentiated thyroid cancer is generally favorable. Actually, appropriate surgical resection of primary tumors and TSH-suppression therapy provide patients with over 90% of 10-year overall survival rate in our institute. In contrast, outcome of patients with primary anaplastic thyroid cancer or anaplastic transformation from well-differentiated thyroid cancer is miserable. A median survival time of these patients from diagnosis is only four months in our institute. Although multidisciplinary treatment modality with surgery, radiation and cytotoxic chemotherapy have been attempted to improve the outcome of these patients, only a small number of patients can survive for over one year. New therapeutic strategies are seriously desired for these patients.

These findings prompted us to investigate antitumor activity of gefitinib, which is one of molecular targeting agents and specifically inhibits HER1 tyrosine kinase activity, in poorly differentiated or undifferentiated thyroid cancer cells. It has been known that these cancer cells secrete several cytokines, such as parathyroid hormone-related protein (PTHrP) [13,14], interleukin (IL)-6 [14,15-19], IL-8 [15,16], vascular endothelial growth factor (VEGF), and that these cytokines induce paraneoplastic syndromes, such as hypercalcemia and cachexia, as well as stimulate tumor angiogenesis. Therefore, the influences of gefitinib on cytokine expression and secretion were also investigated in this study.

Materials and Methods

Thyroid Cancer Cell Lines

We recently established three different thyroid cancer cell lines, KTC-1, KTC-2 and KTC-3 and used them in this study. KTC-1 cells are derived from a patient with poorly differentiated thyroid papillary carcinoma. KTC-2 cells are derived from a patient with anaplastic transformation from thyroid papillary carcinoma. Characteristics of KTC-1 and KTC-2 cell lines were published elsewhere, respectively [14,19].

KTC-3 cells are derived from the malignant pleural effusion of a 76 year-old female patient with anaplastic thyroid cancer. Histological examination revealed that she had primary anaplastic thyroid carcinoma in June 2001. Radiotherapy and chemotherapy with etoposide and carboplatin were given. Massive left pleural effusion appeared in December, 2001. Thoracic drainage was performed to remove the pleural effusion. Cytological analysis showed atypical epithelial cells. Approximately 50 ml of the heparinized effusion was collected for cell culture followed by obtaining informed consent from the patient. After centrifugation, the cell pellet was resuspended with RPMI 1640 medium supplemented with 5% fetal bovine serum (FBS) and cultured. Atypical epithelial cells rapidly grew in a monolayer fashion and have been passed at 1:10 split once or twice a week more than 100 times for over two years. Regrettably, this patient died of cancer in February 2002.

Summarized characteristics of the three thyroid cancer cell lines are shown in Table 1.

Table 1. Characteristics of three thryoid cancer cell lines tested in this study.

	KTC-1	KTC-2	KTC-3
Patient	68 y.o., male	70 y.o., female	76 y.o., female
Histological diagnosis	poorly differentiated papillary cancer	anaplastic cancer	anaplastic cacer
Origin	pleural effusion	pleural effusion	pleural effusion
Passage	over 70	over 80	over 100
In vitro growth	monolayer	monolayer	monolayer
Morphology	cobble stone-like, small in size	cobble stone-like, large in size	cobble stone-like, large/giant in size
Doubling time	48 h	36 h	24 h
Karyotype	46, XY	102-124 (median 109)	140-151 (median 146)
In vivo growth			
tumorigenicity	yes	yes	yes
tumor growth	very slow	regressing	very fast
Differentiation marker			
Tg (mRNA)	weak	weak	weak
Tg (IHC)	weak	weak	negative
Cytokine secretion			
IL-6	small amount	large amount	large amount
PTHrP	small amount	large amount	large amount
IL-8	large amount	small amount	very large amount
VEGF-A	small amount	large amount	very large amount
HER family expression			
HER1	yes	yes	high
HER2	yes	high	high

Cell Culture

Gefitinib was kindly provided by AstraZeneca (Macclesfield, UK) and dissolved with DMSO and added to the medium at a final concentration of 0.1%.

To investigate the effects of gefitinib on the cell growth and secretion of cytokines, thyroid cancer cells (2 X 10^5 cells per well) were seeded in 12-well plates (SB Medical, Tokyo, Japan) and grown in RPMI 1640 medium supplemented with 5% FBS at 37°C in a 5% CO_2-atmosphere for 2 days. After washing with phosphate-buffered saline (PBS), the cells were incubated with phenol red-free RPMI 1640 supplemented with 2% dextran-coated charcoal (DCC)-stripped FBS plus 1 – 20 μM of gefitinib for 2 or 3 days to reduce the influences of impurities in phenol red and unknown factors in FBS on the activity of gefitinib. After the incubation, the culture medium was collected and stored at –80°C until use, and the cells were enumerated with the Coulter counter (Coulter Electronics, Harpenden, UK).

To investigate the effects of gefitinib on mRNA expression levels of cytokines, after washing once with PBS, semi-confluent cells in 6-well plates (SB Medical) were incubated with phenol red-free RPMI 1640 supplemented with 2% DCC-stripped FBS plus 10μM of gefitinib for 1 or 2 days. After the incubation, the cells were collected and stored at –80℃ until use.

Expression of HER1 and HER2

Protein expression levels of HER1 and HER2 were measured by Western blotting using anti-HER1 goat polyclonal antibody (Santa Cruz Biotechnology, Santa Cruz, CA, USA) and anti-HER2 mouse monoclonal antibody (Santa Cruz Biotechnology), respectively [20].

Harvested cells were washed once with cold PBS and lysed by 200 μl per well of cold RIPA buffer (50 mM Tris-HCl [pH7.4], 150 mM NaCl, 1% Nonidet P-40, 1% deoxycholic acid sodium, 0.05% SDS) plus 4 μl per well of protease inhibitor (Sigma Chemical Co., St. Louis, MI, USA). The cell lysate was clarified by centrifugation at 14,000 x g at 4℃ for 10 min. Twenty to 30 μg of protein was heated in Laemmli gel loading buffer for 5 min at 95°C and subjected to electrophoresis on 12.5% polyacrylamide gel (Bio-Rad, Richmond, CA, USA). The protein was transferred to nitrocellulose membranes (Amersham Life Sciences, Buckinghamshire, UK) and immunoblotted with appropriate primary antibodies. For detection, the blots were incubated with the appropriate secondary antibodies conjugated with horseradish peroxidase (Santa Cruz Biotechnology), and developed using ECL Plus Western Blotting Detection Reagents (Amersham Life Sciences), according to the instructions of the manufacturer. Anti-actin monoclonal antibody as internal control was obtained from Santa Cruz Biotechnology. Reproducibility was confirmed in at least two separate experiments.

Expression and Secretion of Cytokines

IL-6 and IL-8 were measured with a Quantikine HS immunoassay kit (R & D SYSTEMS, Minneapolis, MN; sensitivity, 0.16 pg/ml and 2.0 pg/ml, respectively). PTHrP was measured with an immunoradiometric assay kit (Mitsubishi-yuka Co., Tokyo, Japan; sensitivity, 1.0 pM). VEGF was measured with an enzyme-linked immunosorbent assay kit (Otsuka Assay Laboratory, Tokushima, Japan; sensitivity, 0.2 pg/ml). Secretion of each factor per cell was calculated as the product of each concentration X volume of medium divided by mean cell number [14,19].

Expression levels of these cytokines were measured by the multiplex reverse transcription-polymerase chain reaction (RT-PCR) as described previously [14,19]. Oligonucleotide primers were designed using a published sequence of each target gene (Table 2) and synthesized by the solid-phase triester method. To amplify both the internal control gene (β -actin) and one of the target genes in a single reaction, multiplex PCR was carried out. The relative expression levels were calculated as the density of the product of the respective target genes divided by that of the control gene.

Expression of Thyroglobulin

Thyroglobulin was measured with an immunoradiometric assay kit (Sanofi Pharmaceuticals, Inc., Diagnostic Pasteur, Marnes La Conquette, France; sensitivity, 1.5

ng/ml). The mRNA expression level of thyroglobulin was also measured by the multiplex RT-PCR as described above.

Table 2. Oligonucleotide primers and conditions for multiplex RT-PCR.

Target genes	Primer sequences		Annealing	Primer ratio	No. of PCR	Expected
	Forward	Reverse	temperature (℃)		cycles[a]	size (bp)
VEGF	5'-gcagaatcatcacgaagtgg-3'	5'-gcatggtgatgttggactcc-3'	58	2:01	38	212
IL-6	5'-gaactccttctccacaagcg-3'	5'-gaatccagattggaagcatcc-3'	58	2:0.2	40	316
Thyroglobulin	5'-ggctaatgctacatgtcctg-3'	5'-gcttctgttggagatgctgg-3'	57	2:1	35	231
β-actin	5'-tgacggggtcacccaca ctgtgcccatcta-3'	5'-ctagaagcatttgcggtggac gatggaggg-3'	NA[b]	NA	NA	661

[a]Numbers of cycles were determined to amplify both products logarithmically and in relatively similar amounts. [b]Not assessible.

Results

Expression Levels of HER1 and HER2 in Thyroid Cancer Cell Lines

Protein expression levels of both HER1 and HER2 in thyroid cancer cell lines tested were relatively high in comparison with those in breast cancer cell lines (data not shown). Relative expression levels of either HER1 or HER2 were KTC-3 > KTC-2 > KTC-1 (Fig. 1).

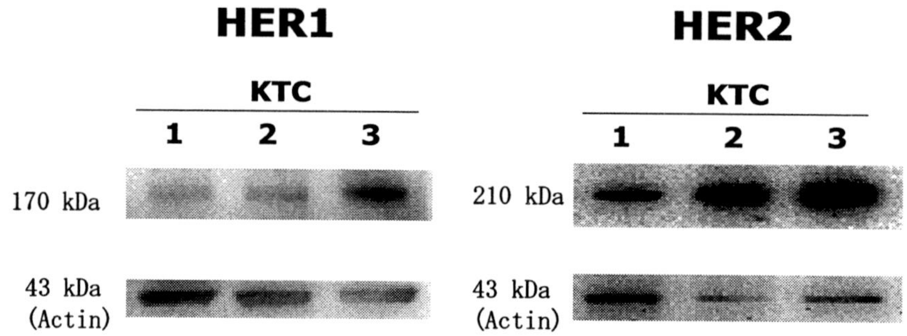

Figure 1. Expression levels of HER1 and HER 2 in three thyroid cancer cell lines by the Western blotting.

Antitumor Effect of Gefitinib on Thyroid Cancer Cell Lines

Gefitinib (1 – 20 μM) dose-dependently inhibited the *in vitro* growth of three thyroid cancer cell lines. The 50%-growth inhibition concentrations (IC_{50}) of gefitinib (2-day-treatment) were 10 μM for KTC-1 cells, 9 μM for KTC-2 cells and 17 μM for KTC-3 cells (Fig. 2). They did not correlate with the relative expression levels of HER1. In addition, gefitinib (10μM) time-dependently inhibited the *in vitro* growth of three thyroid cancer cell lines (Fig. 3).

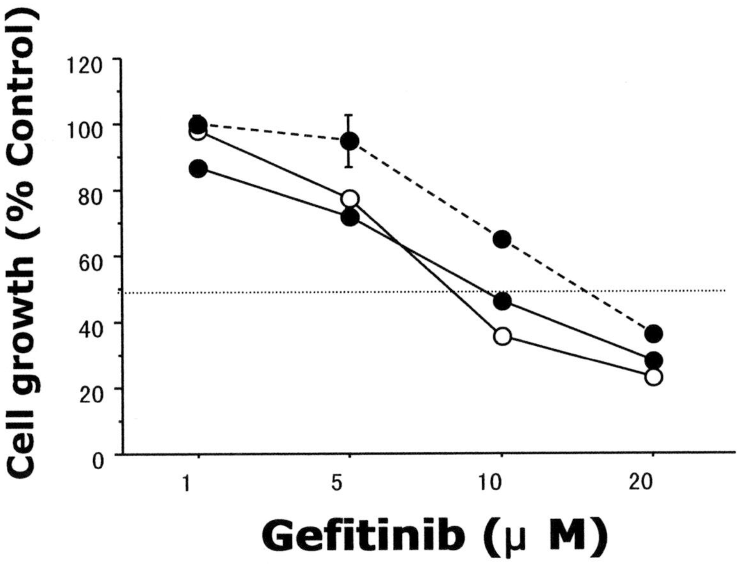

Figure 2. Dose-dependent growth inhibition by gefitinib (1 - 20 μM for 48 hours) on three thyroid cancer cell lines. ●——●, KTC-1; ○——○, KTC-2; ●-----●, KTC-3.

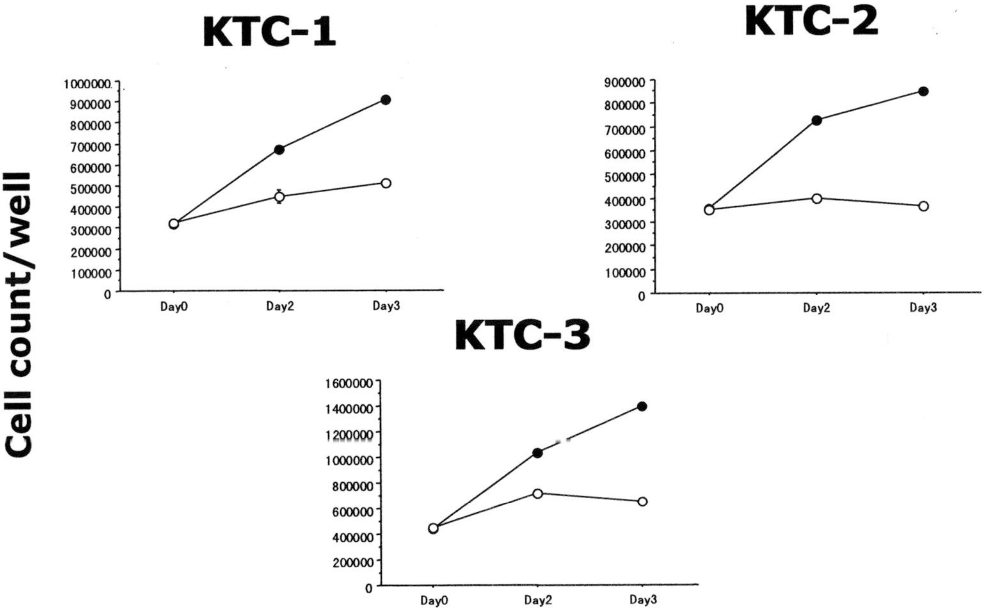

Figure 3. Time-dependent growth inhibition by gefitinib (10 μM for 2 or 3 days) on three thyroid cancer cell lines. ●——●, control; ○——○, gefitinib-treated.

Effects of Gefitnib on Expression and Secretion of Cytokines

All thyroid cancer cell lines tested secreted a large amount of one of angiogenic factors, VEGF into culture medium. Low doses of gefitinib (0.1 μM) did not significantly change VEGF secretion from any cell lines. However, a moderate or high dose of gefitinib (1 or 10 μM) significantly decreased VEGF secretion from KTC-1 and KTC-2 cells but a high dose of gefitinib (10μM) significantly increased VEGF secretion from KTC-3 cells (Fig. 4).

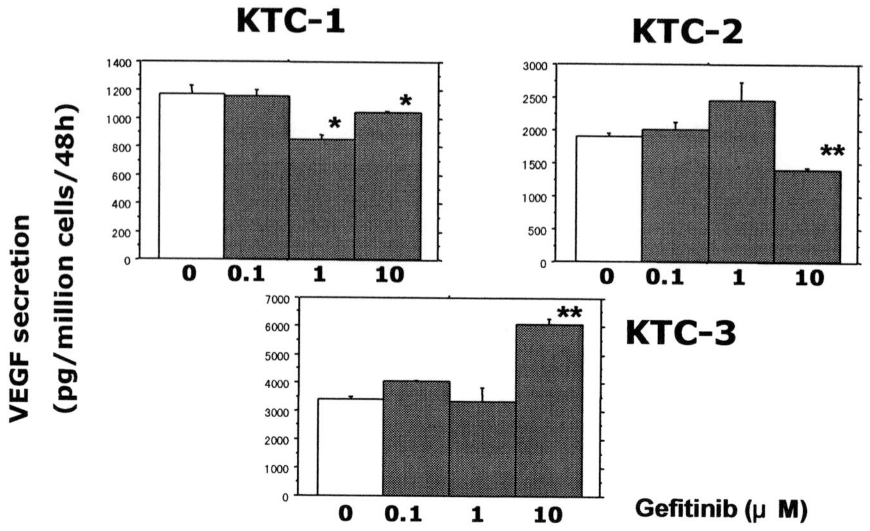

Figure 4. Effects of gefitinib (0.1 to 10 μM for 48 hours) on VEGF secretion from three thyroid cancer cell lines. Secretion was calculated as described in Materials and Methods. *, $P < 0.05$; **, $P < 0.01$.

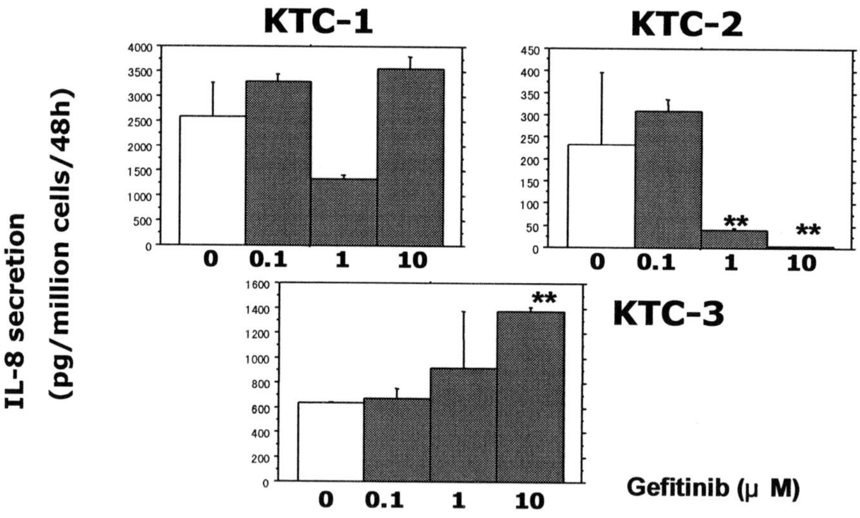

Figure 5. Effects of gefitinib (0.1 to 10 μM for 48 hours) on IL-8 secretion from three thyroid cancer cell lines. Secretion was calculated as described in Materials and Methods. **, $P < 0.01$.

Thyroid cancer cell lines tested secreted a various amount of one of angiogenic factors, IL-8 into culture medium. KTC-1 cells secreted a largest amount of IL-8, and gefitinib did not significantly change IL-8 secretion from KTC-1 cells. KTC-2 cells secreted a smallest amount of IL-8, and gefitnib (1 or 10 μM) significantly decreased IL-8 secretion from KTC-2 cells. KTC-3 cells secreted a moderate amount of IL-8, and gefitinib (10 μM) significantly increased IL-8 secretion from KTC-3 cells (Fig. 5).

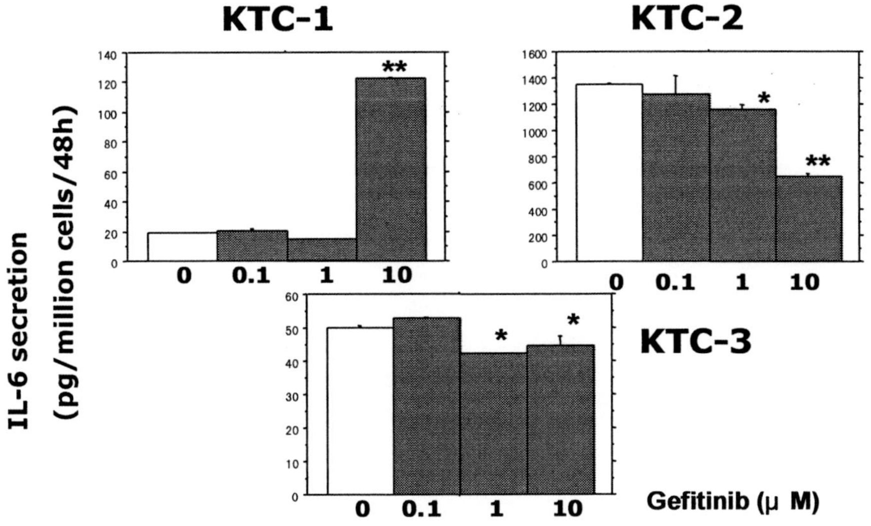

Figure 6. Effects of gefitinib (0.1 to 10 μM for 48 hours) on IL-6 secretion from three thyroid cancer cell lines. Secretion was calculated as described in Materials and Methods. *, $P < 0.05$; **, $P < 0.01$.

Thyroid cancer cell lines tested secreted a various amount of one of cachectic factors, IL-6 into culture medium. KTC-2 cells secreted a largest amount of IL-6, and gefitinib (1 or 10 μM) significantly decreased IL-6 secretion from KTC-2 cells. KTC-1 cells secreted a small amount of IL-6, and gefitinib (10 μM) significantly increased IL-6 secretion from KTC-1 cells. KTC-3 cells secreted a moderate amount of IL-6, and gefitinib (1 or 10μM) significantly decreased IL-6 secretion from KTC-3 cells (Fig. 6).

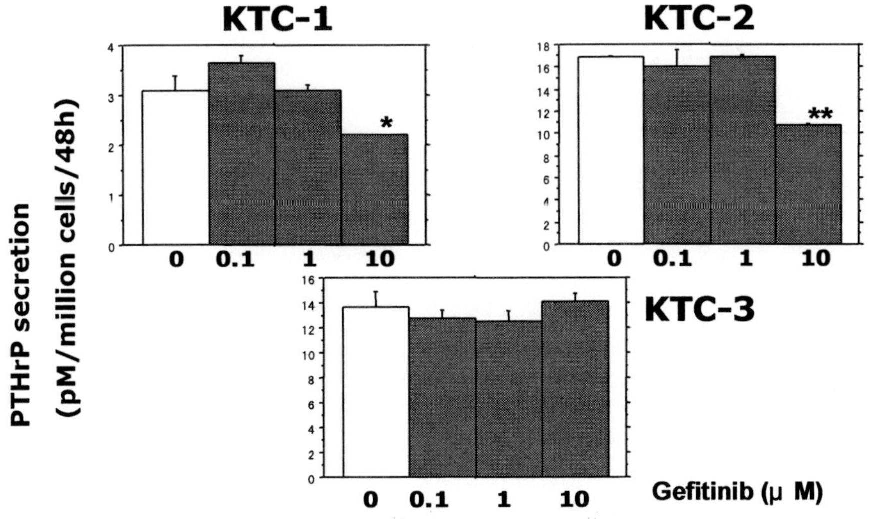

Figure 7. Effects of gefitinib (0.1 to 10 μM for 48 hours) on PTHrP secretion from three thyroid cancer cell lines. Secretion was calculated as described in Materials and Methods. *, $P < 0.05$; **, $P < 0.01$.

Thyroid cancer cell lines tested secreted a various amount of one of hypercalcemic factors, PTHrP into culture medium. Low doses of gefitinib (0.1 or 1 μM) did not significantly change PTHrP secretion from any cell lines. However, a higher dose of gefitinib (10 μM) significantly decreased PTHrP secretion from KTC-1 and KTC-2 cells but did not significantly change PTHrP secretion from KTC-3 cells (Fig. 7).

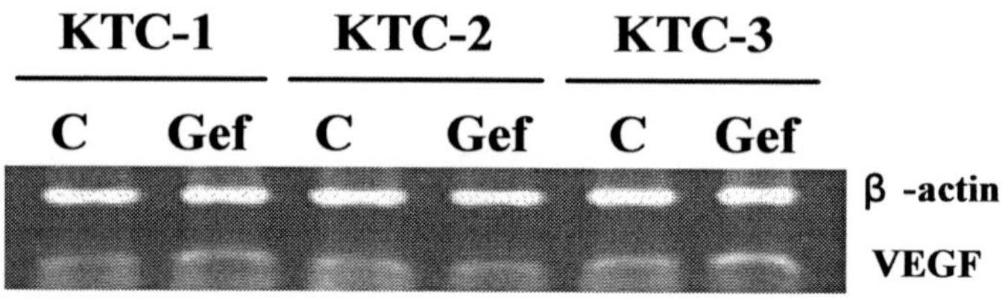

Figure 8. Effects of gefitinib (10 μM for 48 hours) on VEGF mRNA expression in three thyroid cancer cell lines by multiplex RT-PCR. C, control; Gef, gefitinib.

To investigate the effects of gefitinib on mRNA expression levels of two cytokines, VEGF and IL-6 in thyroid cancer cell lines, the semi-quantitative multiplex RT-PCR was applied. Treatments with gefitnib (10 μM) for 48 hours decreased the mRNA expression level of VEGF in KTC-2 cells and increased it in KTC-3 cells (Fig. 8). These findings coincided with the changes in VEGF secretion from KTC-2 and KTC-3 cells, respectively. Treatments with gefitnib (10 μM) for 24 or 48 hours increased the mRNA expression level of IL-6 in KTC-1 cells (Fig. 9). These findings coincided with the changes in IL-6 secretion from KTC-1 cells.

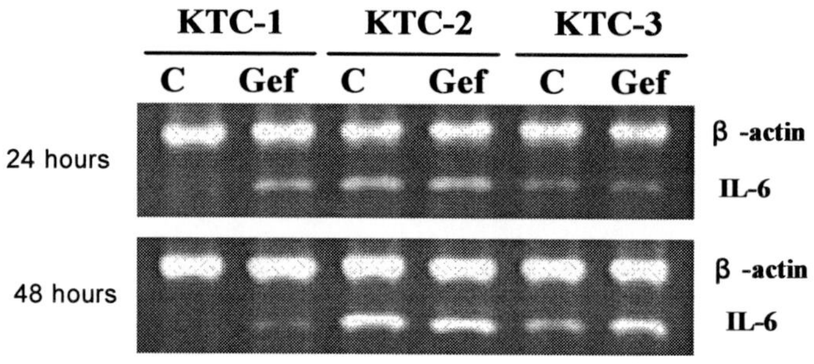

Figure 9. Effects of gefitinib (10 μM for 24 or 48 hours) on IL-6 mRNA expression in three thyroid cancer cell lines by multiplex RT-PCR. C, control; Gef, gefitinib.

Effects of Gefitnib on Secretion and Expression of Thyroglobulin

To clarify whether gefitnib induces differentiation of thyroid cancer cells, secretion and expression of one of thyroid differentiation markers, thyroglobulin were investigated. Thyroglobulin in culture medium was undetectable in all cell lines tested, regardless of gefitinib treatment or not. In contrast, the mRNA expression of thyroglobulin was detectable at various levels in all cell lines tested. No significant change in the expression level of thyroglobulin was observed after gefitinib treatment (10 μM) for 48 hours in any cell lines (Fig. 10).

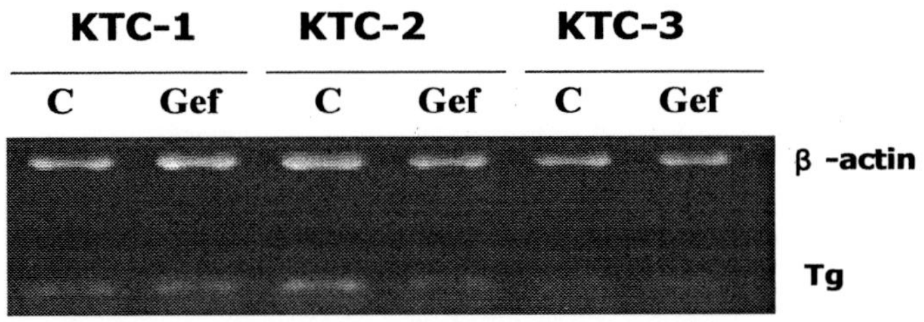

Figure 10. Effects of gefitinib (10 μM for 48 hours) on thyroglobulin (Tg) mRNA expression in three thyroid cancer cell lines by multiplex RT-PCR. C, control; Gef, gefitinib.

Conclusion

HER1 Expression in Thyroid Cancer

Both HER1 and HER2 were highly expressed in all three thyroid cancer cell lines tested in this study. All cell lines are derived from patients with poorly differentiated or anaplastic thyroid cancer associated with distant metastases [14,19]. It seems that all three cell lines are categorized as aggressive types of thyroid cancer, and that they express a high level of both HER1 and HER2.

It has been reported that HER1, although expressed higher levels in anaplastic and differentiated thyroid cancers than normal thyroid tissue, is present in all of the thyroid tissues, but the data in different studies vary widely. In addition, Bergstrom et al. reported that HER1 was highly expressed in all six anaplastic thyroid cancer cell lines tested in their study [6]. Schiff et al. have recently reported that HER1 expression is higher in anaplastic thyroid cancer than differentiated papillary thyroid cancer or normal thyroid tissue [9]. These findings suggest that HER1 expression is increasing associated with malignant progression in thyroid cancer.

Gefitinib and Thyroid Cancer Therapy

During the preparation of this article, Schiff et al. has reported for the first time that a HER1 tyrosine kinase inhibitor, gefitinib, inhibits the growth of anaplastic thyroid cancer [9]. They used six anaplastic thyroid cancer cell lines and revealed that five out of six cell lines express a high level of HER1. The IC_{50} of gefitinib was reported to be 6 μM in one of the cell lines expressing HER1, KAT-4. A modest antitumor effect of gefitinib was also observed in the KAT-4 xenograft model.

In this study, we found that the IC_{50} of gefitinib ranged from 9 to 17μM in three different thyroid cancer cell lines. According to phase I trial of gefitinib, a mean steady-state trough plasma concentration was 1.1 to 1.4 μM for daily oral administration of 400 to 600 mg of gefitinib [21]. The IC_{50}s of gefitinib in Schiff's study and ours are 5-10 times higher than the steady-state plasma concentrations in men. However, it should be noted that the IC_{50}s of gefitinib significantly depend on the duration of drug exposure (Fig. 3), types of culture medium and analyzing system of cell growth. Actually, we used two-day-exposure of gefitinib in this study and Schiff et al. used three-day-exposure. Our preliminary study has shown that the lowest IC_{50} of gefitinib is 2.5 μM in four-day-exposure system using same three cell lines (data not shown).

Action Mechanisms of Gefitinib

Recently, it has been recognized that certain somatic mutations in the HER1 gene play an important role in responsiveness of lung cancer to gefitinib [22,23]. To the best of our knowledge, except for lung cancer there is only one colorectal cancer reported to harbor such a mutation in the HER1 gene [24]. Schiff et al. has reported that their analysis of exons 18, 19, and 21 of the HER1 gene showed no mutations in six anaplastic thyroid cancer cell lines tested [9]. We have not yet done mutation analysis of the HER1 gene in the three thyroid cancer cell lines. It has been reported that lung cancer cells harboring such somatic mutations were very sensitive to gefitinib, and that their IC_{50}s of gefitinib were under 0.1μM [23]. Therefore, it is likely that three thyroid cancer cell lines tested in this study do not harbor such somatic mutations in the HER1 gene.

Experimental studies have suggested that gefitinib is effective not only in cancer cells overexpressing HER1 but also in cancer cells overexpressing HER2 [25]. It has been known that ligand-activated HER1 preferentially binds to HER2, leads to heterodimerization and activates intracellular signaling pathways [1]. Gefitinib has been reported to effectively inhibit HER2 phosphorylation *in vivo* [25]. Therefore, it might be possible that cancer cells expressing both HER1 and HER2 are more likely to respond to gefitinib. Very recently, Amann et al. have suggested that in addition to HER1 mutations, other factors, such as high expression of HER family members, may constitutively activate AKT and sensitize cells to HER1 inhibitors [26]. In this study, relative expression levels of either HER1 or HER2 were KTC-3 > KTC-2 > KTC-1 and the IC_{50}s of gefitinib were KTC-3 > KTC-1 > KTC-2. It could be concluded that the expression levels of HER1 and/or HER2 did not relate to sensitivity to gefitinib in this study (Figs. 1 and 2). However, since it is hard to quantitatively analyze data obtained from the Western blotting, this relation is not definitive.

Cytokine Secretion and Paraneoplastic Syndrome in Thyroid Cancer

Anaplastic cancer or anaplastic transformation from differentiated thyroid cancer sometimes causes a variety of paraneoplastic syndromes such as cachexia, hypercalcemia and leucocytosis. These syndromes significantly worsen the quality of life of patients with advanced thyroid cancer. In the last two decades, action mechanisms responsible for these syndromes have been elucidated. It has been reported that various cytokines secreted by anaplastic thyroid cancer cells induce these syndromes. IL-6, PTHrP, IL-8 and others are responsible for cachexia [27]. PTHrP, IL-6 and others are responsible for humoral hypercalcemia [28]. Granulocyte growth stimulating factor (CSF), macrophage CSF and granulocyte-macrophage CSF are responsible for leucocytosis [14,16,17]. If production and secretion of these cytokines from anaplastic cancer cells are decreased by certain agents, troublesome paraneoplastic syndromes are controllable.

Our previous studies have revealed that a progestin, medroxyprogesterone acetate (MPA) and a glucocorticoid, dexamethasone, significantly decreased the expression and secretion of IL-6 and PTHrP mediated through glucocorticoid receptors in an anaplastic thyroid cancer cell line, KTC-2 [14]. It has been known that glucocorticoid ameliorate hypercalcemia and cachexia in clinics. Since glucocorticoid sometimes causes serious adverse effects, MPA may be an attractive alternate to glucocorticoid in patients with paraneoplastic syndromes.

Effects of Gefitinib on Cytokine Expression in Thyroid Cancer Cells

To test a hypothesis that inhibition of HER1 signaling pathway modifies cytokine secretion from thyroid cancer cells, effects of gefitinib on expression and secretion of four cytokines, VEGF, IL-8, IL-6 and PTHrP from three different thyroid cancer cells were systematically investigated in this study.

Hirata et al. reported that gefitinib decreased the expression level of angiogenic cytokines such as VEGF and IL-8 up-regulated by EGF in an *in vitro* model using squamous or epidermoid cancer cells [29]. In contrast, gefitinib decreased both VEGF and IL-8 secretion in KTC-1 and KTC-2 cells but increased them in KTC-3 cells in this study (Figs. 4 and 5). In addition, the RT-PCR analysis revealed that gefitinib decreased VEGF mRNA expression in KTC-2 cells but increased it in KTC-3 cells (Fig. 8). Differences in types of cancer cells and experimental conditions may explain discordant results between Hirata's study and ours. In the other words, the effect of gefitinib on expression levels of angiogenic factors may differ among various types of cancer cells.

To the best of our knowledge, there is no published data on the effect of gefitnib on IL-6 and PTHrP secretion from cancer cells. In this study, gefitinib differentially modified IL-6 secretion among three thyroid cancer cell lines. A high dose of gefitinib (10μM) drastically increased IL-6 secretion from KTC-1 cells. In contrast, gefitinib significantly decreased IL-6 secretion from KTC-2 and KTC-3 cells (Fig. 6). PTHrP secretion was significantly decreased by gefitinib in KTC-1 and KTC-2 cells but not in KTC-3 cells (Fig. 7). Both IL-6 and PTHrP are recognized as cachectic and hypercalcemic factors. Decrease in their secretion by gefitinib may improve paraneoplastic syndromes, cachexia and hypercalcemia. Since the effects of gefitinib on IL-6 and PTHrP secretion from three thyroid cancer cell lines tested were heterogeneous, it is hard to speculate clinical implication of these experimental results.

Effects of Gefitinib on Thyroglobulin Expression in Thyroid Cancer Cells

Since HER1 signaling pathway plays important roles not only in cell growth and survival but also in cell differentiation, effects of gefitinib on one of thyroid differentiation markers, thyroglobulin were investigated in this study. All three thyroid cancer cell lines tested were poorly or anaplastic types and expressed a very low level of thyroglobulin. No significant change in thyroglobulin mRNA expression was observed after treatment with gefitinib for 48 hours in any cell lines. A longer exposure of gefitinib might influence expression levels of thyroid differentiation makers in thyroid cancer cells.

PART 2: THE EXPRESSION AND ROLE OF THROMBOSPONDIN-1 (TSP-1) IN THYROID CANCER

Introduction

Angiogenesis is essential for tumor progression. Folkman et al. have reported that a tumor requires angiogenesis when grows larger than 2 mm in diameter [30]. Many angiogenic factors have been identified as follows: VEGF [31], basic fibroblast growth factor (bFGF) [32], angiopoietin-2 [33], angiogenin, [34], platelet-derived growth factor [35], proliferin [36], endothelin [37], transforming growth factor (TGF) - α, –β [38,39], tumor necrosis factor-α [40] and insulin-like growth factor -1 [41]. On the other hand, some tumors stop growing and remain at a dormant state. It was reported that distant metastases sometimes grow rapidly after the resection of main tumors [42]. In such situations, hormones or cytokines secreted by tumor cells are assumed to work as anti-angiogenic factors and inhibit the growth of metastases. At present, several anti-angiogenic factors have been identified as follows: angiostatin [43], endostatin [44], proliferin-related protein [45], angioarrestin [46], vasostatin [47], angiopoietin-1 [48], and thrombospondin-1 (TSP-1) [49] and -2 [50].

Among them, TSP-1 has been considered as one of the most potent anti-angiogenic factors in tumors. TSP-1 was identified as a glycoprotein to be secreted by platelet in 1978 [51]. Physiologically, TSP-1 is secreted from various cells such as vascular endothelial cells, fibroblast, monocytes, macrophages, megakaryocytes and smooth muscle cells [52-54]. TSP-1 consists of N- and C-terminal globular domains, a region of sequence with similarity to procollagen and three types of repeated sequence motifs named type 1, type 2 and type 3 repeats [55]. TSP-1 mostly exists on extracellular matrix (ECM) but not in circulation. Therefore, TSP-1 requires the binding of receptors of an integrin family, such as α3β1 integrin [56], α5β3 integrin (CD51/CD61) [57], α6β1 [58], IAP (CD47) [59] and Mr 80,000/105,000 receptor [60]. CD36 has been demonstrated to be the first non-integrin receptor [61].

Previously, we have reported that TSP-1 expression inversely correlated with the degree of invasion of the primary tumor to adjacent organs and microvessel density in patients with papillary thyroid carcinoma [62]. It has been demonstrated that mutated p53 [63-66], p73 [67], mutated ras [68,69], c-jun [70], hypoxia [71] and hepatocyte growth factor [72,73] inhibit TSP-1 expression, and that chemotherapy [74,75] and wild-type p53 [63-66] stimulate it. In this study, we immunohistochemically investigated the relationship between expression levels of p53 and TSP-1 in papillary thyroid carcinomas. Moreover, we examined the effect of TSP-1 on invasion of thyroid carcinoma cell lines using *in vitro* invasion assay.

Materials and Methods

Tissue Samples

Surgical specimens of papillary thyroid carcinoma were obtained from 75 patients. They consisted of 25 patients with recurrent diseases and 50 non-recurrent patients. The median age and primary tumor size were 57 years old and 3.0 cm, respectively. Fifty-one patients were women (68%) and 24 were men (32%). There were 24 patients with pEX2 (infiltrating to adjacent organs except for muscles), and three with poorly differentiated carcinoma. Among the patients with recurrent diseases, metastases were observed in lungs (53.8% of the patients), bones (30.8%), pleura (7.7%), liver (3.8%), and brain (3.8%), respectively. The median disease-free interval and overall survival of patients with recurrent diseases were 24 and 86 months, respectively. The median overall survival of all the patients was 94 months. There was no significant difference in the duration of follow-up between the recurrent and non-recurrent groups. Among all the patients, 47 patients were without evidence of disease, 15 patients were alive with disease and 10 patients died of cancer. Informed consent was obtained from all enrolled patients.

Cell Lines

Six human thyroid carcinoma cell lines (KTC-1, KTC-2, KTC-3, TTA-1, TTA-2 and KTA-4) were used for invasion assay. These cell lines were originated from anaplastic thyroid carcinoma patients except for the KTC-1 cell line, which was originated from poorly differentiated papillary carcinoma. The KTC-1, -2 and -3 cell lines were established in our department, and TTA-1, -2 and KTA-4 cell lines were kindly provided by Dr. A. Yoshida (Kanagawa Cancer Center, Yokohama, Japan). Characteristics of each cell line were shown in Table 3.

Table 3. Characteristics of six thyroid cancer cell lines tested.

Cell line	Histology of original tumor	p53 immunostaining
KTC-1	poorly differentiated papillary thyroid cancer	Negative
KTC-2	anaplastic thyroid cancer	Postive
KTC-3	anaplastic thyroid cancer	Postive
TTA-1	anaplastic thyroid cancer	Postive
TTA-2	anaplastic thyroid cancer	Negative
KTA-4	anaplastic thyroid cancer	Negative

Immunohistochemistry

The samples embedded in paraffin were cut into sections 4 μm in thickness, and fixed on aminopropyltrietoxysilane-coated glass slides (Matsunami, Osaka, Japan). After typical deparaffinization, the slides were autoclaved for 20 min at 121 ℃ in 10 mM citrate buffer (pH 6.0) for antigen retrieval for detection of p53. Then normal rabbit serum was applied and the sections were incubated for 10 min at room temperature to block non-specific binding of the antibody. The slides were incubated for two hours at room temperature with each of the following primary antibodies; anti-p53 antibody, a mouse monoclonal immunoglobulin G2b antibody (DO-7, DAKO Corp., Carpinteria, CA, USA) at a 50-fold diluted concentration, anti-VEGF antibody, a mouse monoclonal immunoglobulin G2a antibody (sc-7269, Santa Cruz, CA, USA) at a concentration of 10 μg/ml and anti-VEGF-C antibody, a mouse polyclonal antibody (sc-9047, Santa Cruz, CA, USA), at a concentration of 20 μg/ml. Anti-

TSP-1 monoclonal antibody (MAB054, Chemicon Int., Inc., CA, USA) was used at 2 μg/ml, and anti-CD36 monoclonal antibody (MAB1204, Chemicon Int., Inc., CA, USA) at a 200-fold diluted concentration.

After incubation, the slides were washed in PBS for 15 min, and each secondary antibody was applied using the LSAB plus kit (DAKO Corp., Carpinteria, CA, USA) according to the manufacturer's protocol. After washing, the color was developed using 5-bromo-4-chloro-3-indoxyl phosphate and nitro blue tetrazolium chloride (BCIP/ NBT) (DAKO Corp., Carpinteria, CA, USA). Then the slides were washed in distilled water for 5 min and mounted. We used normal mouse serum instead of primary antibody in control studies, which were performed for all slides (data not shown).

Analysis of Immunohistochemical Detection

Immunostaining was evaluated by two repeated stainings of the same specimen. We blinded ourselves to the characteristics of specimens and cell lines. Cells of a tissue section were evaluated as positive when they showed a distinctly specific stain when compared with the cells of negative control sections. Then, two investigators independently decided the level of intensity of positive cells in each slide. Only in the case of discordance between two investigators, we each other discussed and decided the intensity.

For these immunohistochemical analyses, except for that of p53, we evaluated both the intensity and proportion of stained cells in each section. For evaluation of the intensity of staining, the intensity was divided into four categories (from 0 to 3). For evaluation of the proportion of stained cells, the proportion was divided into four categories, 0 (absent), 1 (less than 30% of the tumor cells to be positive), 2 (30 - 60%), and 3 (over 60%). Multiplication of both scores resulted in a final quotation ranging from 0 - 9, and they were presented as means ± S.D. For evaluation of p53 expression, we calculated the rate of positively stained nuclei in 1000 cells.

Invasion Assay

We used 24-well BioCoat Matrigel invasion chambers (Becton Dickinson Labware, Franklin Lakes, NJ, USA) with an 8-μm pore polycarbonate filter coated Matrigel to measure chemoinvasion. For control filter, we used Falcon Cell Culture Inserts containing 8-μm pore polycarbonate filter without any coating (Becton Dickinson Labware). Recombinant TSP-1 (TH-200-07, Athens Research and Technology, Georgia, USA, 25 μg/ml in DMEM) and anti-TSP-1 neutralizing antibody (603250, Calbiochem, CA, USA, 100 μg/ml in DMEM) were added to the bottom well of the chambers. Then, we added 5×10^4 cells into the top chambers and incubated for 22 h at 37 °C in triplicate. After incubation, the cells that had passed through the filter into the lower wells were stained with Diff Quick solution (International Reagents Co., Kobe, Japan) and counted the number of invaded cells in three fields of triplicate membranes. Invasion ratio was calculated as follows: the number of invaded cells through the Matrigel membrane/the number of invaded cells through the control membrane.

Statistical Analysis

The F test and Spearman's rank correlation test were used, and $p < 0.05$ was considered significant.

Results

Immunohistochemistry of Tissue Samples

Positive staining for VEGF, VEGF-C, TSP-1 and CD36 was found in the cytoplasm of tumor cells. Strongly positive staining for TSP-1 and CD36 was also observed in endothelium. In the 75 patients tested, the positive rates of VEGF, VEGF-C, TSP-1 and CD36 were 96%, 88%, 100% and 100%, respectively. The immunohistochemical scores for VEGF, VEGF-C, TSP-1 and CD36 were 5.3 ± 2.3, 5.1 ± 2.9, 6.4 ± 1.8 and 5.9 ± 2.0, respectively. Positive staining for p53 was found in the nuclei of tumor cells. It was observed in 17 of the 75 patients (22.7%). It was observed in nine of 25 recurrent patients (36%). Representative immunohistochemical findings using each antibody are shown in Figure 11.

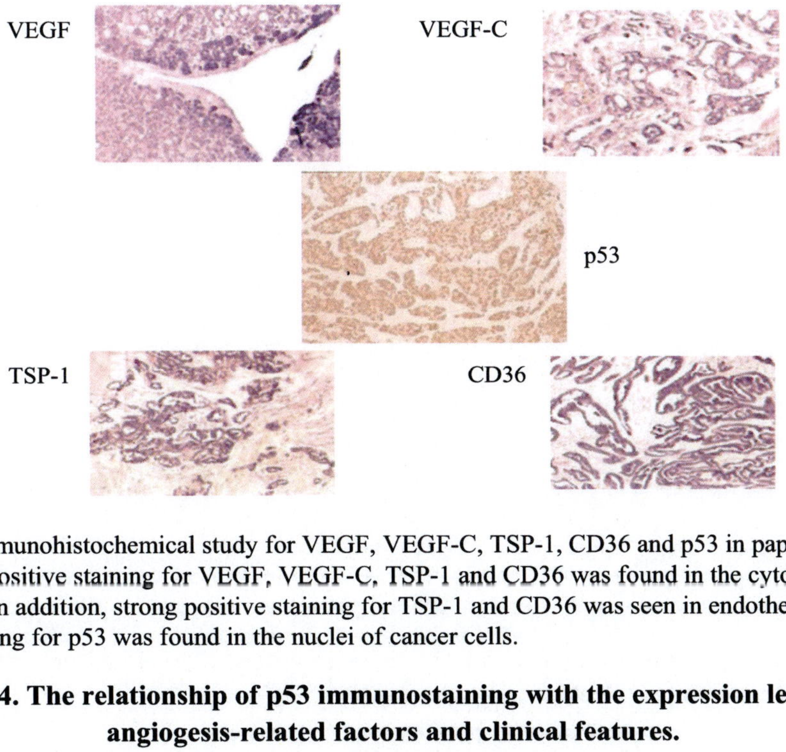

Figure 11. Immunohistochemical study for VEGF, VEGF-C, TSP-1, CD36 and p53 in papillary thyroid carcinomas. Positive staining for VEGF, VEGF-C, TSP-1 and CD36 was found in the cytoplasm of cancer cells. In addition, strong positive staining for TSP-1 and CD36 was seen in endothelium. Positive staining for p53 was found in the nuclei of cancer cells.

Table 4. The relationship of p53 immunostaining with the expression levels of angiogesis-related factors and clinical features.

Factors	p53 immunostaining
VEGF	No correlation
VEGF-C	No correlation
TSP-1	Inverse correlation ($p < 0.01$)
CD36	No correlation
Age	No correlation
Gender	No correlation
Extrathyroidal infiltration	Positive correlation ($p < 0.05$)

Nodal status	No correlation
Recurrence	No correlation
Overall survival	Inverse correlation ($p < 0.05$)

Relationship Between Clinical Data and the Expression Levels of Angiogenesis-Related Factors and p53

Among the angiogenesis-related factors, the expression level of TSP-1 inversely correlated with that of p53 ($p < 0.01$). In clinical data, the expression level of p53 positively correlated with extrathyroidal infiltration, but inversely correlated with overall survival ($p < 0.05$ in either correlation). The other factors had no correlation with the expression level of p53 (Table 4).

Immunohistochemistry of Cell Lines

All cell lines expressed VEGF, VEGF-C, TSP-1 and CD36 at various levels. In the TTA-1 cell line, all of the factors expressed at the lowest level. Table 5 shows the immunohistochemical score for each cell line.

Table 5. Immunohstochemical scores for VEGF, VEGF-C, TSP-1 and CD36 in each cell line.

Factors/Cell line	KTC-1	KTC-2	KTC-3	TTA-1	TTA-2	KTA-4
VEGF	4	6	6	2	4	4
VEGF-C	4	2	9	2	9	4
TSP-1	2	4	4	2	4	4
CD36	2	4	4	2	4	4

Effects of TSP-1 and anti-TSP-1 Antibody on the Invasion of each Cell Line

Fig. 12 shows the effects of TSP-1 and anti-TSP-1 body on the invasive potential of each cell line. Except for the TTA-1 cell line, TSP-1 tended to decrease the invasive potential of all the cell lines in comparison with control. Anti-TSP-1 antibody tended to decrease the invasive potential in the KTC-2 and TTA-2 cell lines, but tended to increase it in the KTC-1, TTA-1 and KTA-4 cell lines. Anti-TSP-1 antibody significantly promoted the invasive potential of the KTC-3 cells.

Table 6. Correlation of changes in the invasive potential by TSP-1 or anti-TSP-1 antibody with the expression level of VEGF, VEGF-C, TSP-1, CD36 or p53.

	TSP-1	Anti-TSP-1 antibody
VEGF	$r = -0.964$, $p = 0.0005$	NS
VEGF-C	$r = -0.964$, $p = 0.0005$	NS
TSP-1	NS	NS
CD36	NS	NS
p53	NS	NS

Relationship between the Effects of TSP-1 and anti-TSP-1 Antibody on the Invasion and Expression Level of Angiogenesis-Related Factors

There was no relationship between the effect of anti-TSP-1 antibody on the invasive potential and expression level of each angiogenesis-related factor. However, there was a significant inverse correlation between the effect of TSP-1 on the invasive potential and expression level of VEGF or VEGF-C. In other words, the exogenous addition of TSP-1 decreased invasive potential of thyroid cancer cells expressing a higher level of VEGF or VEGF-C.

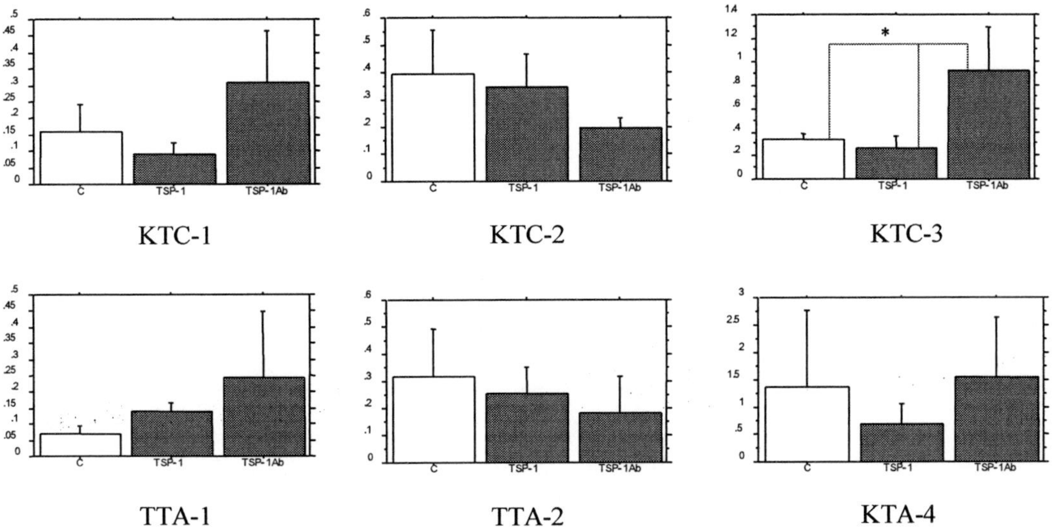

Figure 12. Effects of TSP-1 and anti TSP-1 antibody on the invasive potential in six thyroid cancer cell lines. The invasion assay was performed using 24-well BioCoat Matrigel invasion chambers as described in the Materials and Methods. *, $P < 0.05$.

Conclusion

TSP-1 has been considered as an anti-angiogenic factor [75]. Some investigators have shown that TSP-1 inhibits endothelial cell growth and/or angiogenesis [76,77]. TSP-1 has been reported to affect activity of Srk family kinase, c-JUN through CD36 and inhibit angiogenesis in a TSP-1-null mouse model [78,79]. It is reported that TSP-1 inhibits angiogenesis induced by bFGF by competing for heparin sulfate sites on the cell surface proteoglycans [80]. Although TSP-1 is widely recognized as an inhibitor of angiogenesis, TSP-1 has been shown to have mitogenic and angiogenic effects [81-83]. Recently, it is reported that angiogenesis is stimulated by a low concentration of TSP-1, but inhibited by a high concentration of TSP-1 in a biphasic manner [84].

In human tumors, a majority of studies have shown that TSP-1 acts as an anti-angiogenic factor in thyroid [62], bladder [85], oral squamous cell [86], cervical [87], prostate [88] and colorectal [89] carcinomas. In contrast, it has been reported that TSP-1 acts as an angiogenic factor in melanoma [90], endometrial [91] and gastric [92] carcinomas. No relationship between TSP-1 expression and angiogenesis has been reported in prostate [93], renal cell [94] and basal cell [95] carcinomas. We have reported that TSP-1 is localized in cytoplasm of cancer cells in thyroid cancer [62]. However, other investigators have demonstrated that TSP-1 mainly localizes at adjacent mesenchymal tissues [72,96,97].

Regulatory mechanisms of TSP-1 expression have been investigated by several investigators. It has been reported that TSP-1 expression is up-regulated by wild-type p53 [63-66], EGF [98], TGF-β [99] and some drugs such as methimazole [86] and anticancer agents [73,74]. On other hand, TSP-1 expression has been reported to be down-regulated by TSH in thyroid cells [99], ras mutation [68,69], c-Jun [69], Myc oncoprotein [100], p73 [67], hypoxia [68,70], HGF [71,72] and hypermethylation of the TSP-1 gene [101]. In this study, we have revealed the correlation between expression levels of mutated p53 and TSP-1 in papillary thyroid carcinomas. Among angiogenesis-related factors, VEGF, VEGF-C and TSP-1, only TSP-1 expression had a significant inverse correlation with mutated p53 expression. In clinical studies, it has been reported that there was a negative correlation between expression levels of mutated p53 and TSP-1 in bladder [85] and prostate [88]. However, it has been reported that there was a positive or no correlation of TSP-1 expression with mutated p53 expression in non-small cell lung [102], prostate [93] and gastric [92] carcinomas. These findings suggest that the relationship between expression levels of TSP-1 and mutated p53 varies in originated organs. Nagayama et al. have demonstrated that the induction of wild-type p53 leads to restoration of TSP-1 expression in a thyroid carcinoma cell line [65]. It is unclear that p53 mutation plays a key role in the decrease in TSP-1 expression in papillary thyroid carcinomas, since p53 mutation is not frequent in papillary thyroid carcinomas [103].

We have previously demonstrated an inverse correlation between extra-thyroidal infiltration and TSP-1 expression [62]. Some investigators have reported that serum TSP-1 levels correlate with infiltration of colorectal carcinoma [104] and oral squamous cell carcinoma [86]. In this study, we have investigated the effects of exogenous TSP-1 and anti-TSP-1 antibody on the invasive potential of thyroid carcinoma cell lines. The addition of TSP-1 did not significantly affect the invasive potential in each cell line. However, except for TTA-1, all cell lines showed a decrease in the invasive potential by adding TSP-1. On the other hand, anti-TSP-1 antibody significantly promoted the invasive potential in the KTC-3 cell line. It has been reported that activity of urokinase plasminogen activator and its receptors stimulated by TSP-1 results in increasing invasion [105].

TSP-1 has been also reported to inhibit angiogenesis by binding matrix methaloproteinases (MMPs) and inactivation of MMP-9 [106]. Other investigators have reported that 25kDa fragment of TSP-1 promotes angiogenesis and tumor invasion through activation of MMP-2 and induction of MMP-9 but 140kDa fragment of TSP-1 inhibits angiogenesis [107]. Recently, anti-TSP-1 antibody has been demonstrated to have an inhibitory effect on invasion in thyroid carcinoma cells [108]. These findings indicate that the effect of TSP-1 on invasion is still controversial and further examination is clearly needed.

ACKNOWLEDGEMENTS

These works were supported by Research Project Grants (15-501, 15-504 and 16-501S) from Kawasaki Medical School and by a grant (14571166) from the Ministry of Education, Science, Sports and Culture of Japan. The authors thank Dr. A. Yoshida (Kanagawa Cancer Center, Yokohama, Japan) for providing thyroid carcinoma cell lines KTA-4, TTA-1 and TTA-2.

REFERENCES

[1] Yarden Y, Sliwkowski MX (2001) Untangling the ErbB signaling network. *Nat Rev Mol Cell Biol 2*: 127-137

[2] Arteaga CL (2002) Overview of epidermal growth factor receptor biology and its role as a therapeutic target in human neoplasia. *Semin Oncol 5 Suppl 14*: 3-9

[3] Haugen DR, Akslen LA, Varhaug JE, Lillehaug JR (1993) Demonstration of a TGF-alpha-EGF-receptor autocrine loop and c-myc protein over-expression in papillary thyroid carcinomas. *Int J Cancer 55*: 37-43

[4] Akslen LA, Myking AO, Salvesen H, Varhaug JE (1993) Prognostic impact of EGF-receptor in papillary thyroid carcinoma. *Br J Cancer 68*: 808-812

[5] Akslen LA, Varhaug JE (1995) Oncoproteins and tumor progression in papillary thyroid carcinoma: presence of epidermal growth factor receptor, c-erbB-2 protein, estrogen receptor related protein, p21-ras protein, and proliferation indicators in relation to tumor recurrences and patient survival. *Cancer 76*: 1643-1654

[6] Chen BK, Ohtsuki Y, Furihata M, Takeuchi T, Iwata J, Liang SB, Sonobe H (1999) Co-overexpression of p53 protein and epidermal growth factor receptor in human papillary thyroid carcinomas correlated with lymph node metastasis, tumor size and clinicopathologic stage. *Int J Oncol 15*: 893-898

[7] Bergstrom JD, Westermark B, Heldin NE (2000) Epidermal growth factor receptor signaling activates met in human anaplastic thyroid carcinoma cells. *Exp Cell Res 259*: 293-299

[8] Park JW, Yeh MW, Wong MG, Lobo M, Hyun WC, Duh QY, Clark OH (2003) The heat shock protein 90-binding geldanamycin inhibits cancer cell proliferation, down-regulates oncoproteins, and inhibits epidermal growth factor-induced invasion in thyroid cancer cell lines. *J Clin Endocrinol Metab 88*: 3346-3353

[9] Schiff BA, McMurphy AB, Jasser SA, Younes MN, Doan D, Yigitbasi OG, Kim S, Zhou G, Mandal M, Bekele BN, Holsinger FC, Sherman SI, Yeung SC, El-Naggar AK, Myers JN (2004) Epidermal growth factor receptor (EGFR) is overexpressed in anaplastic thyroid cancer, and the EGFR inhibitor gefitinib inhibits the growth of anaplastic thyroid cancer. *Clin Cancer Res 10*: 8594-8602

[10] Giaccone G (2004) The role of gefitinib in lung cancer treatment. *Clin Cancer Res 15*: 4233s-4237s

[11] Cohen MH, Johnson JR, Pazdur R (2005) U.S. Food and Drug Administration Drug Approval Summary: conversion of imatinib mesylate (STI571; Gleevec) tablets from accelerated approval to full approval. *Clin Cancer Res 11*: 12-19

[12] Dagher R, Cohen M, Williams G, Rothmann M, Gobburu J, Robbie G, Rahman A, Chen G, Staten A, Griebel D, Pazdur R (2002) Approval summary: imatinib mesylate in the treatment of metastatic and/or unresectable malignant gastrointestinal stromal tumors. *Clin Cancer Res 8*: 3034-3038

[13] Yazawa S, Toshimori H, Nakatsuru K, Katakami H, Takemura J, Matsukura S (1995) Thyroid anaplastic carcinoma producing granulocyte-colony-stimulating factor and parathyroid hormone-related protein. *Intern Med 34*: 584-588

[14] Kurebayashi J, Otsuki T, Tanaka K, Yamamoto Y, Moriya T, Sonoo H (2003) Medroxyprogesterone acetate decreases secretion of interleukin-6 and parathyroid hormone-related protein in a new anaplastic thyroid cancer cell line, KTC-2. *Thyroid 13*: 249-258

[15] Fiore L, Pollina LE, Fontanini G, Casalone R, Berlingieri MT, Giannini R, Pacini F, Miccoli P, Toniolo A, Fusco A, Basolo F (1997) Cytokine production by a new undifferentiated human thyroid carcinoma cell line, FB-1. *J Clin Endocrinol Metab 82*: 4094-4100

[16] Asakawa H, Kobayashi T (1999) The secretion of cytokines and granulocyte colony stimulating factor by anaplastic and poorly differentiated thyroid carcinoma cell lines. *Anticancer Res 19*: 761-764

[17] Sato T, Omura M, Saito J, Hirasawa A, Kakuta Y, Wakabayashi Y, Nishikawa T (2000) Neutrophilia associated with anaplastic carcinoma of the thyroid: production of macrophage colony-stimulating factor (M-CSF) and interleukin-6. *Thyroid 10*: 1113-1118

[18] Chang JW, Yeh KY, Shen YC, Hsieh JJ, Chuang CK, Liao SK, Tsai LH, Wang CH (2003) Production of multiple cytokines and induction of cachexia in athymic nude mice by a new anaplastic thyroid carcinoma cell line. *J Endocrinol 179*: 387-394

[19] Kurebayashi J, Tanaka K, Otsuki T, Moriya T, Kunisue H, Uno M, Sonoo H (2000) All-trans-retinoic acid modulates expression levels of thyroglobulin and cytokines in a new human poorly differentiated papillary thyroid carcinoma cell line, KTC-1. *J Clin Endocrinol Metab 85*: 2889-2896

[20] Okubo S, Kurebayashi J, Otsuki T, Yamamoto Y, Tanaka K, Sonoo H (2004) Additive antitumour effect of the epidermal growth factor receptor tyrosine kinase inhibitor gefitinib (Iressa, ZD1839) and the antioestrogen fulvestrant (Faslodex, ICI 182,780) in breast cancer cells. *Br J Cancer 90*: 236-244

[21] Albanell J, Rojo F, Averbuch S, Feyereislova A, Mascaro JM, Herbst R, LoRusso P, Rischin D, Sauleda S, Gee J, Nicholson RI, Baselga J (2002) Pharmacodynamic studies of the epidermal growth factor receptor inhibitor ZD1839 in skin from cancer patients: histopathologic and molecular consequences of receptor inhibition. *J Clin Oncol 20*: 110-124

[22] Lynch TJ, Bell DW, Sordella R, Gurubhagavatula S, Okimoto RA, Brannigan BW, Harris PL, Haserlat SM, Supko JG, Haluska FG, Louis DN, Christiani DC, Settleman J, Haber DA (2004) Activating mutations in the epidermal growth factor receptor

underlying responsiveness of non-small-cell lung cancer to gefitinib. *N Engl J Med 350*: 2129-2139

[23] Paez JG, Janne PA, Lee JC, Tracy S, Greulich H, Gabriel S, Herman P, Kaye FJ, Lindeman N, Boggon TJ, Naoki K, Sasaki H, Fujii Y, Eck MJ, Sellers WR, Johnson BE, Meyerson M (2004) EGFR mutations in lung cancer: correlation with clinical response to gefitinib therapy. *Science 304*: 1497-1500

[24] Barber TD, Vogelstein B, Kinzler KW, Velculescu VE (2004) Somatic mutations of EGFR in colorectal cancers and glioblastomas. *N Engl J Med 351*: 2883

[25] Moulder SL, Yakes FM, Muthuswamy SK, Bianco R, Simpson JF, Arteaga CL (2001) Epidermal growth factor receptor (HER1) tyrosine kinase inhibitor ZD1839 (Iressa) inhibits HER2/neu (erbB2)-overexpressing breast cancer cells in vitro and in vivo. *Cancer Res 61*: 8887-8895

[26] Amann J, Kalyankrishna S, Massion PP, Ohm JE, Girard L, Shigematsu H, Peyton M, Juroske D, Huang Y, Stuart Salmon J, Kim YH, Pollack JR, Yanagisawa K, Gazdar A, Minna JD, Kurie JM, Carbone DP (2005) Aberrant epidermal growth factor receptor signaling and enhanced sensitivity to EGFR inhibitors in lung cancer. *Cancer Res 65*: 226-235

[27] Ramos EJ, Suzuki S, Marks D, Inui A, Asakawa A, Meguid MM (2004) Cancer anorexia-cachexia syndrome: cytokines and neuropeptides. *Curr Opin Clin Nutr Metab Care 7*: 427-434

[28] Esbrit P (2001) Hypercalcemia of malignancy--new insights into an old syndrome. *Clin Lab 47*: 67-71

[29] Hirata A, Ogawa S, Kometani T, Kuwano T, Naito S, Kuwano M, Ono M (2002) ZD1839 (Iressa) induces antiangiogenic effects through inhibition of epidermal growth factor receptor tyrosine kinase. *Cancer Res 62*: 2554-2560

[30] Folkman J (1990) What is the evidence that tumors are angiogenesis dependent? *J Natl Cancer Inst 82*: 4-6

[31] Leung DW, Cachianes G, Kuang W, Goeddel DV, Ferrara N (1989) Vascular endothelial growth factor is a secreted angiogenic mitogen. *Science 246*: 1306-1309

[32] Montesano R, Vassalli JD, Baird A, Guillemin R, Orci L (1986) Basic fibroblast growth factor induces angiogenesis in vitro. *Proc Natl Acad Sci USA 83*: 7297-7301

[33] Maisonpierre PC, Suri C, Jones PF, Bartunkova S, Wiegand SJ, Radziejewski C, Compton D, McClain J, Aldrich TH, Papadopoulos N, Daly TJ, Davis S, Sato TN, Yancopoulos GD (1997) Angiopoietin-2, a natural antagonist for Tie2 that disrupts in vivo angiogenesis. *Science 277*: 55-60

[34] Fett JW, Strydom DJ, Lobb RR, Alderman EM, Bethune JL, Riordanm JF, Vallee BL (1985) Isolation and characterization of angiogenin, an angiogenic protein from human carcinoma cells. *Biochemistry 24*: 5480-5486

[35] Ishikawa F, Miyazono K, Hellman U, Hannes D, Werstadt C, Haiwara K, Utsuki K, Takaku F, Risau W, Heldin CH (1989) Identification of angiogenic activity and thecloning and expression of platelet-derived endothelial cell growth factor. *Nature 338*: 557-562

[36] Jackson D, Volpert O, Bouck N,Linzer DIH (1994) Stimulation and inhibition of angiogenesis by placental proliferin and proliferin-related protein. *Science 266*: 1581-1584

[37] Komuro I, Kurihara H, Yoshizumu M, Takaku F, Yazaki Y (1988) Endothelin stimulates c-fos and c-myc expression and proliferation of vascular smooth muscle cells. *FEBS Lett 238*: 249-252

[38] Schreiber AB, Winker ME, Derynck R (1986) Transforming growth factor-α: a more potent angiogenic mediator than epithelial growth factor. *Science 232*: 1250-1253

[39] Robert AB, Sporn MB, Assoian RK, Smith JM, Rosch NS, Wakefield LM, Heine UI, Liotta LA, Falanga V, Kehrl JH, Fauci AS (1986) Transforming growth factor type β: rapid induction of fibrosis and angiogenesis in vivo and stimulation of collagen formation in vitro. *Proc Natl Acad Sci USA 84*: 4167-4171

[40] Leibovich SJ, Polverini PJ, Shepard HM, Wiseman DM, Shively V, Nuseir N (1987) Macrophage-induced angiogenesis is mediated by tumor necrosis factor-α. *Nature 329*: 631-632

[41] Bar RS, Boes M, Dake BL, Booth BA, Henley SA, Sandra A (1988) Insulin, insulin-like growth factors, and vascular endothelium. *Am J Med 85*: 59-70

[42] Prehn RT (1991) The inhibition of tumor growth by tumor mass. *Cancer Res 51*: 2-4

[43] O'Reilly MS, Holmgren L, Shing Y, Chen C, Rosenthal RA, Moses M, Lane WS, Cao Y, Sage EH, Folkman J (1994) Angiostatin: a novel angiogenesis inhibitor that mediates the suppression of metastases by a Lewis lung carcinoma. *Cell 79*: 315-328

[44] O'Reilly MS, Boehm T, Shing Y, Fukai N, Vasios G, Lane WS, Flynn E, Birkhead JR, Olsen BR, Folkman J (1997) Endostatin: an endogeneous inhibitor of angiogenesis and tumor growth. *Cell 88*: 277-285

[45] Dhanabal M, LaRochelle WJ, Jeffers M, Herrmann J, Rastelli L, McDonald WF, Chillakuru RA, Yang M, Boldog FL, Padigaru M, McQueeney KD, Wu F, Minskoff SA, Shimkets RA, Lichenstein HS (2002) Angioarrestin: an antiangiogenic protein with tumor-inhibiting properties. *Cancer Res 62*: 3834-3841

[46] Pike SE, Yao L, Jones KD, Cherney B, Appella E, Sakaguchi K, Nakhasi H, Teruya-Feldstein J, Wirth P, Gupta G, Tosato G (1998) Vasostatin, a calreticulin fragment, inhibits angiogenesis and suppresses tumor growth. *J Exp Med 188*: 2349-2356

[47] Stoeltzing O, Ahmad SA, Liu W, McCarty MF, Wey JS, Parikh AA, Fan F, Reinmuth N, Kawaguchi M, Bucana CD, Ellis LM (2003) Angiopoietin-1 inhibits vascular permeability, angiogenesis, and growth of hepatic colon cancer tumors. *Cancer Res 63*: 3370-3377

[48] Rastinejad F., Polverini PJ., Bouck NP (1989) Regulation of the activity of a new inhibitor of angiogenesis by a cancer suppressor gene. *Cell 56*: 345-355.

[49] Filleur S, Volpert OV, Degeorges A, Voland C, Reiher F, Clezardin P, Bouck N, Cabon F (2001) In vivo mechanisms by which tumors producing thrombospondin 1 bypass its inhibitory effects. *Gene Dev 15*: 1373-1382

[50] Volpert OV, Tolsma SS, Pellerin S, Feige J-J, Chen H, Mosher DF, Bouck N (1995) Inhibition of angiogenesis by thrombospondin-2. *Biochem Biophys Res Commun 217*: 326-332

[51] Lawler JW, Slayter HS, Coligan JE (1978) Isolation and characterization of a high molecular weight glycoprotein from human blood platelets. *J Biol Chem 253*: 8609-8616

[52] Mosher DF, Doyle MF, Jaffe EA (1982) Synthesis and secretion of thrombospondin by cultured human endothelial cells. *J Cell Biol 93*: 343-348

[53] Jaffe EA, Ruggiero JT, Falcone DJ (1985) Monocytes and macrophages synthesize and secrete thrombospondin. *Blood 65*: 79-84

[54] McLaren KM (1983) Immunohistochemical localization of thrombospondin in human megakaryocytes and platelets. *J Clin Pathol 36*: 197-199

[55] Lawler J, Connolly J, Ferro P, Derick L (1986) Thrombin and chymotrypsin interactions with thrombospondin. *Ann NY Acad Sci 485*: 273-287

[56] Krutzsch HC, Choe BJ, Sipes JM, Guo N-H, Roberts DD (1999) Identification of an α3β1 integrin recognition sequence in thrombospondin-1. *J Biol Chem 274*: 24080-24086

[57] Lawler J, Weinstein R, hynes RO (1988) Cell attachment to thrombospondin: the role of ARG-GLY-ASP, calcium, and integrin receptors. *J Cell Biol 107*: 2351-2361

[58] Calzada MJ, Sipes JM, Krutzsch HC, Yurchenco PD, Annis DS, Mosher DF, Roberts DD (2003) Recognition of the N-terminal modeles of thrombospondin-1 and thrombospondin-2 by α6β1 integrin. *J Biol Chem 278*: 40679-40687

[59] Gao A-G, Lindberg FP, Finn MB, Blystone SD, Brown EJ, Frazier WA (1996) Integrin-associated protein is a receptor for the C-terminal domain of thrombospondin. *J Biol Chem 271*: 21-24

[60] Yabkowitz R, Dixit VM (1991) Human carcinoma cells bind thrombospondin through a Mr 80,000/105,000 receptor. *Cancer Res 51*: 3648-3656

[61] Asch AS, Barnwell J, Silverstein RL, Nachman RL (1987) Isolation of the thrombospondin membrane receptor. *J Clin Invest 79*: 1054-1061

[62] Tanaka K, Sonoo H, Kurebayashi J, Nomura T, Ohkubo S, Yamamoto Y, Yamamoto S (2002) Inhibition of infiltration and angiogenesis by thrombospondin-1 in papillary thyroid carcinoma. *Clin Cancer Res 8*: 1125-1131

[63] Dameron KM, Volpert OV, Tainsky MA, Bouck N (1994) Control of angiogenesis in fibroblasts by p53 regulation of thrombospondin 1. *Science 265*: 1582-1584

[64] Volpert OV, Stellmach V, Bouck N (1995) The modulation of thrombospondin and other naturally occurring inhibitors of angiogenesis during tumor progression. *Breast Cancer Res Treat 36*: 119-126

[65] Nagayama Y, Shigemitsu K, Namba H, Zeki K, Yamashita S, Niwa M (2000) Inhibition of angiogenesis and tumorigenesis, and induction of dormancy by p53-null thyroid carcinoma cell line in vivo. *Anticancer Res 20*: 2723-2728

[66] Harada H, Nakagawa K, Saito M, Kohno S, Nagato S, Furukawa K, Kumon Y, Hamada K, Ohnishi T (2003) Introduction of wild-type p53 enhances thrombospondin-1 expression in human glioma cells. *Cancer Lett 191*: 109-119

[67] Vikhanskaya F, Bani MR, Borsotti P, Ghilardi C, Ceruti R, Ghisleni G, Marabese M, Giavazzi R, Broggini M, Taraboletti G (2001) p73 overexpression increases VEGF and reduces thrombospondin-1 production: implications for tumor angiogenesis. *Oncogene 20*: 7293-7300

[68] Landeroute KR, Alarcon RM, Brody MD, Calaoagan JM, Chen EY, Knapp AM, Yun Z, Denko NC, Giaccia AJ (2000) Opposing effects of hypoxia on expression of the angiogenic inhibitor thrombospondin 1 and the angiogenic inducer vascular endothelial growth factor. *Clin Cancer Res 6:* 2941-2950

[69] Kalas W, Gilpin S, Yu JL, May L, Krchnakova H, Bornstein P, Rak J (2003) Restoration of thrombospondin 1 expression in tumor cells harbouring mutant ras oncogene by treatment with low doses of doxycycline. *Biochem Biophys Res Commun 310*: 109-114

[70] Tenan M, Fulci G, Albertoni M, Diserens A-C, Hamou M-F, Atifi-Borel ME, Feige J-J, Pepper MS, Van Meir EG (2000) Thrombospondin-1 is downregulated by anoxia and suppresses tumorigenicity of human glioblastoma cells. *J Exp Med 191*: 1789-1797

[71] Zhang Y-W, Su Y, Volpert OV, Vande Woude GF (2003) Hepatocyte growth factor/scatter factor mediates angiogenesis through positive VEGF and negative thrombospondin 1 regulation. *Proc Natl Acad Sci USA 100*: 12718-12723

[72] Scarpino S, Di Napoli A, Taraboletti G, Cancrini A, Ruco LP (2005) Hepatocyte growth factor (HGF) downregulates thrombospondin 1 (TSP-1) expression in thyroid papillary carcinoma cells. *J Pathol 205*: 50-56

[73] Bpcci G, Francia G, Man S, Lawler J, Kerbel RS (2003) Thrombospondin 1, a mediator of the antiangiogenic effects of low-dose metronomic chemotherapy. *Proc Natl Acad Sci USA 100*: 12917-12922

[74] Kalas W, Gilpin S, Yu JL, May L, Krchnakova H, Bornstein P, Rak J (2003) Restoration of thrombospondin 1 expression in tumor cells harbouring mutant ras oncogene by treatment with low doses of doxycycline. *Biochem Biophys Res Commun* 310: 109-114

[75] Tanaka K, Sonoo H (2004) Angiogenesis in thyroid cancer. *Res Adv in Cancer 4*: 1-22

[76] Iruela-Arispe ML, Bornstein P, Sage H (1991) Thrombospondin exerts an antiangiogenic effect on cord formation by endothelial cells in vitro. *Proc Natl Acad Sci USA 88*: 5026-5030

[77] Tolsma SS, Volpert OV, Good DJ, Frazier WA, Polverini PJ, Bouck N (1993) Peptides derived from two separate domains of the matrix protein thrombospondin-1 have anti-angiogenic activity. *J Cell Biol 122*: 497-511

[78] Jimenez B, Volpert OV, Crawford SE, Febbraio M, Silverstein RL, Bouck N (2000) Signals leading to apoptosis-dependent inhibition of neovascularization by thrombospondin-1. *Nature Med 6*: 41-48

[79] Jimenez B, Volpert OV, Reiher F, Chang L, Munoz A, Karin M, Bouck N (2000) c-JUN N- terminal kinase activation is required for the inhibition of neovascularization by thrombospondin-1. *Oncogene 20*: 3443-3448

[80] Kanda S, Shono T, Tomasini-Johansson B, Klint P, Saito Y (1999) Role of thrombospondin-1-derived peptide, 4N1K, in FGF-2-induced angiogenesis. *Exp Cell Res 252*: 262-272

[81] Majack RA, Cook SC, Bornstein P (1986) Control of smooth muscle cell growth by components of the extracellular matrix: autocrine role for thrombospondin. *Proc Natl Acad Sci USA 83*: 9050-9054

[82] Tuszynski GP, Gasic TB, Rothman VL, Knudsen KA, Gasic GJ (1987) Thrombospondin, a potentiator of tumor cell metastasis. *Cancer Res 47*: 4130-4133

[83] Taraboletti G, Roberts D, Liotta LA, Giavazzi R (1990) Platelet thrombospondin modulates endothelial cell adhesion, motility, and growth: a potential angiogenesis regulatory factor. *J Cell Biol 111*: 765-772

[84] Qian X, Wang TN, Rothman VL, Nicosia RF, Tuszynski GP (1997) Thrombospondin-1 modulates angiogenesis in vitro by up-regulation of matrix metalloproteinase-9 in endothelial cells. *Exp Cell Res 235*: 403-412

[85] Grossfeld GD, Ginsberg DA, Syein JP, Bochner BH, Esrig D, Groshen S, Dunn M, Nichols PW, Taylor CR, Skinner DG, Cote RJ (1997) Thrmobospondin-1 expression in bladder cancer: association with p53 alternations, tumor angiogenesis, and tumor progression. *J Natl Cancer Inst 89*: 219-227

[86] Yao L, Zhao Y-L, Itoh S, Wada S, Yue L, Furuta I (2000) Thrombospondin-1 expression in oral squamous cell carcinomas: correlations with tumor vascularity, clinicopathological features and survival. *Oral Oncol 36*: 539-544

[87] Kodama J, Hashimoto I, Seki N, Hongo A, Yoshinouchi M, Okuda H, Kudo T (2001) Thrombospondin-1 and -2 messenger RNA expression in invasive cervical cancer: correlation with angiogenesis and prognosis. *Clin Cancer Res 7*: 2826-2831

[88] Mehta R, Kyshtoobayeva A, Kurosaki T, Small EJ, Kim H, Stroup R, McLaren CE, Li K-T, Fruehauf JP (2001) Independent association of angiogenesis index with outcome in prostate cancer. *Clin Cancer Res 7*: 81-88

[89] Miyanaga K, Kato Y, Nakamura T, Matsumura M, Amaya H, Horiuchi T, Chiba Y, Tanaka K (2002) Expression and role of thrombospondin-1 in colorectal cancer. *Anticancer Res 22*: 3941-3948

[90] Straume O, Akslen LA (2001) Expression of vascular endothelial growth factor, its receptors (Flt-1, KDR) and TSP-1 related to microvessel density and patient outcome in vertical growth phase melanomas. *Am J Pathol 159:* 223-235

[91] Seki N, Kodama J, Hashimoto I, Hongo A, Yoshinouchi M, Kudo T (2001) Thrombospondin-1 and –2 messenger RNA expression in normal and neoplastic endometrial tissues: correlation with angiogenesis and prognosis. *Int J Oncol 19*: 305-310

[92] Zhang J, Ito R, Oue N, Zhu X, Kitadai Y, Yoshida K, Nakayama H, Yasui W (2003) Expression of thrombospondin-1 is correlated with microvessel density in gastric carcinoma. *Virch Arch 442*: 563-568

[93] Grossfeld GD, Carroll PR, Lindeman N, Meng M, Groshen S, Feng A-C, Hawes D, Cote RJ (2002) Thrombospondin-1 expression in patients with pathologic stage T3 prostate cancer undergoing radical prostatectomy: association with p53 alternations, tumor angiogenesis, and tumor progression. *Urology 59*: 97-102

[94] Baltaci S, Orhan D, Gorus C, Filiz E, Tulunary Gorus O (2003) Thrombospondin-1, vascular endothelial growth factor expression and microvessel density in renal cell carcinoma and their relationship with mutifocality. *Eur Urol 44*: 76-81

[95] Oh C-K, Kwon Y-W, Kim Y-S, Jang H-S, Kwon K-S (2003) Expression of basic fibroblast growth factor, vascular endothelial growth factor, and thrombospondin-1

related to microvessel density in nonaggressive and aggressive basal cell carcinomas. *J Dermatol 30*: 306-313

[96] Patel VA, Hill DJ, Eggo MC, Sheppard MC, Becks GP, Logan A (1996) Changes in the immunohistochemical localization of fibroblast growth factor-2, transforming growth factor-β1 and thrombospondin-1 are associated with early angiogenic events in the hyperplastic rat thyroid. *J Endocrinol 148*: 485-499

[97] Patey M, Delemer B, Bellon G, Martiny L, Pluot M, Haye B (1999) Immunohistochemical study of thrombospondin and its receptors αvβ3 and CD36 in normal thyroid and in thyroid tumours. *J Clin Pathol 52*: 895-900

[98] Okamoto M, Ono M, Uchiumi T, Ueno H, Kohno K, Sugimachi K, Kuwano M (2002) Up-regulation of thrombospondin-1 gene by epidermal growth factor and transforming growth factor β in human cancer cells-transcriptional activation and messenger RNA stabilization. *Biochimi Biophys Acta 1574*: 24-34

[99] Pellerin S, Croizet K, Rabilloud R, Feige J-J, Rousset B (1999) Regulation of the three-dimensional organization of thyroid epithelial cells into follicle structures by the matricellular protein, thrombospondin-1. *Endocrinology 140*: 1094-1103

[100] Watnick RS, Cheng Y-N, Rangarajan A, Ince TA, Weinberg RA (2003) Ras modulates Myc activity to repress thrombospondin-1 expression and increase tumor angiogenesis. *Cancer Cell 3*: 219-231

[101] Yang Q-W, Liu S, Tian Y, Salwen HR, Chlenski A, Weinstein J, Cohn SL (2003) Methylation-associated silencing of the thrombospondin-1 gene in human neuroblastoma. *Cancer Re 63*: 6299-6310

[102] Fontanini G, Boldrini L, Calcinai A, Chine S, Lucchi M, Mussi A, Angeletti CA, Basolo F, Bevilacqua G (1999) Thrombospondin 1 and 2 messenger RNA expression in lung carcinoma: relationship with p53 alternations, angiogenic growth factors, and vascular density. *Clin Cancer Res 5*: 155-161

[103] Farid NR (2001) P53 mutations in thyroid carcinoma: tidings from an old foe. *J Clin Invest 26*: 536-545

[104] Yamashita Y, Kurohiji T, Tuszynski GP, Sakai T, Shirakusa T (1998) Plasma thrombospondin levels in patients with colorectal carcinoma. *Cancer 83*:2043-2045

[105] Albo D, Tuszynski GP (2004) Thrombospondin-1 up-regulates tumor cell invasion through the urokinase plasminogen activator receptor in head and neck cancer cells. *J Surg Res 120*: 21-26.

[106] Rodriguez-Manzaneque JC, Lane TF, Ortega MA, Hynes RO, Lawler J, Iruela-Arispe ML (2001) Thrombospondin-1 suppresses spontaneous tumor growth and inhibits activation of matrix metalloproteinase-9 and mobilization of vascular endothelial growth factor. *Proc Natl Acad Sci USA 98*: 12485-12490

[107] Taraboletti G, Morbidelli L, Donnini S, Parenti A, Granger HJ, Giavazzi R, Ziche M (2000) The heparin binding 25kDa fragment of thrombospondin-1 promotes angiogenesis and modulates gelatinase and TIMP-2 production in endothelial cells. *FASEB J 14*: 1674-1676

[108] Soula-Rothhut M, Coissard C, Sartelet H, Boudot C, Bellon G, Martiny L, Rothhut B (2005) The tumor suppressor PTEN inhibits EGF-induced TSP-1 and TIMP-1 expression in FTC-133 thyroid carcinoma cells. *Exp Cell Res 304*: 187-201

In: Trends in Thyroid Cancer Research
Editor: Carl A. Milton, pp. 117-135
ISBN 1-59454-627-4

Chapter VI

TELOMERASE ACTIVITY IN THYROID NEOPLASMS

***E. Lerma*[3,*], *J. Mora*[1], *J. Prat*[3] *and A. de Leiva*[2]**
Departments of [1]Clinical Biochemistry, [2]Endocrinology and [3]Pathology,
Autonomous University, Hospital de la Santa Creu i Sant Pau, Barcelona, Spain.

ABSTRACT

In this chapter we will review the role of telomerase in carcinogenesis of thyroid and its potential aplication for the diagnosis of carcinomas. Human telomeres are composed of 5,000 to 15,000 base pairs, with a repeat sequence of TTAGGG. Their role is to protect the end of chromosomes. Under unknown circumstances, cells may become immortal by stabilizing the length of telomeres and this almost always occurs through the activation of telomerase. Telomerase is a ribonucleoprotein that adds the telomeric repeats onto the 3′end of chromosomes. It has two major components: the human telomerase RNA (hTR), which is present in all somatic cells as a template on which telomeric repeats are added to the chromosome, and the catalitic subunit called human telomerase reverse transcriptase (hTERT). Activity of Telomerase (TA) plays a major role in maintaining genetic integrity while the cells are in mitotic cycles and it is normally detected in germ cells, stem cells and lymphocytes. Also, TA has been demonstrated in neoplasms, mainly in those with endocrine differentiation, such as neoplasms of the thyroid, breast, prostate, parathyroid and adrenal gland. Our experience, in agreement with scientific literature, shows that around 50% of papillary carcinomas and 80% of follicular carcinomas had TA, whereas adenomas and other benign lesions rarely express TA. This result could be achieved in frozen tissue and also in material obtained by Fine Needle Aspirate (FNA) of thyroid. It is widely accepted that thyroid FNA is a useful tool in the screening of nodules for surgery, with sensitivity ranging from 65% to 99%, and specificity from 72% to100%. Nevertheless, 15-20% of FNAs are not diagnostic because the distinction

* Correspondence concerning this article should be addressed to Enrique Lerma, Department of Pathology, Hospital Santa Creu i Sant Pau. Avda. Sant Antonio Mª Claret, 167. 08025 Barcelona. Spain. Telf. 34-3-291.92.39 FAX: 34-3-291.93.44; E-mail: elerma@hsp.santpau.es.

between adenomatous nodules and follicular neoplasms could not be achieved. We attempted to determine whether TA could improve the sensitivity of cytology, mainly in this group of lesions with inconclusive cytological diagnosis, for a more accurate selection of patients before thyroidectomy.

1. Telomeres and Telomerase: An Overview

Telomeres are highly conserved structures located at the end of chromosomes for the preservation of the genome integrity. They are composed by repeat sequences of 6 bases, with predominance of G. Telomeres are very important during cell development, differentiation, proliferation and apoptosis of all species [1-6]. The repeated sequence of human telomeres is TTAGGG [2],and the lenght, genetically determined, range from 5000 to 15.000 base pairs [3]. In each división, telomeres are shortened between 50-200 base pairs [4]. The progressive shortering of telomeres in cell cultures induces, after 40-70 sucesive mitosis, the cellular senescence with a final crisis related with cell death [3,5]. The same process is expected to occurs in vivo and preservation of telomeres lenght seems very important to keep alive the tissues and organs. This telomere attrition could be also accelerated by environmental factor like oxidative stress [7].

Human telomeres are though to end in a large t-loop whose structure and stability may depend on a number of proteins, such as TRF1 and 2 (TRF = Telomere repeat factor), pot-1 (protein on telomeres 1), TIN2, RAP1. They are very important in the integrity of the double strand in the t-loop and in the regulation of the telomere length. Pot-1 is very important to telomere capping at the end of the loop. Other poly-ADP ribose polymerases, such as TANK1 and 2, may be associated with the telomere by interaction with TRF1 and 2; Rad 50 interacts with TRF2; and Ku form complexes with TRF1. All these proteins protect telomeres from fusions and help in repair of DNA strands [8,9,10].

Telomerase is a DNA polymerase that add telomeric repeats onto the 3′end of chromosomes [4], and its activity is only present in germ cells, stem cells and lymphocytes as a normal event to maintain the genetic integrity while the cell is in mitosis [5,6,8]. Normaly, conventional DNA polymerases fail to replicate linear chromosome ends completely. Consequently, terminal base pairs of telomeric DNA are lost in each cell division, unless the existence of telomerase activity [6].

Two major components and several associate proteins are essential for the telomerase activity and they must be expressed and correctly assembled into a functional unit that is capable of adding 5'-TTAGGG-3' repeats to the end of a telomere. The first major component is the human telomerase RNA (hTR) which contains an 11 bp sequence that serves as a template on which telomeric repeats are added to the chromosome. The hTR is constitutively present in all somatic cells [11]. The second major component is the human telomerase reverse transcriptase (hTERT), a catalytic subunit that is only present in germ cells, stem cells and some lymphocytes, and that is neccesary to express the telomerase activity [11].

Under diverse circumstances, cells can become immortal and this should be associated with the stabilization of the telomere lenght, generally produce by the activation of the enzyme telomerase [8,12].

2. Telomerase in Human Neoplasia

Telomerase and genome instability: Loss of telomeric sequences or mutations of telomere binding proteins leads to genomic instability, which could alter cell homeostasis, producing, alternatively, the senescence or a cellular proliferation without control called neoplasia. Nevertheless, human senescent cells could overcome senescence, become immortal and finally to be transformed in neoplastic cells. There are two antagonic effects that would be important in the begining of neoplasia:

1. Telomere attrition: during early phases of tumorigenesis promotes aneuploidy and chromosomal aberrations such are "end to end fusions", "double strand breaks" and "genomic instabilities" which may facilitate the accumulation of mutations necessary to establish a transformed or neoplastic phenotype
2. Cell proliferation: requires the activation of telomerase to maintain the minimal length of telomeres necessary for cell division [6,9].

Presence of hTERT is necessary for telomerase activity and it was initially detected in approximately 85% of neoplasms, including samples from breast, prostate, lung, liver, pancreas, colon and endocrine neoplasias such as thyroid, parathyroid and adrenal glands [4,13].

Up-regulation of hTERT is actually considered a crucial step during tumorigenesis to allow immortalization of human cells and a very frequent alteration in most of neoplasias [14,15,16,17,18]. Well known causes of hTERT up-regulation are hormone stimulation, membrane receptors activation, deregulation of transcription factors and presence of viral DNA and proteins. Estrogens, progesterone and even androgens can induce hTERT transcription in several tumors; this effect can be represses by diverse nuclear hormone receptors including Vitamin D and retinoic acid. Dysregulated activity of two families of transcription factors (E-box binding proteins and ETS proteins) sometimes induced by membrane receptors such as EGF and HER-2-neu, can also stimulates hTERT production secondarily [16].

DNA from human papilloma virus (HPV) and hepatitis B virus (HBV) could be integrated in genes neighboring to the hTERT gene, inducing their up-regulation.

Viral proteins such are HPV- E6 could inhibit p53 and then, after c-Myc amplification, increase hTERT transcription. E1A protein from Adenovirus and latency associated nuclear antigen (LANA) of human herpes virus type 8 (HHV-8) could produce the same effect [16].

The promoter hypermethylation of a gene is usually associated with its inactivation and i.e. this mechanism in p16 is very frequent in most types of neoplasias [19]. Paradoxically, the promoter hypermethylation of hTERT could have a stimulative effect on cell growth [20]

Down regulation of hTERT could be produced by viral proteins such are HPV-E2, and oncoprotein Tax from HTL-1 virus, via E-boxes and Sp1. Among the tumor suppressor genes candidates for repression of hTERT are Wilms tumor supressor 1 (WT1), myeloid specific zinc finger protein 2 (MZF-2), p53 that form complexes with Sp1 and prevent their binding with hTERT, pRb which is recruited by E2F, TGFβ and others [16].

Alternative lengthening of telomeres (ALT): Another mechanisms of maintain telomeres length, that could be present in the scanty human tumors lacking telomerase activity, were described in mammalian and other organisms and even in human tumors. There were called "alternative lengthening of telomeres" (ALT) [21-25]. Among the agents that activate this ALT there are the oncogene c-myc, the integration of HBV near the TERT promoter [15] and infection of SV 40 virus (25], and some of these mechanisms have been also previously cited in relation of hTERT up-regulation.

Genetic experiments: Several genetic experiments have also confirmed the important role of hTERT in neoplasias. The introduction of hTERT gene into mortal human cells constitutively activates telomerase expresion [26] and, also, the cloning of the hTERT promoter [27-30] could facilitate the up-regulation of hTERT in tumor cells. In contrast, expression of inactive mutant hTERT in human cancer cell lines with previous telomerase activity undergo subsequent telomeric shortening and apoptosis [31]. Loss of hTERT, opposite to up-regulation of neoplasias, has been recently described as the cause of several diseases associated with accelerated aging such are diverse types of dyskeratosis congenital and ataxia telangiectasia. [32]. Other diseases related with aberrant DNA replication and indirectly related with telomere shortening are ataxia telangiectasia, Nijmegen breakage syndrome and Fanconi anemia [6].

All these observations support the notion that the immortalization of human cells by the up-regulation of *hTERT* is a crucial step during tumorigenesis. Therefore, the high levels of telomerase that are observed in most malignant human cells maintain telomere structure and length and prevent the activation of the senescence or crisis programs.

Surprisingly, neoplasias are not always associated with elongation of telomeres, as recently reviewed by Satyanarayana [15]. Probably, the telomerase activity has the role of elongate the telomere only enough to allow the continuous mitosis and indefinitive viability of neoplastic cells in association with other genetic changes.

Recently, there was defined a set of genetic alterations, sufficient to program the tumorigenic phenotype in most human cells: these alterations include telomerase activity to maintain the telomere length, inactivation of retinoblastoma and p53 tumor supressor pathways, and acquisition of a constutive mitogenic signal provided by RAS or by protein phosphatase 2A (PP2A) by ST from the SV40 virus [33].

3. Detection Procedures

They could be related with the detection of telomerase activity (TA) or with the identification of the telomerase ribonucleoprotein components: the human telomerase reverse transcriptase (hTERT), the integral template or human telomerase RNA (hTR), or with a number of additional proteins subunits and a large variety of proteins contributing to the assembly and maturation of the telomerase enzymatic complex.

3.1. Telomerase Activity Assays

The telomeric repeat amplification protocol (TRAP assay) described by Kim et al [8] has been the standard method of choice in detection of telomerase activity. Several techniques to assess telomerase activity have been developed, in order to improve detection, including quantitative methods.

3.1.1. Telomeric Repeat Amplification Protocol ((TRAP)

The TRAP general procedure is divided into three main steps that consist of an extension step, a PCR amplification and a detection of telomerase products. In the extension step, the telomerase from the cell or tissue lysate adds telomeric repeats to the telomerase substrate. The reaction is carried out in the presence of a DNA polimerase enzyme and nucleotides that may be radioactive or nonradioactive-labeled depending on the method used later in the detection procedure. Following the extension step, the substrate with the extended products is amplified by the polymerase chain reaction (PCR). Finally, the amplified products are detected either by radioactive or by nonradioactive methods that affects the estimate of telomerase activity. Thus an autoradiography mode of detection would provide a semiquantitative estimate of telomerase activity, but a colorimetric, fluorescent or quemiluminiscent reaction would provide a quantitative estimate. The extraction process is a crucial step as the amount of telomerase that can be extracted from cells or tissues affects the estimation of enzyme activity. Suitable lysing agents described are CHAPS, NP-40 and sodium deoxicholate. The presence of RNases in lysates would degrade the template (hTR) of the enzyme whereas the PCR inhibitors would affect the amplification process. The combinatorial use of buffers replaces the dilution of PCR inhibitors by reextraction steps. Most extraction procedures use RNase inhibitors to minimize the possibility of hTR degradation. If the tissues or lysates are not rapidly frozen, RNA can be completely degraded at the time of extraction or tissue handling. The choice of the method needs to be based on the source and the quality of the sample [34].

3.1.2. PAGE-TRAP

The conventional TRAP is suitable for telomerase detection, but its application to large-scale screening is not very practical due to the radioactive/nonradioactive silver staining, phosphoroimaging or fluoroimaging polyacrylamide gel electrophoresis, which can be time consuming [35]. The gel-based methods are affected by excessive amounts of sample used, the presence of cells other than tumor cells and the presence of inhibitory substances in tumor samples as hemoglobin. In a hemorrhagic specimen, a band of approximately 45 bp could be observed and this was not consistent with the typical 6-bp DNA ladder pattern produced by telomerase [36]. However the use of an internal control allow to suspect false-negatives results [37,38]. In order to minimized false negative results due to the presence of a small percentage of telomerase-positive cells in the environment of large amounts of telomerase-negative cells, a magnetic bead retrieval assay has been described. This method consists of the isolation of the extended products by magnetic beads before PCR amplification. The extended products are treated with a biotinylated primer and are separated from nonbiotinylated products by the streptavidin-coated magnetic beads. This method is suitable for the detection of a subpopulation of cells present in small numbers and could be in association with standard TRAP or ELISA-TRAP, enhancing the specificity and the sensitivity of both assays [34].

3.1.3. ELISA-TRAP

A telomerase assay that replaces the electrophoretic step with an ELISA detection system has been described. In this assay the detection of the products are colorimetrically, which provides a semiquantitative estimate of telomerase activity. The telomeric repeats are added to a biotinylated substrate by the telomerase present in the sample, and the extended biotinylated substrate is amplified by PCR. The optimal concentration of protein lysate ranged between 1-3 μg/uL of total protein. The amplification products are denatured, hybridized with a digoxigenin-labeled probe and immobilized on microtiter plates by streptavidin-biotin binding. The complex is treated with a secondary antibody (anti-digoxigenin-conjugated horseradish peroxidase) and after the addition of TMB, absorbance was measured at 450nm with a reference wavelength at 690nm. Samples are regarded as telomerase positives if the difference in absorbance after subtracting the readings of negative controls is higher than 0.2. In comparison with conventional TRAP it is more sensitive and relatively quick, it offers a more quantitative estimate of telomerase activity and it is less affected by the presence of telomerase-negative cells and interfering substances as hemoglobin. However, the lack of an internal control makes it more vulnerable to false-negatives. Samples with atypical electrophoretic patterns should also be tested with ELISA-TRAP assay. When possible it is best to avoid mixed cell populations, because of the potential masking of telomerase expressing tumor cells from the presence of large population of normal cells and the potential contamination of TA from activated lymphocytes [36,39].

3.1.4. RTQ-TRAP

This method is a combination of standard TRAP with real-time PCR and was designed to avoid the deficiencies of conventional PCR. The amplified products generated by PCR are measured exponentially by the intensity of fluorescence. The fluorescence detection of the telomerase products with SYBR Green dye, which is capable of binding to the double-stranded amplicons and generating fluoresence, makes the assay reliable, safe and quantitative [40]. RTQ-TRAP appears to be the method of choice because of its accuracy, sensitivity, speed and reproducibility. One of the major advantages of the RTQ-TRAP is that measurement of the PCR products are performed at the early phase of exponential amplification, when reaction components are not limiting and the accumulation of inhibitory PCR products is unlikely to occur and the chances of primer-dimer formation is reduced. Besides, signals generated by primer-dimers differ from the real amplification products. This ensure the accuracy of the quantification of telomerase activity and prevents potential variations associated with the end-point assay in the conventional TRAP assay. Moreover, RTQ-TRAP is applicable for large-scale detection of telomerase activity [39,41].

3.2. Detection Of Catalytic Subunit Of Telomerase, hTERT

The advantages and limitations of various techniques involved in the detection of telomerase activity have shown that the source and quality of the sample plays an important role in the detection [34]. The expression of telomerase is a direct reflection of the physical association and functional activity of its subunits. hTERT is the catalytic subunit and its expression and upregulation in most cases positively correlates with telomerase activity. The close relationship between hTERT expression and telomerase activity suggests that quantification of the expression of the hTERT gene may be use as an alternative to telomerase activity measurement. hTERT can be detected by in situ hybridization, immunofluorescence-based flow cytometry, reverse-transcriptase polymerase chain reaction (RT-PCR) or a combination of these methods.

3.2.1. In Situ Hybridization

Analysis of telomerase activity measures the activity of telomerase in all cells present in a tumor tissue and represents the collective activity whereas the in situ hybridization produces more specific signals and allows the direct assessment of distribution patterns of the specific mRNA or protein among the different cell types. The most suitable probes that hybridize to the mRNA of interest are small synthetic oligonucleotides that can easily enter the cell for hybridization. The probes are end-labeled either with digoxigenin, biotin, or radioactive isotopes. Digoxigenin-labeled probes offer a high detection with low background signal. Detection of hTERT is therefore a useful marker for identifying cell types and hTERT expression may be used in determining the prognosis of cancer [42].

3.2.2. Immunofluorescence-Based flow Cytometry

In this assay a direct assessment of hTERT expression is provided in a subpopulation of cells without cell disruption. The first step in analyzing the cell types expressing hTERT would be to separate the cells by type from the mixed population using different methods. Kits for the magnetic activating cell sorting are commercially available. Sorted cells are stained with specific antibodies for hTERT. The stained cells are analyzed by flow cytometry, which enables simultaneous identification of the cell type and subunit expression. An elevated level of hTERT expression in tumors could indicate a poor prognosis. The fluorescent values obtained correlate well with telomerase activity.

The detection of hTERT by flow cytometry enables detection of the protein in a subpopulation of cells without disturbing the integrity of the cells [43].

3.2.3. Reverse Transcriptase-Polymerase Chain Reaction (RT-PCR) Detection of hTERT

In RT-PCR assay, RNA extraction is done by disruption of cells, by guanidium isothiocyanate extraction, or by tri-reagent protocol. The isolate RNA is treated with DNase and a fraction is used to reverse transcribe cDNA. Finally, the cDNA is amplified by specific primers either by standard PCR or by quantitative PCR (RTQ-PCR) [38,42]. Because the real time assay only needs a fragment of the hTERT mRNA, it is probably less sensitive than telomerase activity to the presence of RNases. Moreover, it is insensitive to proteases and protein inhibitors [44]. Based on this quantitative detection assay, automated systems have been described which allows for large-scale detection in clinical samples [45].

3.3. Discrepancy between Telomerase Activity and hTERT Expression

Because the telomerase activity assays needs the functional ribonucleoprotein, the presence of protein activity inhibitors, proteases, or RNases in an aggressive medium may complicate detection and subsequently lower sensitivity. To measure telomerase activity, all telomerase components (hTERT and hTR) must be expressed and correctly assembled into functional unit [46]. The quality of the RNA template (hTR) affects telomerase activity; thus, if the hTR is degraded telomerase activity is negative. If the hTR is partially degraded and the crucial regions for binding are not affected enzyme activity will be observed. RNases present in the lysates of tissue samples will degrade hTR, giving false-negative results for enzyme activity. RNA component is also degraded if the samples are not rapidly frozen. These false negatives may also be due to inadequate cellular material and /or protein concentration and that the number of cells required for a positive result with telomerase activity assay is higher than those required for hTERT expression [38]. Also, it has been demonstrated that premalignant lesions and some normal cells may exhibit hTERT gene expression [47]. Some authors found a high level of concordance between in situ telomerase activity results and hTERT expression, showing a heterogeneity of telomerase activity within the tumor tissue [39]. In discordant samples where the hTERT expression was negative and the telomerase activity positive a posttranscriptional modification of the subunit has been appointed; some of these discrepancies may be attibuted to differential splicing of hTERT mRNA [45,48,49].

4. Clinical Utility of Telomerase Activity in Carcinoma: Diagnosis and Treatment

Clinically, a trend for the search of less invasive and more cost-effective method for cancer diagnosis is clearly established. Nevertheless, morphological criteria for cancer diagnosis are, in general, more objective than molecular markers.

Telomerase can be detected in almost all kind of carcinomas with a high positive rate. In some instances, Telomerase Activity could even be detected in preneoplastic or in situ lesions,; then, it would be a useful tool for early detection of cancer, specially in cytology samples including pleural fluid [50], bronchial washing [51], urine washing [52,53] and material obtained by fine needle aspiration (FNA) from diverse organ such are breast [54,55] or thyroid as we will discuss later.

Several studies reviewed by Hyyama et al. [56] tried to demonstrate that telomerase activity or immunohistochemical expression of hTERT have a prognostic value and could be a way to determining appropriate treatments for patients with malignant tumors, but these results were not convincing and they are not commonly used in the routine clinical practice.

Many approaches have been assayed for telomerase inhibition trying to control the cell cancer growth, once established the role of the telomerase in the carcinogenesis [57-60].

Initially, several drugs were used to attack directly the telomeres, such is ethidium bromide and related compounds. Today, other antineoplasic mechanisms in investigation are:

Antisense oligodeoxynucleotides consist in short stretches of DNA that are complementary to a target RNA inhibiting the translation of mRNA by active o passive mechanisms.

Use of hammerhead ribozymes, small RNA molecules with specific endoribonuclease activity, could reduce the telomerase activity, al least temporarily.

Inhibition of hTERT by introduction of cDNA that contains point mutations in the reverse transcriptase motifs of hTERT. This inactive product would also sequester hTR.

Reverse transcriptase inhibitors, such is the AZT used in HIV treatment, have also be used for inhibit hTERT with non conclusive results.

Immunotherapy against proteins located in hTERT have also be used in experimentation.

Small molecules inhibitors, obtained by bioinformatic approaches.

Targets for active sites, such as for the aspartic triad in active hTERT subunit,

Substances that fold the telomeric repeats at and close to the 3′end into a higher DNA structures such are quadruplex. This later way could theoretically inhibit telomerase activity and the alternative elongation of telomeres.

Even more or less promising results, today all these strategies are not applied in the routine oncologic treatments.

5. Results: Telomerase Activity in Thyroid Fine Needle Aspirates

In our laboratories, adequate material had been obtained by fine needle aspiration (FNA) from palpable thyroid nodules in two hundred and sixty seven patients. This material had been processed for conventional cytological studies for TA study. All cases have been followed for 1 to 4 years and the patients with suspicious or positive FNA underwent a total thyroidectomy or lobectomy and isthmusectomy for pathological studies of nodules. Material for TA was obtained after smearing. Briefly, a needle-washing with 2-3 cc of normal saline solution was transferred to microcentrifuge tubes and stored at –70°C for TA analysis. The concentration of protein in each lysate was measured by the Coomassie Brilliant Blue method® (Bio-Rad). Telomerase activity was analyzed by the Telomerase PCR ELISA® (Roche Diagnostics), a method based on the original telomere repeat amplification protocol (TRAP), first described by Kim et al [8]with nonradioactive detection. The TRAP-ELISA method is a PCR-based assay, with a colorimetrical detection of the products.

Cytological diagnosis were positive for malignant tumor cells in 8 cases (confirmed histologically) and TA was positive in 50 % of them.

Diagnosis of follicular cell proliferation suspicious for malignancy was done in 36 cases Five of them were excluded because the presence of lymphoid infiltrate, that would produce a false positive TA determination. The aspirates of the remaining 31 patients with a FNA suspicious for follicular cell tumor constitutes the core of this paper. The histopathological diagnosis of these thyroid lesions were nodular hyperplasia in 16 cases, follicular adenoma in

4, follicular carcinoma in 1, and papillary carcinoma in 10 (Table 1). TA were detected in only one follicular adenoma and three papillary carcinomas.

Table 1. Results of TA in suspicious FNA.

Pathological diagnosis	№	Telomerase Activity +
Hyperplasic nodules	16	0
Follicular adenomas	4	1
Follicular carcinomas	1	0
Papillary carcinomas	10	3

The remaining FNA were negative for malignant tumor cells in the cytology and also telomerase activity was never detected when lymphoid infiltrate was absent.

In conclusion, the detection of TA helped to confirm a neoplasia in 4 of 31 (13%) suspicious thyroid nodules. Although less sensitive than FNA, TA specificity was 100% for neoplasia when cases with lymphoid infiltrate in the cytological smears were excluded. The sensitivity of thyroid FNA increased with the use of TA detection when cytology was non-conclusive for malignancy.

6. Discussion: Telomerase Activity Detection as an Ancillary Tool of FNA in Thyroid Neoplasias

Thyroid carcinomas are fairly uncommon and include disease types that range from indolent localized papillary carcinoma, with a survival rate up to 90%, to the anaplastic carcinoma, with a survival rate of 13% [61,62]. The clinical management of patients with thyroid nodules suspicious of neoplasia present a challenge; only 10-15% of them will be neoplastic, whereas the remaining would have undergo an unnecessary operation. Fine needle aspiration (FNA) cytology of the thyroid gland is widely accepted as a tool in the screening of nodules for surgery, with a sensitivity range from 65% to 99% and a specificity from 72% to100% [63-67]. Based on FNA, up to 60% of the nodules may be diagnosed accurately as benign, sparing unnecessary surgery [68-71], but there is a 10-15% of cases with certain follicular proliferation in which cytological diagnosis is no conclusive [72,73]. Besides cytological diagnosis, there are a considerable number of factors to be considered before surgery, such are cytological diagnosis, size of lesion, studies of thyroid function, CT scans and ultrasonography [72,73]. Furthermore, there are numerous attempts to identify the molecular alterations in thyroid carcinogenesis that could be used as potential markers to improve the cytological diagnosis of thyroid nodules, including thyroid stimulating hormonal receptor (TSHR), thyroglobulin, galectins, thyroid peroxidase, ciclooxigenases, copper and iron binding glipoproteins, serine proteases from cell membrane, intermediate filaments, beta-catenine, tirosin kinases, transcription factors, suppressor genes as PTEN, other nuclear proteins and telomerase [74-76].

Table 2. Telomerase in thyroid nodules (FNA material).

Authors	Method	Papil Carc	Folic Carc	Total Malignancy	Adenoma	Goiter (*)
Aogi et al 1998 [73]	TRAP-PCR	N/A	N/A	6/8	N/A	4/48
Sabesta et al 2001 [85]	TRAP-PCR	N/A	N/A	3/5	N/A	9/14 ¿?
Kamori et al 2003 [78]	TRAP-PCR & FISH	N/A	6/6	6/6	5/15	N/A
Trulsson et al 2003 [87]	TRAP-PCR	4/11	2/5	6/16	0/15	0/15
Mora et al 2004 [82]	TRAP-PCR	2/7	N/A	4/9	0/1	0/57
TOTAL	**TRAP-PCR**			**25/44 (56.8%)**	**5/31 (16.1%)**	**4/120 (3.3%)**
Saji et al 1999 [38]	RT-PCR	7/13	6/6	13/19	2/7	3/11
Zieger et al 1999 [91]	RT-PCR	8/8	5/6	13/14	1/5	0/5
Siddiqui et al 2001 [86]	RT-PCR	11/18	5/6	16/24	3/8	2/7
Liou et al 2003 [79]	RT-PCR	8/8	5/6	13/14	3/6	3/6
Umbrich etal 2004**[89]	RT-PCR	N/A	N/A	42/47	7/19	2/24
TOTAL	**RT-PCR**			**97/118 (82.2%)**	**16/45 (35%)**	**10/53 (18.8%)**

(*) This group includes all non neoplastic nodules (Goiter, hiperplastic nodules and "normal tissue")
(**) Excluding cases with inflammation.
Malignancies includes follicular and papilar carcinomas, as well other rare neoplasms as medullary carcinomas, anaplastic carcinomas and lymphomas.
¿? Mix of 4 adenomas, thyroiditis and nodular goiter make data no valuable.

Telomerase activity in thyroid pathology have been repeteadly studied in material obtained by FNA or from frozen tumors, generally with TRAP-PCR or RT-PCR, but most of these studies include relatively few cases [38,77-95]. In a compilation of several papers and in our own experience, including material obtained by fine needle aspiration (FNA) and from frozen tumoral tissue, TA was detected in 52.3 % of papillary carcinomas, almost 80% of follicular carcinomas, and around 50% of other unfrequent thyroid neoplasias such are medulary carcinomas and anaplastic carcinomas. In contrast, less than 20% of follicular adenomas and less than 10% of other benign thyroid lesions express TA [86]. When this analysis is restricted to results from FNA material, there are several papers that can be classified (Table 2) in two groups: these using TRAP-PCR or variants [77,82,86,89,91], and those that utilizes TR-PCR [38, 83,90,93,95]. Each of the previously cited methods has pros and cons. By TRAP-PCR, mean sensitivity of TA for malignancy was not very high, of 56.8%, but only 16.1% of adenomas and 3.3% of hyperplasic nodules express TA. In contrast, RT-PCR has higher sensitivity for malignancy, but it is accompanied with a decreased specificity: TA was detected in a mean of 82.2% of malignancies, 35% of adenomas and in 18.8% of hyperplasic nodules.

Several authors question if TA determination is a real ancillary tool in the preoperative management of thyroid nodules, in combination with cytology, and the answer varies: Some of them [85,89,91] deny the utility of TA, but in their investigations all of them used the less sensitive method (TRAP-PCR), one of them do not have used FNA material, sensitivity of their study was very low (26%), and also they realizes the existence abundant false positive results, due to the presence of lymphocytes [85]; other study has a very high false positive rate in hyperplasic nodules [89], absolutely discordant with remaining papers of the literature, and the last one paper [91]has also a low sensitivity.

In contrast, others papers, in general with higher sensitivity for TA determination, either by TRAP-PCR of mostly RT-PCR and more accurate correlation with the cytological findings support the value of TA as an ancillary tool for cytological diagnosis of thyroid neoplasias [38,77,82,83,86,90,93,95], although it is restricted to cases of thyroid FNA with marked follicular proliferation in which cytological diagnosis is no conclusive [86,93].

Relationship between TA and the diverse categories of thyroid neoplasias would be described as follows:

1. Follicular carcinomas and adenomas: follicular carcinoma constitutes 25% of thyroid malignant neoplasms and citologically they are characterized by scanty colloid, crowding of cells with frequent formation of a microfollicular structures, variable atypia and prominent nucleoli; nevertheless, these features are not specific and do not appears in all cases. It makes frequently impossible the differentiation between follicular carcinomas, follicular adenomas and from hyperplasic nodules of goiters [92]. This diagnostic problem may occurs up to 15% of cytologies and it could be the principal utility for detection of telomerase activity, but with limited value due to a low specificity: TA can be detected in almost 80% follicular carcinomas but also in 10% of hyperplastic goiterous nodules, and 20% of adenomas, or even 30% by RT-PCR. In relation with the presence of TA in some adenomas, it should be stated that the differentiation between adenomas and carcinomas could be histologically impossible. Adenomas could be considered as carcinomas that have nor yet infiltrate capsule or metastasized. For all these reasons, TA could be considered a diagnostic help but only in correlation with the clinical impression and size of the nodule, and according to Umbrich et al [93], TA could be very useful as a negative predictor(87%) when tumors are smaller than 3 cm.

Hurthle cell neoplasia is a variant of follicular one, and have similar problems in cytological diagnostic [62,96]. The cytological differences with conventional follicular tumors are the presence larger cells with of abundant finely granular cytoplasm and nuclear enlargement with prominent nucleoli. Detection of TA occurs in a percentage almost equal than conventional follicular neoplasms (around 80%) and utility should be the same.

2. Papillary carcinoma is the most frequent malignant neoplasm of thyroid and constitutes approximately 70% of malignancies, including cases of the follicular variant of papillary carcinoma. The most important cytological criteria for diagnosis are presence of fronds and sheets of cells with intranuclear inclusions, nuclear grooves and psammoma bodies and these features allow the correct diagnosis in 90% of cases [96]. Other minor cytological criteria for diagnosis are presence of multinucleated cells, dense colloid and squamous metaplasia. Because TA was detected by TRAP-PCR only in half of these tumors [86], it was considered that this is not very useful method; nevertheless, the sensitivity for detect TA increases to the 90-94% of papillary carcinoma in a recent study with RT-PCR [93]. This finding gives new support to this use as an ancillary diagnostic tool when cytology is no conclusive for malignacy.

3. Other neoplasms: Detection of TA have been describe in other unfrequent thyroid neoplasms such are medullary carcinoma, anaplastic carcinoma or lymphomas. These tumors are so unfrequent than the experience collect is very scanty to obtain conclusion. Medullary carcinoma includes 5% of thyroid neoplasms and it is characterized by disperse cellularity with variable size and shape and granular cytoplasm; amiloid and calcitonin detection could help in diagnosis [96]. Calcitonin is much more specific that TA which is only expressed in half of medullary carcinomas [75,86].

One of the main causes of false positive TA in thyroid FNA is related with the presence of abundant lymphocytes, which constitutively express TA. Presence of TA in around 30% of follicular adenomas by RT-PCR [93] remains the main limitation for their use. As previously stated, positivity of some of these cases could be related with the presence of lymphoid infiltrate [85,86,93]. Also, it is well known that 10 to 46% of thyroid carcinomas may have lymphocytic infiltration [97,98], and abundance of normal lymphocytes can appears in benign process such are Hashimoto (lymphocytic) thyroiditis and Graves disease [38,87,88,94]. This would explain some of the false positives results when TA is considered alone, without FNA. Nevertheless, cytology has the advantage that lymphocytes can easily be differenciate from cells of the suspected epithelial neoplasia. Even more the posibility to deteminate TA in material from cytological smears, after destaining the samples, could help to precise if TA appears in lymphocytes or in other cells suspicious of a thyroid neoplasia as Siddiqui et al did [90].

In summary, TA can be studied in material obtained by FNA. We believe that TA could help to increase the sensitivity of thyroid FNA in cases of follicular cells proliferation with inconclusive cytological diagnosis.

REFERENCES

[1] Bekaert S, Derradji H, Baatout S. (2004). Telomere biology in mammalian germ cells and during development. *Developmental Biology 274*: 15-30.

[2] Morin GB. (1989) The human telomere terminal transferase enzyme is a ribonucleoprotein that synthesizes TTAGGG repeats. *Cell, 59:* 521-9.

[3] Holt SE, Shay JW. (1999) Role of telomerase in cellular proliferation and cancer *J Cell Physiol 180*: 10-18.

[4] White LK, Wright WE, Shay JW. (2001) Telomerase inhibitors. *Trends on Biotechnology 19*:114-120.

[5] Shay JW, Wright WE. (2001) Haylick, his limit, and cellular aging. *Nature Review: Mol Cell Biol 1*: 72-76.

[6] Harvey CB. (2002) Telomerase is not an oncogene. *Oncogene 21*:494-502.

[7] Von Zglinicki T, Pilger R, Sitte R. (2000) Accumulation of single-strand breaks is the major cause of telomere shortening in human fibroblast. *Free Radic Biol Med. 28*: 64-74.

[8] Kim NW, Piatyszek MA, Prowse KR, Harley CB, West MD, Ho PL, Coviello GM, Wright WE, Weinrich SL, Shay JW. (1994) Specific association of human telomerase activity with immortal cells and cancer. *Science 266*:2011-15.

[9] Kim SH, Kaminker P, Campisi J. (2002) Telomeres, aging and cancer: In search of a happy ending. *Oncogene 21*:503-511.

[10] Saldanha SN, Andrews LG, Tollefsbol TO. (2003) Assessment of telomere length and factors that contribute to its stability. *Eur J Biochem 270*:389-403.

[11] Feng J, Funk WD, Wang SS, Weinrich SL, Avilion AA, Chiu CP, Adams RR, Chang E, Allsopp RC, Yu J. (1995) The RNA component of human telomerase. *Science 269*.1236-41.

[12] Wright WE, Shay JW. (1992) The two-stage mechanism controlling cellular senescence and immortalization. *Exp Gerontol 27*:383-389.

[13] Shay JW and Bacchetti S. (1997) A survey of telomerase activity in human cancer. *Eur J Cancer 33*: 787-791.

[14] Orlando C, Gelmini S. (2001) Telomerase in endocrine and endocrine-dependent tumors. *J Steroid Biochem Moll Biol 78*: 201-14.

[15] Satyanarayana A, Manns MP, Rudolph KL. (2004) Telomeres and telomerase: A dual role in hepatocarcinogenesis. *Hepatology 40*:276-283.

[16] Janknecht R. (2004) On the road to immortality: hTERT upregulation in cancer cells. *FEBS letters 564*:9-13.

[17] Wong JM, Collins K. (2003) Telomere maintenance and disease. *Lancet 362*:983-988.

[18] Sharpless NE, DePinto RA. (2004) Telomeres, stem cells, senescence and cancer. *J Clin Invest 113*:160-168.

[19] Herman JG, Graff JR, Myohanen S, Nelkin BD, Baylin SB. (1996) Methylation-specific PCR: a novel PCR assay for methylation status of CpG islands. *Proc Natl Acad Sci U S A. 93*:9821-9826.

[20] Guilleret I, Yan P, Grange F, Braunschweig R, Bosman FT, Benhattar J. (2002) Hypermethylation of the human telomerase catalytic subunit (hTERT) gene correlates with telomerase activity. *Int J Cancer 101*:335-341.

[21] Prescott JC, Blackburn EH. Telomerase: DR Jekyll or Mr Hyde? (1999) *Curr Opin Genet Dev 9*:368-373.

[22] Bryan TM, Englezou A, Dalla-Pozza L et al. (1997) Evidence for an alternative mechanism for maintaining telomere lenght in human tumors and tumor-derived cell lines *Nature Med 3*:1271-1274.

[23] Colgin LM, Kaminker P, Campisi J. (1999) Telomere maintenance mechanisms and cellular inmortalization. *Curr Opin Genet Dev 9*:97-103.

[24] Stewart SA, Hahn WC, O'Connor BF, Banner EN, Lundberg AS, Modha P, Mizuno H, Brooks MW, Fleming M, Zimonjic DB, Popescu NC, Weinberg RA. (2002) Telomerase contributes to tumorigenesis by telomere lenght independent phenotype. *Proc Natl Acad Sci USA 99*:12606-12612.

[25] Scheel C, Poremba C. (2002) Telomere lengthening in telomerase-negative cells: the ends are coming together. *Virchows Arch 440*;573-582.

[26] Bodnar AG, Ouellette M, Frolkis M, Holt SE, Chiu CP, Morin GB, Harley CB, Shay JW, Lichtsteiner S, Wright WE. (1998) Extension of life span by introduction of telomerase into normal human cells. *Science 279*:349-352.

[27] Cong YS, Wen J, Bacchetti S. (1999) The human telomerase catalytic subunit hTERT: organization of the gene and characterization of the promoter. *Hum. Mol. Genet. 8*:137–142.

[28] Horikawa I, Cable PL, Afshari C, Barrett JC. (1999) Cloning and characterization of the promoter region of human telomerase reverse transcriptase gene. *Cancer Res. 59*:826–830.

[29] Takakura M, Kyo S, Kanaya T, Hirano H, Takeda J, Yutsudo M, Inoue M. (1999) Cloning of human telomerase catalytic subunit (hTERT) gene promoter and identification of proximal core promoter sequences essential for transcriptional activation in immortalized and cancer cells. *Cancer Res. 59*:551–557.

[30] Wick M, Zubov D, Hagen G. 1999) Genomic organization and promoter characterization of the gene encoding the human telomerase reverse transcriptase (hTERT). *Gene 232*:97–106.

[31] Hahn WC, Stewart SA, Brooks MW, York SG, Eaton E, Kurachi A, Beijersbergen RL, Knoll JH, Meyerson M, Weinberg RA. (1999) Inhibition of telomerase limits the growth of human cancer cells. *Nat Med 5*:1164-1170.

[32] Collins K, Mitchell JR. (2002) Telomerase in the human organism. Oncogene 21:564-579.

[33] Zhao JJ, RobertsTM, Hahn WC. (2004) Functional genetics and experimental models of human cancer. *Trends in molecular medicine 10*:344-350.

[34] Saldanha SN, Andrews LG, Tollefsbol TO. (2003) Analysis of telomerase activity and detection of its catalytic subunit, hTERT. *Anal Biochem 315*: 1-21.

[35] Nemos C, Remy-Martin JP, Adami P, Arbez-Gindre F, Schaal JP, Jouvenot M, Delage-Mourroux R. (2003) Improved TRAP-silver staining versus conventional radioactive TRAP assys: quantification of telomerase activity during immortalization and in pathological human endometrium. *Clin Biochem 36*: 621-628.

[36] Wu YY, Hruszkewycz AM, Delgado RM, Yang A, Vortmeyer AO, Moon YW, Weil RJ, Zhuang Z, Remaley AT. (2000) Limitations on the quantitative determination of telomerase activity by the electrophoretic and ELISA based TRAP assays. *Clin Chim Acta 293*: 199-212.

[37] Kim NW, Wu F. (1997) Advances in quantification and characterization of telomerase activity by the telomeric repeat amplification protocol (TRAP). *Nucleic Acids Res 25*: 2595-2597.

[38] Saji M, Xydas S, Westra WH, Liang CK, Clark DP, Udelsman R, Umbricht CB, Sukumar S, Zeiger MA. (1999) Human telomerase reverse transcriptase (hTERT) gene expression in thyroid neoplasms. *Clin Cancer Res 5*:1483-1489.

[39] Longchampt E, Lebret T, Molinie V, Bieche I, Botto H, Lidereau R. (2003) Detection of telomerase status by semiquantitative and in situ assays, and by real-time reverse transcription-polymerase chain reaction (telomerase reverse transcriptase) assay in bladder carcinomas. *BJU 91*: 567-572.

[40] Wege H, Chui MS, Le HT, Tran JM, Zern MA. (2003) SYBR Green real-time telomeric repeat amplification protocol for the rapid quantification of telomerase activity. *Nucleic Acids Research 31*: 1-7.

[41] Hou M, Xu D, Björkholm M, Gruber A. (2001) Real-time quantitative telomeric repeat amplification protocol assay for the detection of telomerase activity. *Clin Chem 47*: 519-524.

[42] Harada K, Yasoshima M, Ozaki S, Sanzen T, Nakanuma Y. (2001) PCR and in situ hybridization studies of telomerase subunits in human non-neoplastic livers. *J Pathol 193*: 210-217.

[43] Ali AS, Chopra R, Robertson J, Testa NG. (2000) Detection of hTERT protein by flow cytometry. *Leukemia 14*: 2176-2181.

[44] de Kok JB, Ruers TJ, van Muijen GN, van Bokhoven A, Willems HL, Swinkels DW. (2000) Real-Time Quantification of human telomerase reverse transcriptase mRNA in tumors and healthy tissues. *Clin Chem 46*: 313-318.

[45] Yu HP, Xu SQ, Lu WH, Li YY, Li F, Wang XL, Su YH. (2004) Telomerase activity and expression of telomerase genes in squamous dysplasia and squamous cell carcinoma of the esophagus. *J Surg Oncol 86*: 99-104.

[46] Hess JL, Highsmith E. (2002) Telomerase detection in body fluids. *Clin Chem 48*: 18-24.

[47] Kolquist KA, Ellisen LW, Counter CM, Meyerson M, Tan LK, Weinberg RA, Haber DA, Gerald WL. (1998) Expression of TERT in early premalignant lesions and a subset of cells in normal tissues. *Nat Genet 19*: 182-186.

[48] Malaska J, Kunicka Z, Borsky M, Sklenickova M, Novotna M, Fajkusova L, Zaloudik J, Fajkus J. (2004) Telomerase as a diagnostic and predictive marker in colorectal carcinoma. *Neoplasma 51*: 90-96.

[49] Kirkpatrick KL, Clark G, Ghilchick M, Newbold RF, Mokbel K. (2003) hTERT mRNA expression correlates with telomerase activity in human breast cancer. *Eur J Surg Oncol 29*: 321-326.

[50] Hiyama K, Hiyama E, Ishioka S, Yamakido M, Inai K, Gazdar AF, Piatyszek MA, Shay JW. (1995) Telomerase activity in small cell and non-small-cell lungh cancers. *J Natl Cancer Inst 87*: 895-902.

[51] Yahata N, Ohiyashiki K, Ohiyashiki JH, , Iwama H, Hayashi S, Ando K, Hirano T, Tsuchida T, Kato H, Shay JW, Toyama K. (1998) Telomerase activity in lung cancer cells obtained from bronchial washing. *J Natl Cancer Inst 90*:684-690.

[52] Yoshida K, Sugino T, Tahara H, Woodman A, Bolodeoku J, Nargund V, Fellows G, Goodison S, Tahara E, Tarin D. (1997) Telomerase activity in bladder carcinoma and

its implication for non invasive diagnosis by detection of exfoliated cancer cells in urine. *Cancer 79*:362-369.

[53] Kavaler E, Landman J, Chang Y, Droller MJ, Liu BC. (1998) Detecting human bladder carcinoma cells in voided urine samples by assaying for the presence of telomerase activity. *Cancer 82*:708-714.

[54] Sugino T, Yoshida K, Bolodeoku J, Tahara H, Buley I, Manek S, Wells C, Goodison S, Ide T, Suzuki T, Tahara E, Tarin D. (1996) Telomerase activity in human breast cancer and benign breast lesions: diagnostic applications in clinical specimens, including fine needle aspirates. *Int J Cancer 69*:301-306.

[55] Villa R, Zaffaroni N, Folini M, Martelli G, De Palo G, Daidone MG, Silvestrini R. (1998) Telomerase activity in benign and malignant breast lesions: a pilot prospective study on FNA. *J Natl Cancer Inst 90*:537-539.

[56] 56.Hiyama E, Hiyama K. (2002) Clinical utility of telomerase in cancer. *Oncogene 21*: 643-649.

[57] Neidle S Parkinson G. (2002) Telomere maintenance as a target for anticancer drug discovery. *Nature Reviews 1*: 383-393.

[58] White LK, Wright WE, Shay JW. (2001) Telomerase inhibitors. *TRENDS in biotechnology. 19*:114-120.

[59] Palumbo M. (2004) Anticancer agents: towards the future. *Curr Med Chem Anti-Canc Agents. 4*: 425-427.

[60] Chang JY. (2004) Telomerase: A potential molecular marker and therapeutic target for cancer. *J Surg Oncol 87*: 1-3.

[61] Sherman SI. (2003) Thyroid carcinoma. *Lancet 361*: 501-511.

[62] Endocrine neoplasms (2004) WHO Lyon .

[63] Akerman M, Tennvall J, Bioklund A, Mastersson H, Moller T. (1985) Sensitivity and specificity of fine needle aspiration cytology in the diagnosis of tumors of the thyroid gland. *Acta Cytol 29*:850-855.

[64] Bakhos R, Selvaggi SM, DeJong S, Gordon DL, Pitale SU, Herrmann M, Woijcik EM. (2000) Fine needle aspiration of the thyroid: rates and causes of cytohistopathologic discordance. *Diagn Cytopathol 23*:233-237

[65] Caraway NP, Sneige N, Samaan NA. (1993) Diagnostic pitfall in thyroid fine-needle aspiration: a review of 394 cases. *Diagn Cytopathol 9*:345-350.

[66] Ravetto C, Colombo L, Dottorini ME. (2000) Usefulness of fine needle aspiartion in the thyroid carcinoma. A retrospective study of 37.895 patients. *Cancer 90*:357-363.

[67] Sidawy MK, Del Vecchio DM, Knoll SM. (1997) Fine needle aspiration of thyroid nodules: correlation between cytology and histology and evaluation of discrepant cases. *Cancer 81*:253-259.

[68] Gharib H, Goellner JR. (1993) Fine needle aspiration cytology of the thyroid. An appraisal *Ann Inter Med 118*: 282-289.

[69] Lowhagen T, Granberg PO, Lundell G, Skinnari P, Sundblad R, Willems JS. (1979) Aspiration biopsy cytology (ABC) in nodules of the thyroid gland suspected to be malignant. *Surg Clin N Am 59*:3-18.

[70] Willems JS, Lowhagen T. (1981) Fine needle aspiration cytology in thyroid diseases. *Clin Endocrinol Metab 10*:247-266.

[71] Willems JS, Lowhagen T. (1981) The role of fine needle aspiration cytology in the management of thyroid diseases. *Clin Endocrinol Metab 10*:267-273.

[72] Schlinkert RT, Van Heerden JA, Goellner JR et al. (1997). Factors that predict malignant thyroid lesions when fine-needle aspiration is "suspicious for follicular neoplasm". *Mayo Clin Proc 72*:913-916.

[73] Baloch ZW, Fleisher S, Li Volsi VA, Gupta PK. (2002) Diagnosis of "follicular neoplasm": a gray zone in thyroid fine-needle aspiration cytology. *Diagn Cytopathol 26*:41-44

[74] Segev D, Clark DP, Zieger M, Umbricht C. (2003) Beyond the Suspicious Thyroid Fine Neddle Aspirate. *Acta Cytol. 47*:709-722.

[75] Alvarez-Nuñez F, Mora J, Matias-Guiu X y grupo de estudio de marcadores tumorales de neoplasias tiroideas, hospital de Sant Pau. Carcinoma tiroideo del epitelio folicular: marcadores tumorales y oncogenes. *Med Clin (Barc)* 2003; 121:264-9.

[76] Segev D, Umbrich C, Zieger M. (2003) Molecular patogénesis of thyroid cancer. *Surg Oncol 12*: 69-90.

[77] Aogi K, Kitahara K, Buley M, Backdahl M, Tahara H, Sugino T, Tarin D, Goodison S.(1998) Telomerase activity in lesions of thyroid: application to diagnosis of clinical samples including fine needle aspirates. *Clin Cancer Res 4*: 1965-70.

[78] Aogi K, Kitahara K, Urquidi V, Backdahl M, Tahara H, Sugino T, Tarin D, Goodison S. (1999) Comparison of telomerase and CD 44 expression as diagnostic tumor markers in lesions of the thyroid. *Clin Cancer Res 5*: 2790-2797.

[79] Brousset P, Chaouche N, Leprat F, Branet-Brousset F, Trouette H, Zenou RC, Merlio JP, Delsol G. (1997) Telomerase activity in human thyroid carcinomas originating from follicular cells. *J Clin Endocrinol Metab 82*:4214-4216.

[80] Cheng AJ, Lin JD, Chang T et al. (1998) Telomerase activity in benign and malignant thyroid diseases. *Br J Cancer 77*: 2177-2180.

[81] Haugen BR, Nawaz S, Markham N, Hashizumi T, Shroyer AL, Werness B, Shroyer KR. (1997) Telomerase activity in benig and malignant thyroid tumors. *Thyroid 7*: 337-342.

[82] Kammori M, Takubo K, Nakamura K. (2000) Telomerase activity and telomere lenght in benign and malignant human thyroid tissues. *Cancer Lett 159*:175-181.

[83] Liou MJ; Chan EC; Lin JD; Liu FH; Chao TC. (2003) Human telomerase reverse transcriptase (hTERT) gene expression in FNA samples from thyroid neoplasms. *Cancer Lett 191*:223-227.

[84] Lo CY, Lam KY, Chan KT, Luk JM. (1999) Telomerase activity in thyroid malignancy. *Thyroid 9*: 1215-1220.

[85] MatthewsP, Jones CJ, Skinner J, Haughton M, de Micco C, Wynford-Thomas D. (2001) Telomerase activity and telomere length in thyrois neoplasia: biological and clinical implications. *J Pathol 194*:183-193.

[86] Mora J, Lerma E and Thyroid Study Group. (2004) Telomerase Activity in Thiroid Fine Needle Aspiration. *Acta Cytol 48*:818-824.

[87] Okayasu I, Osakabe T, Fujiwara M, Fukuda H, Kato M, Oshimura M.. (1997) Significant correlation of telomerase activity in thyroid papillary carcinoma with cell differentiation, proliferation and extrathyroid extension. *Jpn J Cancer Res 88*:965-970.

[88] Saji M, Westra WH, Chen H, Umbricht CB, Tuttle RM, Box MF, Udelsman R, Sukumar S, Zeiger MA. (1997) Telomerase activity in the differential diagnosis of papillary carcinoma of the thyroid. *Surgery 122*:1137-1140.

[89] Sebesta J, Brown T, Williard W, Dehart MJ, Aldous W, Kavolius J, Azarow K. (2001) Does telomerase activity add to the value of fine needle aspiration in evaluating thyroid nodules?. *Am J Surg. 181*:420-422.

[90] Siddiqui MT, Greene KL, Clark DP, Xydas S, Udelsman R, Smallridge RC, Zieger MA, Saji M. (2001) Human telomerase reverse transcriptase expression in Diff-Quik stained FNA samples from thyroid nodules. *Diag Mol Pathol 10*:123-129.

[91] Trulsson LM, Velin AK, Herder A, Söderkvist P, Rüter A, Smeds S. (2003) Telomerase activity in surgical specimens and fine needle aspiration biopsies from hyperplastic and neoplastic human thyroid tissues. *Am J Surg 186*:83-88.

[92] Umbricht CB, Saji M, Westra WH, Udelsman R, Zeiger MA, Sukumar S. (1997) Telomerase activity: a marker to distinguish follicular thyroid adenoma from carcinoma. *Cancer Res 57*:2144-2147.

[93] Umbricht CB, Conrad GT, Clark DP, Westra WH, Smith DC, Zahurak M, Saji M, Smallridge RC, Goodman S and Zeiger MA. (2004) Human Telomerase Reverse Transcriptase Gene Expression and the Surgical Management of Suspicious Thyroid Tumors. *Clinical Cancer Research 10*:5762-5768

[94] Yashima K, Vuitch F, Gazdar AF, Fahey TJ. (1997) Telomerase activity in benign and malignant thyroid diseases. *Surgery 122*: 1141-1145.

[95] Zieger MA, Smallridge RC, Clark DP, Liang CK, Carty SE, Watson CG, Udelsman R, Saji M. (1999) Human telomerase reverse transcriptase gene expression in FNA samples from thyroid neoplasms. *Surgery 126*:1195-1199.

[96] Gray W, Mckee GT. Diagnostic cytopathology (2 ed.) Churchill Livingstone. London 2003.Pp.577-601.

[97] Hirabayashi RN, Linsday S. (1965) The relation of thyroid carcinoma and cronic thyroiditis. *Surg Gynecol Obstet 121*:243-252.

[98] Walker RP, Paloyan E. (1990) The relationship between Hashimoto´s thyroiditis, thyroid neoplasia and primary hyperparathyroidism. *Otolaryngol Clin North Am 23*:291-302.

In: Trends in Thyroid Cancer Research
Editor: Carl A. Milton, pp. 137-153
ISBN 1-59454-627-4

Chapter VII

MALIGNANCES IN SOLITARY THYROID GLAND NODULES: DIAGNOSTIC AND SURGICAL TREATMENT

Dragos Lj. Stojanovic[1]*, Zorica V. Caparevic[2], Predrag D. Stevanovic[3], Mirjana M. Stojanovic[4], Branislav Lj. Dakovic[1], Ivan R. Paunovic[1], Dragan L. Radovanovic[1] and Lalosevic J. Djordje[4]

[1]University Clinic for General Surgery, Department of Endocrine Surgery,
[2]University Clinic for Internal Medicine, Department of Endocrinology,
[3]University Clinic for General Surgery, Department of Anestesiology,
[4]Clinical Hospital Centre, Department of Radiology,
University of Belgrade, 11050 Belgrade, Serbia and Montenegro.

ABSTRACT

Malignant alterations in thyroid gland, especially carcinoma, can occur in solitary nodules, diffuse enlarged gland or in gland with multiple nodules, and they are of special interest in diagnosis and treatment because of uncertain clinical evaluation as well as their frequency and malignant potential.

Finding of malignances in solitary thyroid gland nodules represent an entity itself in thyroid surgery and endocrinology because of frequency in occurrence and differential diagnosis of thyroid diseases.

* Correspondence concerning this article should be addressed to Dr. Dragos Lj. Stojanovic, assistant professor Clinical Hospital «Dr Dragisa Misovic» - Dedinje, University Clinic for General Surgery, Department of Endocrine Surgery, School of Medicine, University of Belgrade, H.M. Tepica 1, 11050 Belgrade, Serbia and Montenegro. Tel.: +381 11 3442 693; +381 63 244 004; Fax: +381 11 3086 984; E-mail: dragoss@net.yu.

Similarities in clinical characteristics and differences in the histological structure and development of the disease, request quick and adequate application of all available diagnostic procedures in evaluation of disease.
After all clinic methods of examination, surgery includes necessary range of extraction of tissue at benign changes while at malignant changes radical intervention of the gland is suggested and if it is necessary on the surrounding structures of the neck.
"Biopsio Ex Tempore" still represents vital method in histological diagnosis and help in making decision about extensiveness of operative procedure.
Because of that, surgery represents both a diagnostic and therapeutic procedure.
Data analysis shows the presence of carcinoma in solitary thyroid gland nodules in 15% of all cases.
The aim of this study is to point out validity of diagnostic procedures, frequency of occurrence and types of changes as well as principles in treatment of thyroid gland carcinoma with emphasis on solitary nodules where carcinoma is the most frequent.

Keywords: carcinoma, solitary nodule, thyroid gland.

INTRODUCTION

Malignant alterations in thyroid gland, especially carcinoma, can occur within solitary nodular lesions, diffuse enlarged gland or in gland with multiple nodules and are of special interest in diagnosis and treatment because of uncertain clinical evaluation, as well as their frequency and malignant potential. They account for about 1% of all malignant tumors in human population. [2,6,9,18,20,26,29,35,40,51,57,67,69,72]

Solitary nodules are clinical orientation for asymmetric range of tumor growth within normal or pathologically altered thyroid gland. Frequency of diagnosed solitary nodules shows lately a permanent increase both because of an increasing number of the diseased and because of advancement of diagnostic methods of examinations and more adequate plan of selection of thyroid gland alterations. Solitary thyroid gland nodules are present in about 1% of the general population, while in the regions with endemic struma they are present in as much as up to 50% of the mentioned population. They are three to six times more frequent in females than in males. [2,6,7,9,17,24,29,35,40,44,51,57,63,67,69,72]

Clinical presentation of solitary thyroid gland nodular lesions in the tissue structure (as per sequence of frequency) takes most frequently the following forms:

1. Solitary solid adenoma,
2. Cyst,
3. Carcinoma,
4. Hyperfunctional adenoma,
5. Hashimoto's thyroiditis,
6. Riedel's thyroiditis [6,7,10,34,35,40,51,57,61,67,69]

Malignances have been described in all forms of pathologically altered thyroid gland, thus there are no specific thyroid gland conditions that exclude them. Here, we can only speak about thyroid gland alterations with lower or higher malignance incidence. According to studies conducted so far, it is uncontestable that solitary nodules are the most frequent site of carcinoma in thyroid gland (4–23 %). [6,7,10,18,20,26,29,34,35,40,51,57,61,67,69]

Malignant tumors most frequently found in thyroid gland tissue belong mostly to the class of well-differentiated neoplastic alterations having lower level of malignant potential:

- Papillary carcinomas (occult, intrathyroid, and extrathyroid);
- Follicular carcinomas (with minimum and/or marked capsular invasion). [2,4,5,7,12,15,18,23,26,27,29,30-32,38,43,47,51,55,58,59,61,64,74]

Less frequent forms of neoplastic alterations with more marked level of malignant potential include the following:

- Hurthle cell carcinoma;
- Medullary carcinoma;
- Anaplastic carcinoma;
- Lymphoma;
- Metastatic tumors. [6,7,10,11,22,26-29,33-35,39,40,45,46,49,51,57,61,65,68]

Although not much knowledge is available about thyroid gland malignance etiopathogenesis, like the other malignant tumors in human population, based on the results of studies conducted so far, certain factors and conditions have been established that contribute to carcinogenesis, so risk groups associated with them have been defined accordingly for thyroid malignance:

1. Group of patients with previous history of low-dose irradiations of the head and neck regions; [1,13,17,20,44,53,60]
2. Group of patients from the population with iodine deficiency, through negative hormonal «feed back» mechanism; [2,20,72]
3. Genetic predisposal (family history); [7,17,20,28,33,44,45,49,72]
4. Sudden alterations and fast growth in the clinical status. [9,20]

Diagnosis of a large number of alterations in solitary thyroid gland nodules, particularly when being aware that the malignance incidence in them is high, requires application of a large number of diagnostic methods and studies:

- Anamnesis, includes knowledge about specific diseases and surgeries on the thyroid gland, association of the thyroid with other systemic diseases, data on possible irradiation of the head and neck regions, general symptoms, gender, and age group. Knowledge about time of occurrence of the developed changes is also important, as well as the growth progressivity and development of local symptoms. [1,7,9,13,17,26,53,60]
- Epidemiological survey, about place of birth, residence, profession practiced by the patient, as well as family history of the disease. [7,9,17,26,44]
- Physical finding, with presence of systemic changes (close and distant), syndromes and signs, as well as findings of local alterations in the thyroid gland itself and in the local regions. [7,9,26,62]

- Laboratory analyses, blood count and biochemical findings, urine, specific hormonal status, antithyroid antibodies, calcitonin immunohistochemical tests, carcinoembryonic antigen markers, etc. [7,9,26,28,49,54,56]

- Laryngoscopy, direct and indirect, for evaluation of vocal cords status, because of possible development of their paresis or paralysis, both in diagnosis and evaluation of the level of local invasion, as idirect signs of the expansion of pathological process. [7,9,26,62]

- X-ray diagnosis of the thyroid gland (Ro), (localization, relations and repercussions for surrounding structures), the neck organs (because of possible dislocation or infiltration of the neck organs by expansive process, with dysphagic, dyspneic and circulatory complications), the thorax (retrosternal or intrathoracic localization of a part of or entire thyroid gland), the lungs (due to possible finding of metastatic alterations). [7,9,26]

- Ultrasound diagnosis (ECHO), is very important because it indicates the size, localization and consistency of the examined thyroid gland alterations, which, according to the tissue density, may have hypo- , iso- , or hyperechogenic properties. [7,9,26,71]

- Computerized tomography (CT), enables insight into anatomical continuity of the thyroid gland tissue and pathologically altered tissue, as well as anatomical-pathological relations between the neck region organs. [7,9,11,22,26,73,75]

- Nuclear magnetic resonance (NMR), enables insight into structural and functional status of thyroid gland, alterations in it and in the surrounding organs, with presentation in transversal, sagittal and circular sections; it is the most precise technique in localizing potentially malignant thyroid gland neoplasia, in the group of noninvasive diagnostic methods. [7,9,11,22,26,73,75]

- Scintigraphy, used for morphologic and functional visualization of tyroid gland tissue by means of competitive binding of certain contrasting radionuclides known for their poorly binding to malignantly altered thyrocytes, showing cold fields in the scan. Its application is of vital importance also in postoperative scanning of the entire body aimed to localize metastatic alterations or remaining («rest») tissue after total thyroidectomy due to malignant process. [5,7,9,11,22,26,73]

- Needle biopsy (FNA) of alterations in thyroid gland and their cytopathological analysis, is of vital importance in differential diagnosis, but there are also silend zones where certain alterations remain undefined, both for impossibility to make a reliable histological differentiation, and also for uncertain findings in biopsied representative specimen (1 – 4 % false positive and false negative findings). [9,16,26,52,66,73]

- «Biopsio Ex Tempore», represents a hard and responsible analysis because of short time it is performed in, differentiation and atypicality of thyroid lesions encountered, as well as because of the decision by which the alteration is declared benign or malignant, based on which the principle of treatment is directly defined; therefore, the pathologists recommend biopsy of the entire alteration, and not only a part of it, with impeccable technical conditions of processing and examination, and professional experience. [8,9,11,14,16,22,26,36,37,43,], [47,48,50,73]

Regardless of availability of all these diagnostic procedures, a reliable histopathologic diagnosis of thyroid gland alterations is only possible during the surgical intervention by application of «Biopsio Ex Tempore» (97 % in the histological type) or by analysis of permanent preparations (postoperatively), so that surgical intervention represents both a diagnostic and therapeutic procedure. [8,9,11,14,16,22,26,36,37,43]

Solitary thyroid gland nodules and possible malignant alterations in them, represent an important entity in the endocrine surgery and require special attention both in evaluation of the disease, and in establishing indications for surgery and range of surgical intervention, in view of possible operative and postoperative complications. In view of the fact that, because of the specific character of the disease, the decision about the type of treatment is made during surgical intervention itself, while the patient is anesthetized and lying on the surgical table, upon receipt of Biopsio Ex Tempore findings, it is necessary to adequately implement certain preoperatively brought attitudes in principle, and adapt them to each individual case. In the entire method, of high importance is also a preoperative medicamentous preparation of patient for the planned surgical intervention aimed to achieve euthyroid status with quality homeostatic mechanisms, mental tranquillity, and stability. In order to perform a safe surgical intervention in the general anesthesia, it is necessary, by means of endotracheal intubation by reinforced tube, to ensure and preserve an adequate free passage of air through airways and pulmonary ventilation, which may be very difficult and associated with serious complications in the cases of advanced expansive neoplastic process with stenosis, dislocation or infiltration of airway (trachea). [3,6,8,14,16,21,26,35-37,39,43,46,47,48,50,57,62,67-69]

Thyroid gland surgery has been developed for more than one century. Contemporary surgical technique is characterized by minutial preciseness of surgical procedure where it is necessary to ensure certain specific conditions:

- Thorough knowledge of anatomy and structures of the neck region;
- Experience and adequate surgical technique;
- Adequate instruments;
- Adequate patient's posture;
- Adequate preoperative preparation;
- Adequate anesthesia and relaxation;
- Adequate analysis of frozen preparation sections;
- Adequate range of surgical intervention;
- Complete removal of pathological alterations;
- Prevention and preservation from injury of close neck structures and organs. [3,8,11,14,22,24,25,36,37,50,62]

Depending on the histopathologic analysis finding, surgical strategy is defined, which includes the range of surgical intervention on the thyroid gland, per the following types:

- unilateral partial lobe resection;
- unilateral subtotal lobectomy;
- unilateral total extracapsular lobectomy;
- unilateral lobectomy and resection of isthmus (unilateral lobe-isthmectomy);
- subtotal thyroidectomy;
- total extracapsular thyroidectomy;
- dissection of the neck lymph nodes;

- modified dissection of the neck organs;
- radical dissection of the neck organs. [5,8,11,14,15,22,36,37,47,48]

Possible postoperative complications may be early or late, depending on the type and extensiveness of the process, as well as on the type and range of surgical intervention. Most frequent forms include obstruction of respiratory ways, larynx edema, postoperative bleedings, tracheal collapse, as a result of intraoperative lesion of laryngeal nerves and parathyroid glands, thyrotoxic crisis, hypothyreosis or tracheomalacia, which all should be taken into account at the preparation and surgical treatment of the patient. [3,8,14,36,41,62]

As for choice of surgical procedure in the treatment of thyroid gland carcinoma, the attitudes are very clear and are based on the principles of active radical treatment comprising total extracapsular thyroidectomy with modified or radical dissection of the neck (as needed), should the conditions allow the mentioned radical approach.[4,5,7,11,14,15,22,23,30-32,36,37,47,48,55,58,59,64]

In view of the role of thyroid gland in the metabolism of iodine, proteins, carbohydrates, lipids, vitamins, calorigenesis, as well as of its important effects on the hormonal hypothalamus-hypophysis-thyroid axis, it is essential to make a reliable histopathologic differentiation between benign and malignant alterations in the conditions where the body remains deprived of such an important organ's function. [8,9,26]

Postoperative treatment of the patients in whom surgical intervention has been performed because of malignant process on the thyroid gland, is based on the fact that a radical surgical invervention has been made including total extracapsular thyroidectomy, and, as needed, also dissection of lymph glands in the neck region. This method of treatment is a precondition for performing, in the postoperative period, scintigraphic examination of the entire body for the detection of distant metastases or «rest» gland tissue. Depending on the type of malignant alteration and extensiveness of the process, measures of postoperative treatment of ablation by Radioactive 131-I may be applied, mainly in well-differentiated carcinoma, or transcutaneous irradiation therapy (prophylactic or palliative) in poorly - differentiated malignances. [7,8,11,12,14,15,21,22,36-39,41-43,46-48,68,70,74]

The objective of the study is to point out reliability of certain diagnostic procedures, incidence, types of alterations, as well as attitudes in princle in the operative and postoperative treatment of thyroid gland carcinoma with a special review of solitary nodules where they are most frequently sited.

MATERIAL AND METHODS

In the paper, data analysis is made of the representative sample of 131 operated patients whose clinical diagnosis indicated presence of solitary thyroid gland nodules, and in 20 patients carcinoma in solitary nodules was found. The conducted study includes analysis of results in operated patients in the 5 year period at Clinical Hospital «Dr Dragisa Misovic» - Dedinje, University Clinic for General Surgery, Belgrade. In the mentioned period, a total number of 295 patients were operated at the Clinic due to different pathological thyroid gland alterations. In all patients, the following preoperative examinations were uniformly performed: anamnestic data from the personal anamnesis and disease anamnesis, as well as epidemiological survey, in order to establish causal correlation already in the first phase of evaluation; physical examination established the signs of general and specific local pathological alterations of the thyroid gland and the surrounding neck structures; general and specific laboratory analyses were made, as well as those aimed to define hormonal status; indirect laryngoscopy was performed aimed to determine the extent of compression or infiltration of laryngeal nerves; radiological diagnosis of sellae turcicae, heart, lungs, trachea and esophagus; ultrasound diagnosis of thyroid gland alterations (solitary nodules, polynodous alterations, diffuse enlargements, solid or cystic), as well as the conditions of regional lymph glands and the neck organs; scintigraphy of the gland with presentation of non-functional, hypofunctional, functional or hyperfunctional alterations and other specific examinations for more precise diagnosis (CT, NMR, FNA). "Biopsio ex tempore" was performed in all patients during the surgical intervention itself, and later also a definitive histopathologic analysis of permanent preparations, as a reliable method in differentiation between benign and malignant alterations. The range and type of surgical intervention on the thyroid gland due to pathological alterations, depended on the correlation between clinical examination findings, patient's biohumoral status, intraoperative macroscopic finding, histopathologic finding, as well as on biological potential of the detected alteration, so that surgical intervention included the range of partial gland resection, lobectomy, lobe-isthmectomy, subtotal thyroidectomy, total thyroidectomy, and, as needed, modified or more radical neck dissection. When malignance was found, the basic principle of radical surgical intervention was observed. In the immediate postoperative period, vital and thyroid functions were monitored, and in the subsequent five-year period, follow-up examinations were performed and therapy was administered depending on histopathologic finding, range of surgical intervention and patient's status.

The obtained data were processed by application of biomedical statistic package program SPSS, results of this research were analyzed and, after comparison with other authors' findings, certain conclusions were made.

RESULTS

Among all operated patients (295), solitary nodules were present in 131 cases (100%), histopathologic finding of carcinoma within solitary thyroid gland nodule was made in 20 patients (15,27%), while benign alterations were found in 111 patients (84,73%). (Chart 1, Chart 2).

Female patients with solitary nodule finding accounted for 101 of the cases (77,1%), while solitary nodules were found in 30 male patients (22,9%), (Chart 3).

Carcinoma finding in solitary thyroid gland nodules was made in 11 cases in female patients (8,39% of all solitary nodules, i.e. 10,89% of all female patients, i.e. 55% of all carcinoma cases), while carcinoma finding in solitary thyroid gland nodules was made in 9 male patients (6,87% of all solitary nodules, i.e. 27% of all male patients, i.e. 45% of all carcinoma cases), (Chart 4).

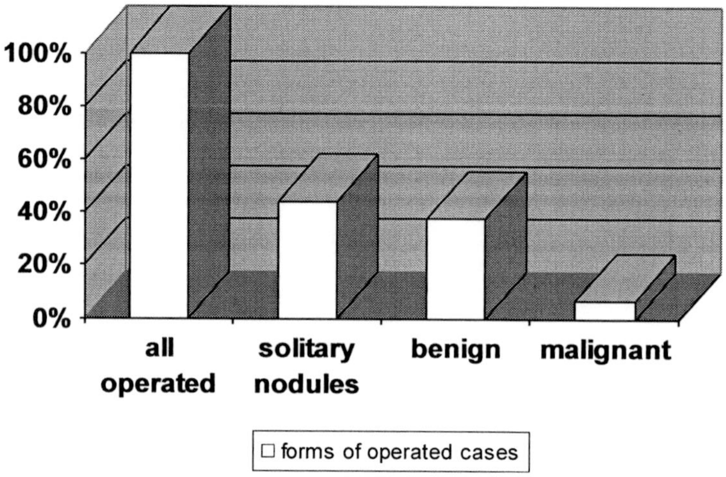

Chart 1.

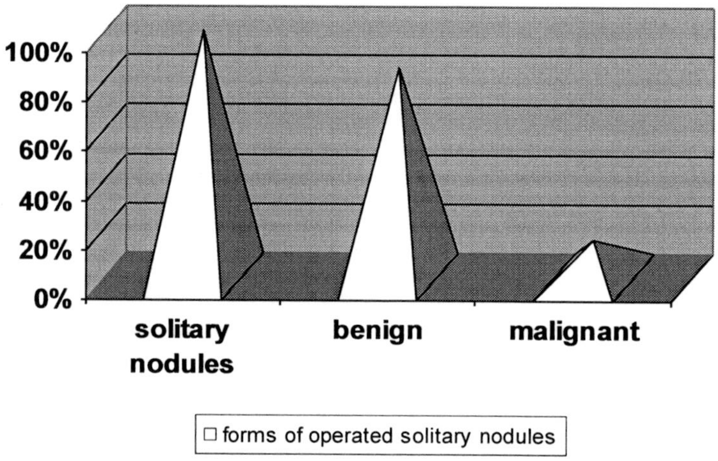

Chart 2.

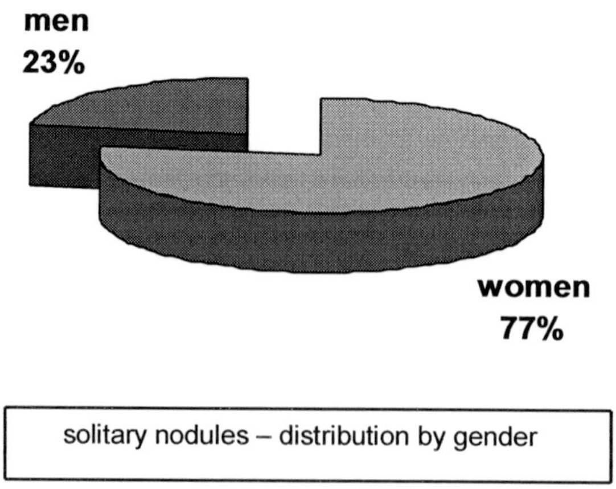

Chart 3.

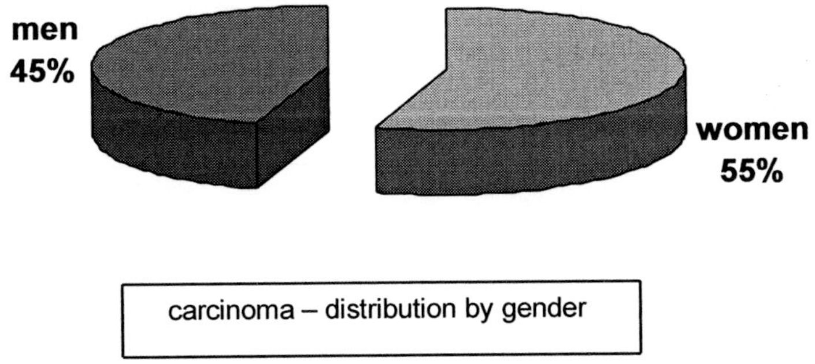

Chart 4.

The youngest patient was aged 37, and the oldest 75, while the highest incidence of carcinoma was found in the group of patients aged 50 to 59.

Carcinoma finding in solitary nodules was made in 6 patients coming from strumogenic regions (4,58% of all solitary nodules, i.e. 33,33% of all carcinoma cases), and also in 6 patients (4,58% of all solitary nodules, i.e. 33,33% of all carcinoma cases) there existed family predisposal. Apart from the mentioned ones, there were no specific anamnestic data that would indicate the nature of alterations in thyroid gland. As for physical status, in 5 patients (3,81% of all solitary nodules, i.e. 25 % of all carcinoma cases) finding was made of a fixed, enlarged, poorly movable nodal alteration with enlarged regional lymph glands. Not a single case showed any cardinal disorders in the values of laboratory analyses and hormonal status. Apart from nodal alterations in the gland and minor dislocations of the neck organs, X-ray examination did not discover any significant pathological metastatic alterations in any of the cases. Ultrasound examination established solitary nodules of solid consistency in all cases of malignance, while in 4 mentioned cases alterations and enlargements of regional lymph glands were verified. In all patients with carcinoma in solitary thyroid gland nodules, non-functional ("cold") nodules were found by scintigraphic examination. Comparation of findings of histopathologic examinations made by Biopsio ex tempore and definitive examinations of preparations, established that reports about carcinoma finding in solitary thyroid gland nodules were identical, therefore, there was no need for any subsequent interventions due to discrepancy between the intraoperative and postoperative histopathologic findings.

In 20 patients (100%), carcinoma finding in solitary thyroid gland nodules was made by histopathologic verification by means of Biopsio ex tempore during surgical intervention. In 17 patients (85%), alterations were of the "well-differentiated" carcinoma type, while in 1 case each (5%), established alterations were of the Medullary carcinoma type, Hurthle cell carcinoma type and Anaplastic carcinoma type, respectively. In the group of well-differentiated carcinoma, 12 patients (60% of all carcinoma cases, i.e. 70,58% of the well-differentiated ones) had the Papillary carcinoma type, while 5 patients (25% of all carcinomas, i.e. 29,42% of the well-differentiated ones) had alteration of the Follicular carcinoma type. (Chart 5).

In 3 patients with Papillary carcinoma (15% of all carcinoma cases, i.e. 17,64% of the well-differentiated ones) it was the Occult type with multicentric occurrence.

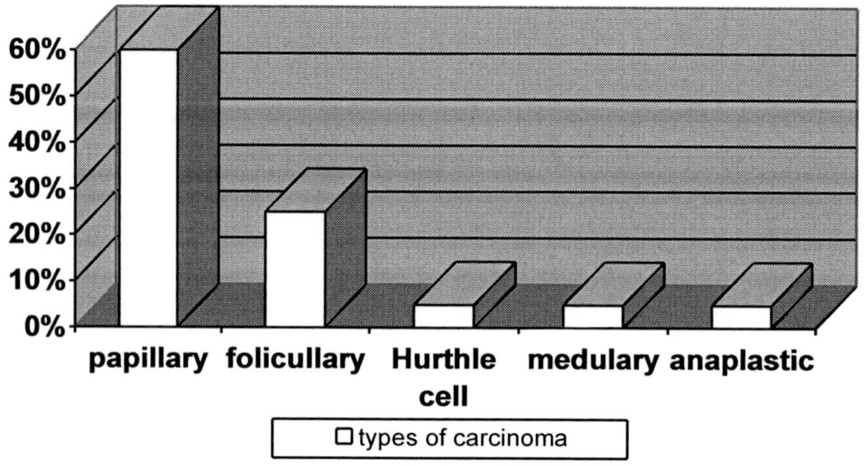

Chart 5.

Intraoperative, macroscopic finding and measuring established that thee size of thyroid gland nodule with malignant alterations was in the range of 10 to 40 mm. Nodules sized up to 10 mm were found in 5 cases (25%), up to 20 mm in 4 cases (20%), up to 30 mm in 5 cases (25%), up to 35 mm in 1 case (5%), and up to 40 mm in 5 cases (25%).

Range of surgical intervention in 19 cases (95%) comprised Total extracapsular thyroidectomy, which in 4 patients (20%) was extended to include modified dissection of lymph nodes of the neck organs, while in 1 case (5%) (Anaplastic type of carcinoma) after Biopsio ex tempore and exploration of the alteration, the decision was made to administer palliative and irradiative treatment due to extension of the process.

In the immediate postoperative period, in 4 patients (20%) signs of hemiparetic changes on vocal cords occurred, while in the subsequent period, in 2 (10%) of these patients the «rest» irreversible sequelae were found. Also in the immediate postoperative period, in 4 patients (20%) secondary signs of peripheral hypoparathyroidism occurred.

In the case of the patient with Anaplastic carcinoma, lethal outcome occurred 2 months after the surgery.

In the five-year follow-up period, apart from the mentioned case with Anaplastic carcinoma, lethal outcome occurred in another 4 patients (20%). In 2 cases (10%), these were the patients with alterations developed due to advancement of Medullary and Hurthle cell carcinoma, respectively, while in the other two cases (10%), the reason of lethal outcome were malignant alterations of the group of well-differentiated Papillary occult carcinoma type with multicentric diffusion.

Conclusion

Analysis of the obtained data considered the levels of statistical significance of individual characteristics and their relations in the differentiation between benign and malignant alterations. Total incidence of solitary nodules in female patients was almost 3.5

times higher than that in male patients, but not in the observed groups with benign, i.e. malignant alterations (significant difference $p = 0.01$). In the group of patients with the finding of carcinoma, number of male and female patients was almost identical (statistical significance $H_0 = 0.62$). Also, no significant differences were found depending on the age group ($p = 0.29$), place of birth ($p > 0.05$) and hereditary factor ($p > 0.05$). Significant differences ($p < 0.01$) of the types were observed in physical finding of solid and fixed alteration with enlarged regional lymph glands in the local status of carcinoma (statistical significance $H_1 = 0.01$). As for laboratory and hormonal analysis results, and radiological examinations, no significant differences were established in the differentiation between benign and malignant alterations ($p > 0.05$). Analysis of ultrasound findings showed significant differences ($p < 0.01$) in solid solitary nodules in the group of patients with carcinoma; almost identical result was obtained at scintigraphic examination in non-functional («cold») nodules (statistical significance $H_1 = 0.046$). High statistical significance and significant differences in differentiation between benign and carcinoma-related alterations were obtained by the analysis Biopsio ex tempore ($p < 0.01$).

In the group of well-differentiated carcinoma, distribution according to the gender was almost identical, and incidence was the highest in the age group from 50 to 59 years. In most patients with the finding of well-differentiated carcinoma, data were obtained about longterm existence of alterations in the thyroid gland which, for various reasons, caused them complaints in the preoperative period. From the anamnestic data, in a relatively small percentage of patients, genetic and endemic predisposal was established, but in the immediate preoperative period, there were relatively frequent reports of minor suffocations, breathlessness and fatigue, difficult swallowing, insomnia, palpitations, sometimes also hoarseness, and body mass loss. In the physical local status, predominant were signs of alterations of solid consistency, painfully sore at palpation, with the finding of moderately enlarged or not at all enlarged regional lymph glands. As for general laboratory analyses, in most patients accelerated sedimentation was found and also elevated values of alkaline phosphatase and fibrinogen. Values of the thyroid gland hormone were in the range of normal. Predominance of incidence in certain blood groups was found in A+ and B+ blood groups. X-ray examination of the neck organs did not discover any significant movement and dislocations of the neck organs, nor any infiltrative changes. Along with solid solitary nodular lesions, ultrasound examination established diffuse enlargement of thyroid gland in small number of patients. All cases of well-differentiated carcinoma manifested themself at the scintigraphuc examination as non-functional («cold») nodules. In the Papillary carcinoma type, histopathologic diagnosis was based on the finding of papillary formations, finding of hypochromic nuclei, sandy bodies, and the squamous metaplasia type, while in the Follicular carcinoma type, diagnosis was based on histological finding of follicular structures covered by neoplastic cells. Papillary carcinoma cases were found in the occult and intrathyroid types, with no finding of extrathyroid form of dissemination, with multicentric localization in three cases. In the group of Follicular carcinoma, all alterations corresponded to the solitary – encapsulated malignance type. According to TNM classification and division as per the disease stages, in the group of well-differentiated carcinoma, findings were in the range up to T2, N1, Mo, i.e. up to the second stage in the clinical finding. By histopathologic analysis, along with the finding of Papillary carcinomaa, as a rarity, in one case, in the altered gland tissue, components of lymphocytic infiltration of parenchyma of the Hashimoto's thyroiditis type were found. Hurthle cell and Medullary types of thyroid gland carcinoma were found in one case each. They were both found in female patients, belonging to the age group from 40 to 49 years. In the anamnestic data, along with accompanying symptoms like in the previous group, the patient with the Medullary carcinoma type pointed out family predisposal to thyroid gland disease. In the local status, in both cases predominant were signs of moderate unilateral painful soreness, poorly movable, solid alteration which corresponded to solitary thyroid gland nodular lesion, without finding of enlargement of regional lymph glands. In the case of the patient with Medullary carcinoma, values of Ca-C 50 were elevated, while in the patient with Hurthle cell carcinoma, values of antithyroglobuline antibodies were elevated. At ultrasound examination, both alterations had characteristics of solid solitary nodular alteration, and at scintigraphic examination they manifested themselves as non-functional («cold») nodules. Histopathologic analysis in Medullary carcinoma was based on microscopic funding of oval cells of eosinophilic cytoplasm with minor mitoses and amyloid in stroma, while in Hurthle cell carcinoma diagnosis was based on the finding of Hurthle cells which are larger than the follicular ones, with abundant eosinophilic granulated cytoplasm with irregular hyperchromatic nuclei. In view of closely related histopathologic finding of Hurthle cell adenoma and Hurthle cell malignance, analysis of the preparation was difficult and required longer duration of examination than usual. Both belonged to T1, No, Mo malignance group, i.e. I group clinical stage. In both cases radical surgical intervention was performed comprising total extracapsular thyroidectomy with additional dissection of the regional lymph nodes. In the five-year follow-up period, in both patients lethal outcome occurred, as a result of late complications of the malignant disease.

Occurrence of Anaplastic carcinoma in one patient was characterized by advanced form with all accompanying significant features of fast progression of disease, physical finding in the local status and regional organs, diagnostic procedures, operative and histopathologic fundings. Preoperative punction biopsy of the alteration produced cytopathological finding most corresponding to malignance of the Papillary carcinoma type, while Biopsio Ex Tempore established the «Giant cell» anaplastic carcinoma type which, according to TNM classification corresponded to T2, N2b, Mo group, and to II group clinical stage. In view of the intraoperative biopsy finding, the disease stage and expansive growth of malignant disease, it was decided to administer irradiation therapy to the patient. Two months after the diagnosis was made and the treatment started, lethal outcome occurred with signs of fast progression and local and systemic dissemination of the malignant process.

Incidence of thyroid gland carcinoma is the highest in solitary nodules. [2,6,15,29,35,40,51,57]

Comparison of the recent literature data with the earlier studies, leads to the conclusion that incidence of carcinoma in solitary thyroid gland nodules is increasing, both because of increased number of factors for their development, and because of more adequate plan of selection of patients in the diagnostic procedure. [2,6,15,20,24,26,29,35,40,57]

Patients whose anamnestic data include their coming from the strumogenic regions and their family predisposal to the disease, if for any reason subjected to low-dose irradiation, with clinical finding of solitary nodule of dense consistency, which shows solid structure at ultrasound examination, and is non-functional at scintigraphic examination, with enlarged regional lymph glands or without them, may have the finding of carcinoma. [1,13,15,17,20,26,29,44,47,48,53,60,63]

However, thyroid gland carcinoma does not always occur with such a clinical status. [7,10,20,26,29,34,51,65]

It is precisely the reason why any finding of asymmetric field of tumor growth within normal or pathologically altered thyroid gland requires special attention and evaluation by means of all available diagnostic methods. [7,9,29,51]

In view of the fact that Biopsio ex tempore is still the crucial method of histopathologic differentiation between benign and malignant alterations, surgical intervention represents both a diagnostic and therapeutic procedure. [8,9,14,26,36,37]

Type and range of surgical intervention are defined by histopathologic and intraoperative macroscopic finding of thyroid gland and the surrounding neck organs. [8,10,14,29,36,37,47,48,65]

Finding of thyroid gland carcinoma requires surgical intervention of the total extracapsular thyroidectomy type (sometimes extended to include the surrounding structures), which is highly delicate in terms of performing, and requires thorough knowledge of anatomical structures and relations of the neck organs, their patho-anatomical variations, as well as experience and skill in surgical practice. [3,5,8,10,14,25,34,36,37,47,50,62,65]

Such a radical attitude and principle of treatment are based on findings that even well-differentiated thyroid gland carcinomas which are of low malignant potential may alter into poorly - differentiated carcinomas with high malignant potential, and in local status they may produce distant metastases. [2,4,5,7,11,15,18,22,23,26,28,30-33,39,45-48,51,55,58,59,64], [68,70]

Awareness that postoperative scintigraphy of the entire body for the detection of distant metastases is only possible after total thyroidectomy supports this finding. [2,5,7,11,12,22,38,41,42,47,51,70,74]

REFERENCES

[1] Abelin, T., Averkin, JI., Egger, M. et al. Thyroid cancer in Belarus post Chernobil: improved detection or increased incidence. *Soz Praventiv Med* 1994; 39: 189-97.

[2] Al Salamah, SM., Khalid, H., Bismar, HA. Incidence of differentiated cancer in nodular goiter. *Saudi Med J* 2002; 23 (8): 947-52.

[3] Attie, JN., Khafif, RA. Preservation of parathyroid glands and laringeal nervs durin total thyroidectomy. *Am J Surg* 1975; 130: 399-404.

[4] Baloch, ZW., Gupta, PK., Yu, GH., Sack, MJ., Li, Volsi VA. Follicular variant of papillary carcinoma. Cytologic and histologic correlation. *Am J Clin Pathol* 1999; 111 (2): 216-22.

[5] Briant, T.D. & Wax, M.K.(1992). Completion thyreoidectomy in the management of well-differentiated thyroid carcinoma. *Otolaryngol Head-Neck Surg*; 107 (1): 63-8.

[6] Bona, G., Bozzola, M., Buzzi, F. et al. Thyroid nodules. *Minerva Pediatr* 2002; 54(3): 263-9.

[7] Byar, DP., Green, SB., Dor, P. A prognostic index for thyroid carcinoma. *Eur J Canc* 1979; 15: 1033-9.

[8] Cady, B. & Rossi, R. (1991). *Surgery of the thyroid and parathyroid glands*. Saunders, Philadelphia.

[9] Capri, A., Toni, MG., Di Coscio, G., Nicollini, A., Sagripant, A. The thyroid nodule: diagnostic strategy. *Thyroid Clin Exp* 1991; 3 (1): 17-23.

[10] Chen, H. & Udelsman, R. (1997). Hurthle cell adenoma and carcinoma. U: Clark OH, Duh QY (eds): *Textbook of Endocrine Surgery*. Saunders, Philadelphia; 103-7.

[11] Chen, H., Nicol, TL., Udelsman, R. Clinicaly significant, isolated metastatic disease of thyroid gland. *World J Surg* 1999; 23: 177-81.

[12] Chow, SM., Law, SC., Mendenhall, T. et al. Papillary thyroid carcinoma: prognostic factors and the role of radioiodine and external therapy. *Int J Radiat Oncol Biol Phys* 2002; 52 (3): 784-95.

[13] Clark, DE. Association of irradiation with cancer of the thyroid in children and adolescents. *JAMA* 1955; 159: 1007-9.

[14] Davis, C.(1993). *Surgery of thyroid cancer*. Butterworth, London; 240-57.

[15] De Groot, LJ., Kaplan, EL., Mc Cormick, M., Straus, FH. Natural history, treatment and corse of papillary thyroid carcinoma. *J Clin Endocrinol Metab* 1990; 71: 414-24.

[16] Duek, SD., Goldenberg, D., Linn, S. The role of fine needle aspiration and intraoperative frozen section in the surgical management of solitary thyroid nodules. *Surg Today* 2002; 32 (10): 857-61.

[17] Ezaki, H. Thyroid cancer: epidemiological study of thyroid cancer in A bomb survivors from extended life span study cohort in Hiroshima. *J Radiat Res* 1993; 32: 193-200.

[18] Fluge, O., Haugen, DR., Lillehaug, JR., Varhaug, JE. Difference in patterns of Met expression in papillary thyroid carcinomas and non neoplastic thyroid tissue. *World J Surg* 2001; 25 (5): 623-31.

[19] Gagel, RFR., Goepfert, H., Callender, DL. Changing concepts in the pathogenesis and management of thyroid carcinoma. *CA-Cancer J Clin* 1996; 46: 261-83.

[20] Gharib, H. A strategy for the solitary thyroid nodule. *Hosp Pract* 1992; 27 (9): 53-8.

[21] Gharib, H., James, EM., Charboneau, JW. et al. Supressive therapy with levothyroxine for solitary thyroid nodules. A double blind controlled clinical study. *N Engl J Mes* 1987; 317: 70-6.

[22] Grebe, SKG., Hay, IC. Thyroid cancer nodal metastases, biologic significances and therapeuthic considerations. *Surg Oncol Clin North Am* 1996; 5: 43-63.

[23] Haigh, PI. Follicular thyroid cancer. *Curr Treat Options Oncol* 2002; 3 (4): 349-54.

[24] Hamdy, RC. The thyroid gland: A brief historical perspective. *South J Med* 2002; 95 (5): 471-3.

[25] Harness, JK., van Heerden, JA., Lennquist, S. Future of thyroid surgery and training surgeons to meet the expectations of 2000 and beyond. *World J Surg* 2000; 24 (8): 976-82.

[26] Hay, ID., Klee, CD. Thyroid cancer – diagnosis and management. *Clin Lab Med* 1993; 13: 275-9.

[27] Hedinger, C., Williams, ED. & Sobin, LH. (1988). Histological typing of thyroid tumors. WHO International Histological Classification of Tumours, 2nd ed., Berlin, Springer Verlag.

[28] Hoerman, R., Quadbeck, B. Medullary thyroid carcinoma. *Oncol Pract* 1999; 1: 8-10.

[29] Hundahl, SA., Fleming, ID., Fremgen, AM., Menck, HR. A national data base report on 53856 cases of thyroid carcinoma in the United States: 1985 – 1995. *Cancer* 1998; 26: 38-48.

[30] Jorda, M., Gonzales, CR., Mora, J., Herrero, ZA., Otal, C., Gavera, H. Prognostic factors in follicular carcinoma of the thyroid. *Arch Pathol Lab Med* 1993; 117: 631-5.

[31] Jossart, GH., Clark, OH. Vell differentiatedthyroid cancer. *Curr Prob Surg* 1994; 31: 935-1001.

[32] Kebebew, E., Clark, OH. Differentiated thyroid cancer: «complete» rational approach. *World J Surg* 2000; 24 (8): 942-51.

[33] Kebebew, E., Ituarte, PH., Siperstein, E. et al. Medullary thyroid carcinoma: clinical characteristics, treatment, prognostic factors and a comparison of staging systems. *Cancer* 2000; 88 (5): 1139-48.

[34] Lazzi, S., Spina, D., Als, C., Tosi, P., Muzzuchelli, L., Kraft, R., Laissve, JA. & Cottier, H. (1999).Oncotic (Hurthle cell) tumors of the thyroid: distinct growth patterns compared with clinico-pathological features. *Thyroid*; 9 (2): 97-103.

[35] Lennquist, S. The thyroid nodule – diagnosis and surgical treatment. Surg *Clin of North Am* 1987; 67 (2): 213-32.

[36] Lennquist, S. Surgical strategy in thyroid carcinoma. Acta Chir Scand 1996; 152: 321-9.

[37] Lenquist, S. (1997). Thyroidectomy. U: Clarck OH, Duh QY. (eds): *Textbook of endocrine surgery*. Saunders, Philadelphia; 147-53.

[38] Li Volsi, VA. Papillary neoplasms of the Thyroid. Pathologic and prognostic features. *Am Clin Pathol* 1992; 97: 426-32.

[39] Lo, CY., Lam, KY., Wan, KY. Anaplastic carcinoma of the thyroid. *Am J Surg* 1999. 177 (4): 337-9.

[40] Mazzaferri, EL. Managementof the solitary thyroid nodule. *N Engl J Med* 1993; 328: 553-9.

[41] Mazzaferri, EL., Jhiang, SM. Long term impact of initial surgical and medical therapy on papillary and follicular thyroid cancer. *Am J Med* 1994; 97: 418-28.

[42] Maxon, HR., Smith, HS. Radioiodine – 131 in the diagnosis and treatement of metastatic well differentiated thyroid cancer. *Endocrinol Metab Clin North Am* 1990; 19: 685-718.

[43] Miki, H., Oshima. K., Inove, H. et al. Diagnosis and surgical treatment of small papillary carcinomas of the thyroid gland. *J Surg Oncol* 1993; 54: 78-81.

[44] Mizukami, Y., Michigishi, T., Nonomura, A., Nochuchi, M., Nakamura, H. Thyroid carcinoma: Clinical and pathologic corelations. *Crit Rev Oncol Hematol* 1995; 18: 67-102.

[45] Modigliani, E., Franc, B., Niccoli, P. Diagnosis and treatment of medullary thyroid cancer. *Baillieres Best Practic Res Clin Endocrinol Metab* 2000; 14 (4): 631-49.

[46] Nilsson, O., Lindeberg, J., Yedenius, J. et al. Anaplastic giant cell carcinoma of the thyroid gland. *World J Surg* 1998; 22: 725-30,

[47] Noguchi, M., Kumaki, T., Taniya, T., Miyazaki, I. Billateral cervical lymph node metastasis in well differentiated thyroid cancer. *Arch Surg* 1990; 125: 804-6.

[48] Noguchi, S., Murakami, N. The value of lymph node dissection in patients with differentiated thyroid cancer. *Surg Clin of North Am* 1987; 67: 251-61.

[49] Ozgen, AG., Hamulu, F., Bayraktar, F. et al. (1999) Evaluation of routine basal serum calcitonin measurment for early diagnosis of medullary thyroid carcinoma in seven hundred seventy three patients with nodular goiter. *Thyroid; 9 (6):* 579-82.

[50] Pasieka, JL. The Surgeon as a prognostic factor in endocrine surgical diseases. Surgical techniques and outcomes. *Surg Oncol Clin North Am* 2000; 9: 13-20.

[51] Paunovic, I., Krgovic, K., Todorovic, M. Carcinoma of thyroid gland in solitary and dominant nodules. *ACI* 1998; (1): 268.

[52] Pisani, T., Bononi, M., Nager, C., Agelini, M., Bezzi, M., Vecchione, A. Fine needle aspiration and core needle biopsy techniques in the diagnosis of nodular thyroid pathologies. *Anticancer Res* 2000; 20 (5): 3843-7.

[53] Ron, E., Modan, B., Preston, D. et al. Thyroid neoplasia following low dose radiation in childhood. *Radiat Res* 1989; 120: 516-31.

[54] Rubello, D., Casara, D., Girelli, ME., Piccolo, M., Busnardo, B. Clinical meaning of circulating antithyroglobulin antibodies in differentiated thyroid cancer: a prospective study. *J Nucl Med* 1992; 33: 1478-80.

[55] Schlumberger, M. Papillary and follicular thyroid carcinoma. *N Engl J Med* 1998; 338: 297-306.

[56] Schlumberger, M., Baudin, E. Serum thyroglobulin determination in the follow up of patients with differentiated thyroid carcinoma. *Eur J Endocrinol* 1998; 138: 249-52.

[57] Shaha, AR. Controversis in the management of Thyroid Nodule. *The Laringoscope* 2000; 110: 183-193.

[58] Shah, JP., Loree, TR., Dharker, D. et al. Prognostic factors in differentiated carcinoma of thyroid gland. *Am J Surg* 1992; 164: 658.

[59] Singer, PA., Cooper, DS., Daniels, GH., Ladenson, PW., Greenspan, FS., Levy, EG., Braverman, LE., Clark, OH., Mc Dougall, IR., Ain, KV., Dorfman, SG. Treatment guidelines for patients with thyroid nodules and well differentiated thyroid cancer. *Arch Intern Med* 1996; 156: 2165-72.

[60] Sloan, R., Newcombe, EW., Pellicer, A. Ionizing radiation and RAS oncogene activation. *J Cancer Res Clin Oncol* 1990; 116: 808.

[61] Sobrinho, S.M., Soares, AP., Rocha, AS., Fonseca, E., Papotti, M., Komminoth, P. Bussolati, G. Divergent differentiation in thyroid tumors. *Rev Esp Pathol* 1999; 32 (3): 468-9.

[62] Souza, JW., Williams, JT., Ayoub, MM., Jerles, ML., Dalton, ML. Billateral recurrent nerve paralysis associated with multinodular substernal goiter: a case report. *Am Surg* 1999; 65: 456-9.

[63] Stefanović, Lj. Malignant tumors of Thyroid gland. *Oncol Arh* 1994; 2: 55-7.

[64] Steinmuller, T., Klupp, J., Rayes, N. et al. Prognostic factors in patients with differentiated thyroid carcinoma. *Eur J Surg* 2000; 166 (1): 29-33.

[65] Stojadinovic, A., Hoos, A., Ghossein, RA. et al. Hurthle cell carcinoma: a 60-years experience. *Ann Surg Oncol* 2002; 9 (2): 197-203.

[66] Suen, KC. Fine needle aspiration biopsy of the thyroid. *CMAJ* 2002; 167 (5): 491-5.

[67] Takashima S, Matsuzuki F, Nagareda T, Tamiyama N, Kozuka T: Thyroid nodules. *Radiology* 1992; 185 (1): 125-30.

[68] Tan, RK., Finley, RK., Driscoll, D., Bakamsian, V., Hisks, WL. Jr, Shedd, DP. Anaplastic carcinoma of the thyroid a 24 year experience. *Head Neck* 1995; 17 (1): 41-7.

[69] Thompson, NW. The thyroid nodule – surgical management. *Endocryn Surg* 1993; 4 (1): 14-24.

[70] Utiger, RD. Follow up of patients with thyroid carcinoma. *N Engl Med* 1997; 337: 928-30.

[71] Voutilainen, PE., Haapiainen, RK., Haglund, CH. Ultrasonically activated shears in thyroid surgery. *Am J Surg* 1998; 175: 491-3.

[72] Wahner, HW., Cuello, C., Correa, P., Uribe, LF., Gaitan, E. Thyroid carcinoma in an endemic goitre area. Cali, Colombia. *Am J Epidemiol* 1996; 40: 58-66.

[73] Woeber, AK. Cost effective evaluation of the patient with a thyroid nodule. *Surg Clin of North Am* 1995; 75 (3): 357-63

[74] Yim, JH., Doherty, GM. Papillary thyroid cancer. *Curr Treat Options Oncol* 2000; 1 (4): 328-9.

[75] Youserm, DM., Huang, F., Loevner, LA. et al. Clinical and economic imapct of incidental thyroid lesions found with CT and NMR. *Am J Neuroradiol* 1997; 18: 1423-28.

In: Trends in Thyroid Cancer Research
Editor: Carl A. Milton, pp. 155-181
ISBN 1-59454-627-4

Chapter VIII

INTERNAL DOSIMETRY FOR THYROID CANCER TREATMENT: A CLINICAL PERSPECTIVE

A. S. M. Sabbir Ahmed*

Bangladesh Atomic Energy Commission, Nuclear Medicine Center,
P.O. Box # 47, Mymensingh 2200, Bangladesh,
Nukleer Tip ABD, I.U. Cerrahpasa Tip Fakultesi, 34303 Cerrahpasa, Istanbul, Turkey.

ABSTRACT

Radioiodine-131 is used in differentiated thyroid cancer (DTC) for ablation of post surgical thyroid remnants and destruction of metastasis. As it is commonly accepted that repeated RAI treatments in metastatic DTC with lower doses are less effective, so large doses of I-131 are routinely administered to patients for this purpose. The dose limiting toxicity of radioiodine treatment on the bone marrow and the absorbed doses in the subsequent organs (act as platform during iodine excretion) are great concern in internal dosimetry. The dosimetric calculations to determine the radiation doses in different organs involve many factors; e.g. percent uptake, effective half life, tumor size, turnover of activity etc. An extensive study has been performed on 29 thyroid cancer patients with the following objects: To calculate i) the effective half lives of iodine for different organs, ii) the absorbed doses in major organs act as platform during excretion process, iii) to find a relation between drinking water and bladder dose, iv) to determine the effective dose equivalent due to uptake of iodine in the therapeutic as well as secondary organs (act as platform of iodine uptake during excretion) and v) to find the phase wise absorbed doses to the remnant thyroid-tissue.

Total twenty-nine patients (all female, age ranged from 40-60 y, mean 50 y) were treated with I-131 (dose-range 3700-7400 MBq, mean 5550 MBq) for thyroid cancer. The radioiodine uptake was measured at 1cm distance from three organs (previously marked by ultrasonography): thyroid, thigh-muscle and stomach by a calibrated Eberline ESP-2

* Correspondence concerning this article should be addressed to Dr. A.S.M. Sabbir Ahmed, Nukleer Tip ABD, I.U. Cerrahpasa Tip Fakultesi, 34303 Cerrahpasa, Istanbul, Turkey. Email: asahmed@ksu.edu.

GM counter under special arrangement of each patient. Urine sample was collected 12 hourly for first 72 h and then 24 hourly for the next 96 h. The individual biologic half-life of excreted urine was calculated using individual effective half-life. Absorbed doses were calculated for an adult female phantom using dynamic bladder model of MIRDOSE 3 program.
The effective half lives were calculated in two phases for the urine sample and it was found (24.81± 0.74) h for the first 72 h and (73.25±0.64) h for the next 96 h. (87±0.9)% of total activity passed through the urinary tract within first 72 h and the amount was (9±0.05)% for the next 96 h. The absorbed doses were calculated in groups of patients at different voiding intervals. The absorbed dose increased around 100% when the voiding interval was changed from 1 h to 2 h. This dose increased by 50% for the next hour and 33% for one more hour consecutively. The effective half lives for thyroid, thigh and stomach were found 39±0.85, 31.50±0.40 and 33.11±0.70 h consecutively. The correlation coefficient (r) among the measured uptakes was found very significant ($p<0.001$) for thyroid-thigh and stomach-urine, fairly significant ($p<0.01$) for thigh-stomach and non-significant for thyroid-stomach and thyroid-urine ($p<0.1$). The effective dose equivalent (EDE) for different target organs (sensitive for fatal occurrences) was calculated separately using MIRDOSE 3 program depending on absorbed doses to three source organs (Thyroid, Stomach and Urine bladder). The doses for stomach are found remarkably highest among the three source organs. The absorbed dose per unit mass (Gy/g) of remnant tissue (calculated using nodule-module protocol of MIRDOSE 3) is found as high as 1.72E+05 Gy and as low as 1.22E+04 Gy.
Extra water drinking in first few days after giving I-131 to the thyroid cancer patients reduces the absorbed doses to bladder. This study indicates that the subsequent uptake of radioiodine in stomach and urine bladder of thyroid cancer patients undertakes some extra burden of probabilistic fatal occurrence than other organs. The long-term post therapeutic follow up of the concerned organs is necessary to reduce the occurrences. The target-absorbed dose strongly depends on the size and mass of the remnant tissue and smaller tissue spot (radius<0.75 cm) shows high uncertainties in dose calculation.

Keywords: Internal dosimetry, differentiated thyroid cancer, MIRDOSE 3, radioiodine therapy

1. Introduction

A radioactive nucleus decays with emission of energy in the form of x-ray, gamma-photons or energetic charged particles. The form and energy of radiation depend on the type of radionuclide and may vary from decay to decay for radionuclides that have multiple decay pathways. Charged particles traveling in a medium slow down quickly because of interactions between the electric charge of the charged particles and orbital electrons and the nuclei of the medium. The photons may be transmitted through or attenuated by the medium due to its charge-less properties. Absorption of energy from ionizing radiation can cause damage to living tissues. This phenomenon is used as an advantage in radionuclide applications for diagnostic and therapeutic purpose. But the application of radiation in diagnostic and therapeutic purpose requires proper caution and planning to minimize the subsequent hazard. Internal dosimetry is the subject that deals the deposition of energy from radiation/charged particles to cells/organs through interactions inside living body during radionuclide treatment.

The interaction of radiation inside living-body occurs by different mechanisms. Though there are different types of interactions between radiation and any interacting medium, but radiation internal dosimetry in nuclear medicine mainly involves two interaction phenomena; - photoelectric effect and Compton scattering.

Different radioactive materials placed in the human body (called as radiotracers) distribute through the human body following the rules of one's pharmacokinetics - including pathology, chemical properties and basic physical properties as well. In general, the distribution varies with time and is spatially non-uniform on both the macroscopic and cellular levels. Internal radiation dosimetry requires knowledge of the time-varying radioactive concentrations in different organs of the body. In general, absorbed dose to certain organ (called target organ) is calculated depending on the tracer distribution over one or more source organs (contained radioactive concentration higher than average concentration in the body). The source and target may be the same organ, and generally the most important contributor to radiation dose is radioactivity contained within the target organ itself. Each radionuclide is assumed to be an isotropic radiation emitter; i.e. the radiation is emitted from the source in all direction with equal probability and has no preferred direction. This fact causes regions near radionuclide concentrations to receive a larger radiation flux than more distant locations. The radiation dose delivered to a medium increases with higher radiation flux. Attenuation and absorption in intervening tissues prevents radiation from reaching distant sites.

1.1. General Concept for Internal Radiation Dose Calculation

Radiation dose measurement for a target organ from radioactivity in source organs follows following steps;

- Measuring amount and duration of activity in the source organs
- Measuring energy emitted by the source organs and
- Measuring fraction of emitted energy deposited by the target organs.

The first step directly related to the amount of activity used during application. Though in clinical purpose, known amount of activity is used, but the duration of stay of the radionuclide in any source organ generally differs from person to person depending on the metabolic and physiologic condition of individual. The second step involves the physical characteristics of the radionuclide (energy, type, decay mode, radiation weighting factor etc). The third step includes anatomy of the concerned person and attenuating properties of the target organs.

1.1.1. Units and Terminology

i) Absorbed dose (D): Absorbed dose is defined as the amount of energy deposited per g in an absorber. SI (System International) unit of absorbed dose is Gy (Gray).

$$1\ \text{Gy}=1\ \text{J/kg} = \frac{10^7\, ergs}{10^3\, gm} = 10^4\, ergs/gm$$

The basic unit of radiation dose is rad (*R*adiation *A*bsorbed *D*ose).

1 rad = 100 ergs/g 1 Gy=100 rad

The integral dose for a volume of tissue mass is calculated as the product of absorbed dose to the mass of tissue.

ii) Cumulated activity ($\tilde{A}$): Cumulated activity measures time-activity relation for a particular radioactive distribution inside body. Consider a source organ in which the time-varying activity distribution A(t) is present. The cumulated activity in the source organ is, $\tilde{A} = \int_t A(t)dt$ is the area under the time-activity curve (figure-1a).

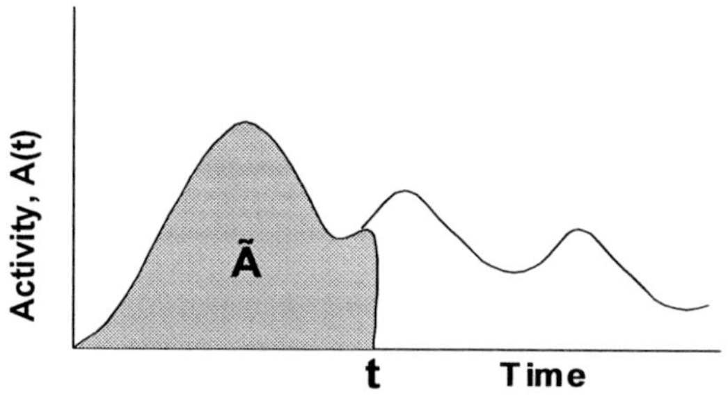

Figure 1a: Cumulated activity

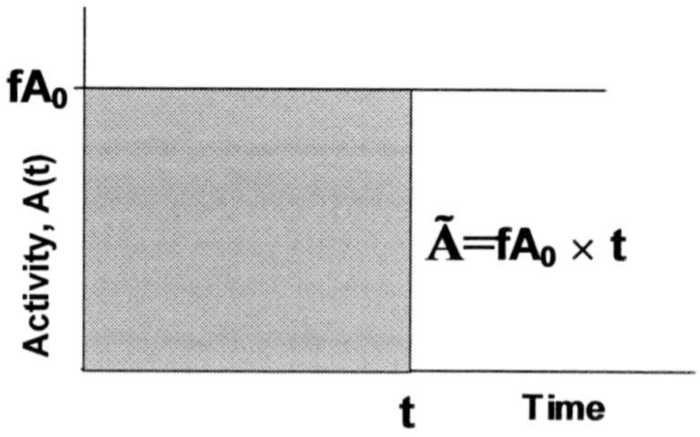

Figure 1b: Cumulated activity ($T_{1/2}=\infty$)

Cumulated activity differs from case to case depending on the distribution of activity inside patient's body. Another expression for cumulated activity calculation can be used considering initial time t=0, for entire span of radioactive decay (t=∞),

$$\tilde{A}=\int_{0}^{\infty} A(t)dt \tag{1}$$

The SI unit of cumulated activity is MBq.sec (or μCi.hr).

From decay calculation, the amount of activity A(t), for a radionuclide after a certain time t with initial activity A_0, and decay constant λ can be expressed as,

$$A(t)= A_0e^{-\lambda t} \tag{2}$$

If $T_{1/2}$ is the time required for a certain nuclei decay down to half of its initial nucleons, then

$$T_{1/2} = 0.693/\lambda \qquad \lambda = 0.693/T_{1/2} \tag{3}$$

In general, the decay factor is expressed as,

$$Df= e^{-\lambda t} = e^{-0.693t/T_{1/2}} \tag{4}$$

The average lifetime for a certain radionuclide,

$$\tau=1/\lambda \tag{5}$$

From equations 3 and 5,

$$\tau=1.44\ T_{1/2} \tag{6}$$

Finally equation (1) becomes,

$$\tilde{A}= 1.44 \times A_0 \times T_{1/2} \tag{7}$$

For practical purposes, time-activity curves for any particular radioactive material are analyzed in different ways under different assumptions depending on the distribution of tracer inside human body.

•) Consider f is the fraction of a long-lived radionuclide ($T_{1/2}\rightarrow\propto$), having initial activity (A_0), accumulated in a certain body. If time of interest (t) is short (i.e. $T_{1/2}>>t$), then cumulated activity is simply (*figure-1b*),

$$\tilde{A}= 1.44 \times fA_0 \times t \tag{8}$$

•) If the accumulated activity (fA_0) is removed from the source organ exponentially, then cumulated activity for a time t is (*figure-1c*),

$$\tilde{A} = 1.44 \times fA_0 \times T_{1/2} \left(1 - e^{-\frac{0.693}{T_{1/2}}} \right) \quad (9)$$

•) If the accumulated activity (fA_0) excretes or decays for infinite time ($t \rightarrow \infty$), then cumulated activity is (*figure-1d*),

$$\tilde{A} = 1.44 \times fA_0 \times T_{1/2} \quad (10)$$

The accumulated activity in the source organ is removed from the body by two simultaneous mechanisms; physical decay and biological washout. If T_p is the physical half-life, and T_b is biologic half life, then the effective half life is expressed as,

$$\frac{1}{T_e} = \frac{1}{T_p} + \frac{1}{T_b} \qquad T_e = \frac{T_p T_b}{T_p + T_b} \quad (11)$$

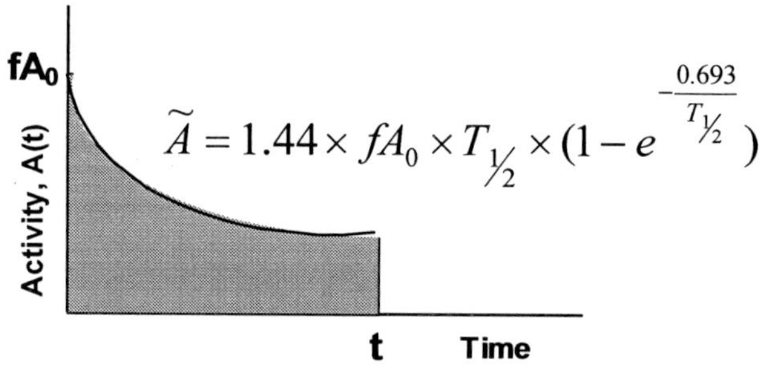

Figure 1c: Cumulated activity after a time t for the activity decaying exponentially.

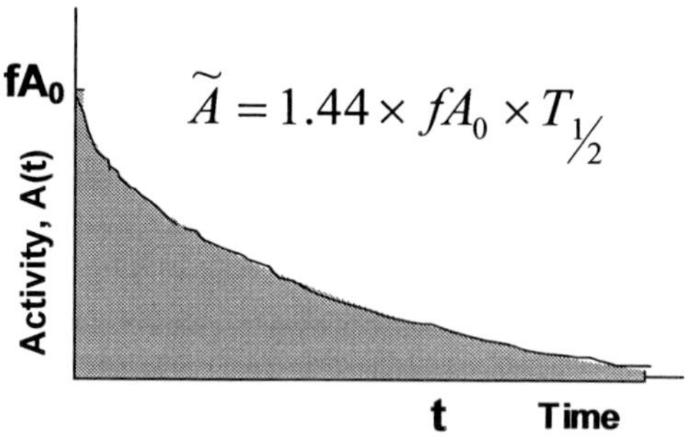

Figure 1d: Cumulated activity for $t=\infty$ for the activity decaying exponentially.

iii) Equilibrium absorbed dose constant (Δ): This parameter equals to the mean energy per nuclear transition and can be defined as the average energy emitted per unit of cumulated activity (Ã). This factor is dependant on the radionuclide and its various decay pathways [1].

Calculation of Δ: Consider for a certain radionuclide, 1Mev energy is released per disintegration.

$$1\ \text{Mev/disinteg} = \frac{1.602\times10^{-13}\,J}{1}\times\frac{3.7\times10^{4}}{\mu Ci.\sec}\times\frac{3600\sec}{hr}$$

$$= \frac{1.602\times10^{-13}\times10^{7}\,erg}{1}\times\frac{3.7\times10^{4}}{\mu Ci.\sec}\times\frac{3600\sec}{hr}$$

$$= \frac{1.602\times10^{-6}\times10^{-2}\,g.rad}{1}\times\frac{3.7\times10^{4}}{\mu Ci.\sec}\times\frac{3600\sec}{hr}$$

$$= 2.13\frac{g.rad}{\mu Ci.hr}$$

Now equilibrium absorbed dose constant,

$$\Delta_i=2.13\times N_i\times E_i\times\frac{g.rad}{\mu Ci.hr}$$

Where, E_i is the average energy (in MeV) of the ith emission having a relative frequency N_i.

iv) Absorbed fraction ϕ: The fraction of radiation energy emitted from the source organ that is deposited in the target organ is the absorbed fraction ϕ, with paired argument (source→target). For weakly penetrating radiations (alpha particle, low energy beta particle), all of the emitted radiation are absorbed locally in the source organ, for which ϕ=1. The absorbed fraction ϕ is zero for target organs distant from the source.

The absorbed fraction ϕ depends on the following factors:

*) Amount of radiation energy reaching the target organ (tissue and distance attenuation between source and target organs).

*) Volume and composition of target organ.

*) Type and energy of the emitted radiation

*) Anatomic relationship of source-target pair

The specific absorbed fraction (Φ), is defined as ϕ divided by the mass of the target organ.

1.2. MIRD Method for Dose Calculation

Although estimate of the absorbed dose can be quite complicated, the most commonly encountered problems can be solved by some elementary operations using the MIRD (*Medical Internal Radiation Dosimetry*) method. This calculates a mean absorbed dose ($\overline{D}$) for one target organ due to the presence of radioactivity in one or more source organs. This method is based on assumption of uniform time varying radioactive concentration in source organs or regions [2]. The MIRD technique groups all penetrating and nonpenetrating radiations together. The source organ typically receives the largest radiation dose in the body. In MIRD method, the geometries of the source and target organs and the attenuating properties of the tissues in the body are presumed on the basis of standard models. But in practical purpose, very rare number of adults and children match these basic assumptions.

According to MIRD parameters, the average energy deposited in the target organ due to a radioactive decay in the source organ is the product of average energy per decay (Δ), and the absorbed fraction (ϕ). If the mass of the target organ is m, then the radiation dose to this target organ per decay in the source organ is, $\phi\Delta/m = \Phi\Delta$.

The conversion of activity to energy emitted, and the amount of energy absorbed per unit mass (absorbed dose) can be put together into a single value called the S-value. Tabulated S values published by MIRD committee are available [1,2,3] for almost all radionuclides used in nuclear medicine for different body-organs.

S value for each source-target pair can be expressed as [3,4]:

$$S(O_t \leftarrow O_s) = \sum_{All-decay-path} [\varphi(O_t \leftarrow O_s)\Delta / m]$$

This term is also known as dose per cumulated activity (O_t →Taget organ, O_s→Source organ).

The total dose to the target organ due to radioactivity in the source organ is equal to the product of S and cumulated activity (Ã). If τ is 'residence time' and A_0 be the initial activity administered to the patient, then the final equation for the dose to the target organ is,

$$D(O_t \leftarrow O_s) = \tilde{A} \times S(O_t \leftarrow O_s)$$
$$= A_0 \times \tau \times S(O_t \leftarrow O_s)$$

Residence time may be thought of as the "effective time" that the administered activity stays in the source organ.

1.2.1. MIRDOSE 3

The MIRD committee of the American Society of Nuclear Medicine (SNM) has developed a standardize method (MIRDOSE 3 software program) to study the internal dosimetry for nuclear medicine. The types and energies of radiations emitted in the decay of nuclear medicine radionuclides were tested and reviewed.

MIRDOSE 3 has a wide range of option to choose a radionuclide from a list of all possible elements. As MIRDOSE 3 does not have the capability to calculate doses from alpha emissions, these nuclides were excluded from the database.

Only one radionuclide of an element may be chosen for a particular study. The program has phantom libraries, which permit the calculation of doses for individuals of different age and size, and for women at different stages of pregnancy. Proper choice of phantom is essential during dose calculation for certain organs (e.g. fetus and/or placenta; not available for adult female phantom) [5].

MIRDOSE 3 calculates radiation dose using the MIRD principle once the residence time(s) are provided for source organ(s) during a radionuclide study. The program doesn't contain any library of residence time. There are 25-28 source organs available depending on the type of phantom used. It is essential to explain carefully the assumptions used for dose calculation [6].

Special features and models of MIRDOSE 3

i. Dynamic bladder model:

The dynamic bladder model of MIRDOSE 3 was first defined by Cloutier et al [7]. This model has been using to calculate the residence time for the urinary bladder, whose time-activity curve is quite irregular because of the filling and voiding. This bladder model requires two values as input: i) fraction of injected activity that enter the bladder and ii) biologic half-life with which urine enters the bladder. Once these two values are provided, this module can calculate the bladder residence time using the exponential series approximation of Cloutier et al. The module cannot be used for an irregular bladder-voiding schedule.

ii. Bone marrow dose calculation

The bone and marrow model in MIRDOSE 3 calculates absorbed fractions for electrons as a function of energy in different bones for marrow or trabecular or cortical bone sources depending on type of distribution (whether distributed on the bone surface or throughout the volume of the bone) of radioactive material [8]. Bone marrow dose report can be obtained in the output file if it is asked for or if trabecular / cortical bone are selected as source organs. 15 skeletal regions [4] are included in this model.

iii. Effective dose equivalent (EDE) and Effective Dose (ED)

The effective dose equivalent (EDE) as defined by ICRP 30 [9] and effective dose (ED) as defined by ICRP 60 [10] assign dimensionless weighting factors for certain organs or organ systems those are functions of their assumed relative radio-sensitivity for expressing fatal cancers or genetic defects. EDE is accomplished by multiplying the doses (actually dose equivalents) for a given organ by a stochastic risk-weighting factor, which is related to overall radiation risk. The assumed radio-sensitivities were derived from the observed rates among various populations exposed to radiation. These numbers should not be used for cases of nonstochastic effects as in situations involving radiation therapy [10].

MIRDOSE 3 calculates effective doses for a list of target organs; - gonads, colon, red marrow, lungs, stomach, urine bladder, breasts, liver, thyroid, bone surface and remainder tissues of the body. It is not necessary that all the target organs in the list show non-zero value all the time. Some target organs might show zero values for an input data set. Zero/non-zero value of a target organ depends on selection of radioisotope, phantom and source organ(s).

iv. Gastrointestinal (GI) tract model

According to ICRP 30, the GI tract is divided into four segments; stomach, small intestine, upper large intestine (ascending colon) and lower large intestine (descending colon) [9]. The user has to select the part of the tract, which acts as an entry organ (e.g. stomach for oral administration; small intestine in case of biliary clearance) and the fraction of activity entering that organ. In case of oral administration, the user also needs to define the fraction of the activity absorbed to the blood from the small intestine.

As the GI transit rates for children are considerably faster than adults, so ICRP 30 GI tract kinetic parameters are not reasonable to apply for the children. A modified GI tract model for children is included in the MIRDOSE 3 program.

v. Nodule-module:

This model allows the user to calculate dose for spheres (masses ranges from 0.01 gm to 6000 gm) composed of unit density material. This feature of this program provides doses for soft tissue spheres such as tumors. For very small spheres, S-values are obtained as being for electron and beta dose; no photon-absorbed fraction is available [11].

1.3. Internal Dosimetry for Thyroid Cancer Patients

Radioactive iodine therapy (^{131}I) is an efficient treatment and good medical practice for therapy of adult patients in case of functional thyroid carcinoma [12]. When a histoligically differentiated tumor is found by biopsy or at surgery for any patients, it is now common surgical practice to attempt a total thyroidectomy as well as total removal of recognizable thyroid tissue. Large doses of ^{131}I are routinely administered to patients for ablation of tumor/cancerous cells/ tissues following the surgery, until all clinical and serum evidence of remaining tumor tissue is abolished. The dosimetric calculations to determine the observed radiation dose per MBq (mCi) administered need percent uptake, effective half-life, tumor size and turnover of activity [13].

The patients treated for differentiated thyroid carcinoma are hypothyroid and the biochemical distribution of iodine within their body is different than that of the hyperthyroid patients. When patients are rendered hypothyroid before treatment, their renal clearance is reduced, which increases the dose to the blood and bone marrow [14]. The body compartments that would retain iodine are relatively small and the effective half-life of the ^{131}I combining physical decay and biological elimination could be quite short [15].

There are lots of different models and methods of calculating therapeutic radioiodine dose for successful ablation of residual thyroid tissues. Maxon et al. [16] suggested that, administrations of ^{131}I that will deliver 300 Gy (30,000 rad) to residual thyroid tissue or 100±20 Gy (10,000±2000 rad) to lymph node metastases will ablate them successfully 80% of the time, and bone marrow depression that is severe enough to require specialized treatment will be avoided if the whole blood dose from a single administration does not exceed 2 Gy (200 rad). Applying biologic dosimetry to thyroid cancer patients, it was found that, repeated administrations of ^{131}I deliver the same dose each time, resulting in a cumulative dose from 1-3.5 Gy (100–350 rad) in the patients who had two to seven treatments [14].

Zanzonico [17] reported that, though the external radiation hazard from the radioiodide-treated thyroid cancer patients is lesser in comparison to that of the hyperthyroid patients because of low uptake (typically <2%) and short biologic and resulting effective half-life (typically 24 h), the absorbed doses to other relevant organs are found remarkable. For 7400 MBq (200 mCi) radioiodide dose to a typical 1g of thyroid cancer-tissue, the absorbed dose to urinary bladder (considering 4-h voiding interval) was 300 rad considering 0.1% uptake with 2 days effective half-life [17].

A case-control study among Swedish thyroid cancer patients was conducted to evaluate the possible influence of ^{131}I treatment and external radiotherapy on the risk of developing a subsequent cancer. Thirty-six breast, 13 stomach, 12 kidneys and 5 bladder cancers were found in more than 2 years after ^{131}I treatment/thyroid cancer diagnosis [18].

The present work is based on a dosimetric study performed on clinical perspective. The uptake of radioiodine in different parts of the body was measured by external monitoring and the amount of radioiodine passed through urinary tract was quantified from urine samples. Effective half-lives were calculated from uptake of iodine in different organs. MIRDOSE 3 was used to calculate the absorbed doses for the concerned organs. The amount of doses absorbed to bladder wall was quantified depending on different drinking/voiding schedule. Effective dose equivalent was also calculated using MIRDOSE 3 to find an impact of post therapeutic risks of the thyroid cancer patients due to uptake of iodine in the therapeutic as well as secondary organs (act as platforms of deposition in excretion process). A model was developed to calculate the absorbed doses for target organs (remnant thyroid tissues) and to find how tissue-size and mass relates to absorbed dose in order to proper ablation.

2. Materials and Methods

2.1. Patients' Selection and Preparation

Twenty-nine female thyroid cancer patients treated with ^{131}I were included in this study. The age range was 40-60 y; mean age 50 y. The patients were accumulated consecutively over a period of 12 months. The therapy doses ranged from 3700-7400 MBq (100-200mCi) of ^{131}I, the mean dose was 5550 MBq (150mCi). All patients had undergone total thyroidectomies and thyroid hormone replacement therapy had been discontinued for appropriate periods to assure adequate hyperthyroidism prior to administered ^{131}I. They had a tracer 24 h thyroid uptake, neck and chest scan before giving tracer and a whole body scans after therapy upon hospital discharge. The patients were checked for any documented kidney diseases or other medical conditions that would decrease urine excretion.

The patients included in this study were restricted to radiation isolation in the hospital for 7 days under their consent. The long-term post therapeutic observation was especially designed to quantify the uptake of radiotracer to different organs and to calculate the effective and biologic half-lives for the entire period of observation. None of the patients' external exposure rate at one meter was more than 2 mR/hr during departure, what is considered the acceptable criterion for resuming contact [19].

2.2. Patients' Isolation Unit

The isolation unit of Cerrahpasa hospital (the place where the study was performed) is designed with two rooms along with attached bath and toilet for each one. The patients included in this study, were asked to release urine in a separate lead tank (designed as a commode) placed inside the toilet. The conventional commode was also available inside the toilet for general purposes as well. The special lead-tank arrangement allowed monitoring the excreted urine-volume of the patients during the time of study. The capacity of the tank was to contain 10 liter at a time and it was scaled in ml that was easily readable. The entire process was described to the patients before giving dose (^{131}I) and they were trained up to collect same volume urine sample by a long pipette in a vial placed inside a lead pot. The patients were asked to collect urine sample, and to note urine volume in a chart twelve-hourly for the first 72 h (3 days) and twenty-four hourly for the next 96 h (4 days). The patients were also asked to monitor the drinking water in a separate chart. After collecting sample and noting volume, they were allowed to flash the tank with sufficient water. The entire procedure along with the schedule of intake-water, collecting sample and flashing the tank was written down clearly for patient's convenience and was attached to the wall both in the room and toilet.

2.3. Collection of Data

External exposure rate measurement with GM (Geiger Muller) counter is a recognized way of measuring distribution and tracer uptake inside body [15,20]. The exposure rate (R/h) can be converted to activity (MBq/Ci) using exposure rate constant Γ (R.cm^2/mCi.h) by the following relation [21]:

$$Exposure = {(Activity \times \Gamma)}\big/{d^2}$$

Where, d is the distance between source organ and GM head. The exposure rate constant (Γ) for iodine (^{131}I) is 2.16 R.cm^2/mCi.h.

Direct data collection from the patients is always a challenging issue for this type of study. Extra shielding facilities are essential in order to maintain the intake dose minimum as much as possible for the radiation personnel. For this study, a temporary wall made of lead-block was arranged near the exit of the isolation unit providing three narrow holes on it. The height, width and thickness of the wall were 180 cm, 90 cm and 15 cm. The narrow holes were arranged to place the GM detector inside keeping the main body (display meter) of the counter outside the wall. The person engaged in measuring stayed out side the wall and holding the GM counter and passed the detector inside through holes.

During exposure measurement at a certain location of the body, the net counting was affected by the activity in surrounding body-part. The GM detector-head was collimated with a small piece of hollow lead pipe before placing upon ROI to minimize extra counting from surroundings.

The patients were previously directed/trained to place the detector within 1cm of thyroid, stomach and thigh those were located by ultrasound and duly marked with deep ink earlier. The exposure rates were collected 12 hourly for the first 72 h and then 24 hourly for the next 96 h. The GM counter (Eberline ESP-2) was calibrated half yearly in the SSDL (Secondary standard dosimetry laboratory) of cekmece nuclear research and study center, Turkish atomic energy commission, Istanbul. The energy response of the meter was checked as 0.97 for ^{131}I and 0.96 for ^{137}Cs. Three trained personnel were engaged in cyclic order to collect the urine sample and in measurement of exposure rate and they were monitored by pocket dosimeter. The average intake dose was (1.50±0.25) mSv for each patient. Special care was taken for these workers so that the total dose was within 20msv/y [10].

In cases where more than one measuring devices are used for same purpose, it is common practice to check all the devices with the same sample to get same result. Each urine sample (1mL) collected for each patient time to time was measured by GM counter at 1cm distance and then by a gamma counter (Atomlab 900). These two sets of readings showed very good correlation ($p<0.005$) and hence proved the authenticity of other readings.

2.4. Dose Calculation and Analysis for Body Organs

2.4.1. Attenuation Correction for Collected Data

The collected data (activity) was corrected for attenuation multiplying by the factor ($1/e^{-\mu d}$), where, tissue attenuation coefficient, μ_{tissue}=0.110 cm^{-1} and d is the average depth of the lesions inside body.

2.4.2. Input form of MIRDOSE 3

During dose calculation with MIRDOSE 3, the parameters selected from the input form were: i) radionuclide $^{131}_{53}$I, ii) adult female non-pregnant phantom and iii) four source organs (thyroid, muscle, stomach and urinary bladder contents). The effective half life for individual organ for each patient was calculated from the time-activity curve drawn from the patients' data. The biologic half life for ^{131}I was calculated from its relation with effective and physical (known) half lives. These quantities were used to calculate the residence times for thyroid, thigh-muscle and stomach [22]. The residence time of urinary bladder was calculated using dynamic bladder model of MIRDOSE 3 program providing fractions of dose passing 0.87 and 0.09 with biologic half-lives 28.5 h and 118.43 h consecutively along with an average voiding interval 3 h.

2.4.3. Patients' Groups

All the patients were divided into four groups depending on the dose administered. The doses for different groups were; Group-a: 3700 – 4625 MBq (100-125 mCi), Group-b: 4626 – 5550 MBq (126-150 mCi), Group-c: 5551 – 6475 MBq (151-175 mCi), Group-d: 6476 – 7400 MBq (176-200 mCi).

The absorbed doses were calculated for individual group at different voiding intervals. All the patients were advised to drink as much water/liquid as possible to reduce the voiding interval and hence absorbed dose.

In the second phase, the patients were divided into four groups depending on the amount of water drunk individually; Gr-A: 10-12 L (first 3 days) & 12-14 L (next 4 days), Gr-B: 13-15 L (first 3 days) & 15-17 L (next 4 days), Gr-C: 16-18 L (first 3 days) & 18-20 L (next 4 days), Gr-D: 19-21 L (first 3 days) & 21-23 L (next 4 days).

To calculate the effective dose equivalent, three organs (thyroid, stomach and bladder) were selected consecutively as source organ and depending on the residence time over these organs, the effective doses were calculated by MIRDOSE 3 program for all the assigned organs (except thyroid). The average group dose was multiplied with this value to find a total effective dose equivalent for each group in mSv. Thyroid dose was not included during dose calculation as that was the therapeutic organ.

The patients were also divided depending on the size of remnant tissue-spot (table-5).

2.4.4. Statistical Analysis

Correlation Coefficient (r) among the measured uptakes for different organs were (thyroid, thigh-muscle, stomach, urine) were calculated using MS Excel and corresponding level of significance was determined (degrees of freedom for n-2 = 27) from the standard table of correlation coefficient [23]. The highest level of significance was considered for $p<0.001$.

2.5. Dose Calculation for Target-Tissues

In this study, the target-tissue dosimetry was performed analytically using MIRDOSE 3 depending on the uptake of ^{131}I in thyroid with time measured at phases (total six months time period; section 2.5.2). Total 57 tissue spots (1.1<diameter<2.58 cm) were selected from 21 patients. The remnant tissues were identified by scintigraphy. The size and depth of the spots were measured by ulatrasonography and were duly marked. For simplicity, the sizes of the remnant tissue spots were considered as spherical shape. The radius of each sphere was measured by ultrasound machine (Philips SONOS 2000). As the diameter of GM counter's head was 3.2 cm, so the bigger remnant tissues (radius>1.6 cm) were not included for this dosimetric calculation.

The steps for dose calculation were as follows:

2.5.1. Selection of Spots and Calculation of Effective Lesion-Activity:

Small spots (spherical radius<1.6 cm) were taken into account. The number of spots of different patients was within 2-4 (table-5). A model was developed to calculate the contribution of each lesion during uptake calculation for individual patient. The collected data was corrected for attenuation ($1/e^{-\mu d}$).

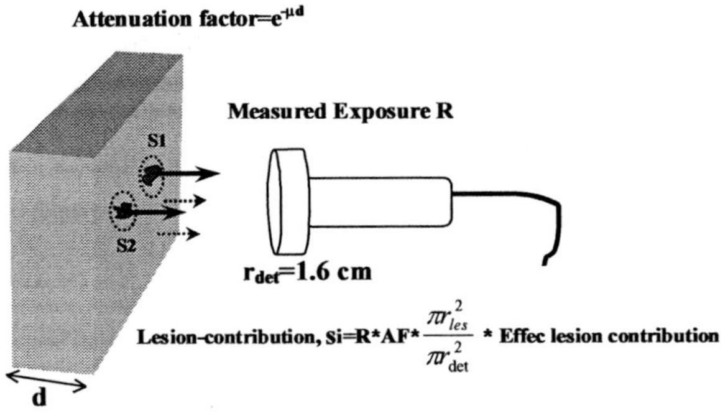

Determination of effective area of individual lesion:

Each lesion effective-area to detector head $= \dfrac{\pi r_{les}^2}{\pi r_{\det}^2}$.

To discard the surrounding contribution rather than lesion, another factor was calculated from the ratio:

$$\text{Lesion-contribution} = \frac{\text{Radiation coming from lesion}}{\text{Total radiation coming from lesion and surrounding}}.$$

This factor was calculated using a neck phantom with some hot spots inside it. Hence, individual effective lesion-activity (ELA) for each patient was calculated taking the products of four factors; - Measured uptake (activity in terms of MBq) $\times \dfrac{1}{(e^{-\mu d})} \times$ lesion effective area $\times$ lesion-contribution factors to the measured activity. Activity-time product (MBq.s) for individual lesion for each phase was calculated multiplying each ELA (MBq) with corresponding average phase-time (s) (described in section 2.5.2).

The volume of spherical spot ($\frac{4}{3}\pi r^3$) was calculated from the measured radius and was converted to mass multiplying by soft tissue density (ρ=1.03g/cm^3). The absorbed-dose per cumulated activity (mGy/MBq.S) corresponding to the measured mass of individual lesion was calculated using log-log graph (fig-5) drawn from nodule-module protocol of MIRDOSE 3.

Finally, individual lesion-absorbed dose for each phase was calculated multiplying activity-time product (MBq.s) with absorbed dose per cumulated activity (mGy/MBq.s). The total absorbed dose for individual lesion was found from the sum of all phase-doses.

2.5.2. Dose Calculation Layout

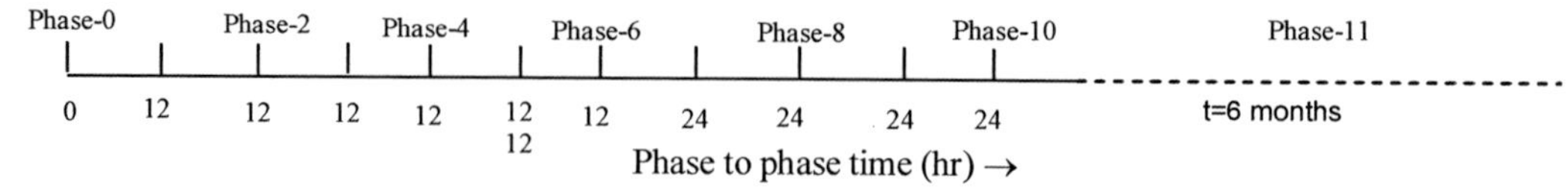

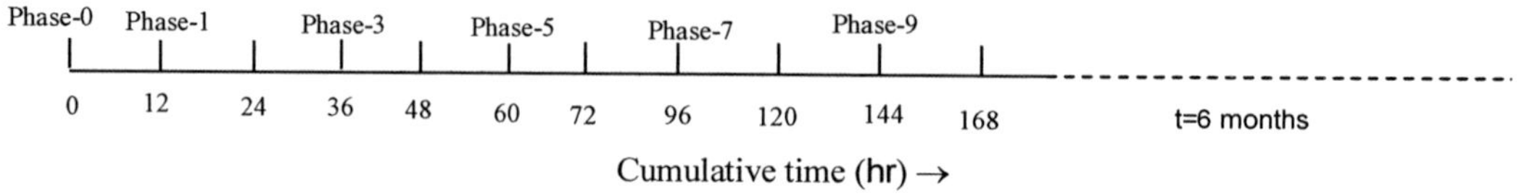

Phase to phase average time $(T_i) = (T_{Phase(i)} + T_{Phase(i-1)})/2$
Average activity (A_i) between two consecutive phase $= (A_{Phase(i)} + A_{phase(i-1)})/2$

Time-activity product for each phase

$$(MBq.s)_i = \frac{\left(A_{Phase(i)} + A_{phase(i-1)}\right)}{2} \times \frac{\left(T_{Phase(i)} + T_{phase(i-1)}\right)}{2}$$

Lesion-absorbed dose for each phase $AD_{(i)}$ = Absorbed dose per unit cumulated activity (mGy/MBq.S) × Time-activity product (MBq.s).

Total lesion-absorbed dose (Gy) =

$$\sum_{i=1}^{10} AD_{(i)} + \text{[Abs. dose per cumulated activity (mGy/MBq.s)]} \times \int_0^t (Activity)_{phase-10} e^{-\lambda t} dt$$

The last term was calculated analytically considering phase-10 activity as reference [at time t=0] with upper limit as [t=6 months]. Activity was decreased with effective decay constant λ ($\frac{\ln 2}{T_{1/2}}$). Considering an average effective half life for all the patients ($T_{1/2}$) ≅ 39.18 hr; $\lambda = 4.92 \times 10^{-6}$ sec^{-1}.

2.5.3. Block Diagram of Different Steps:

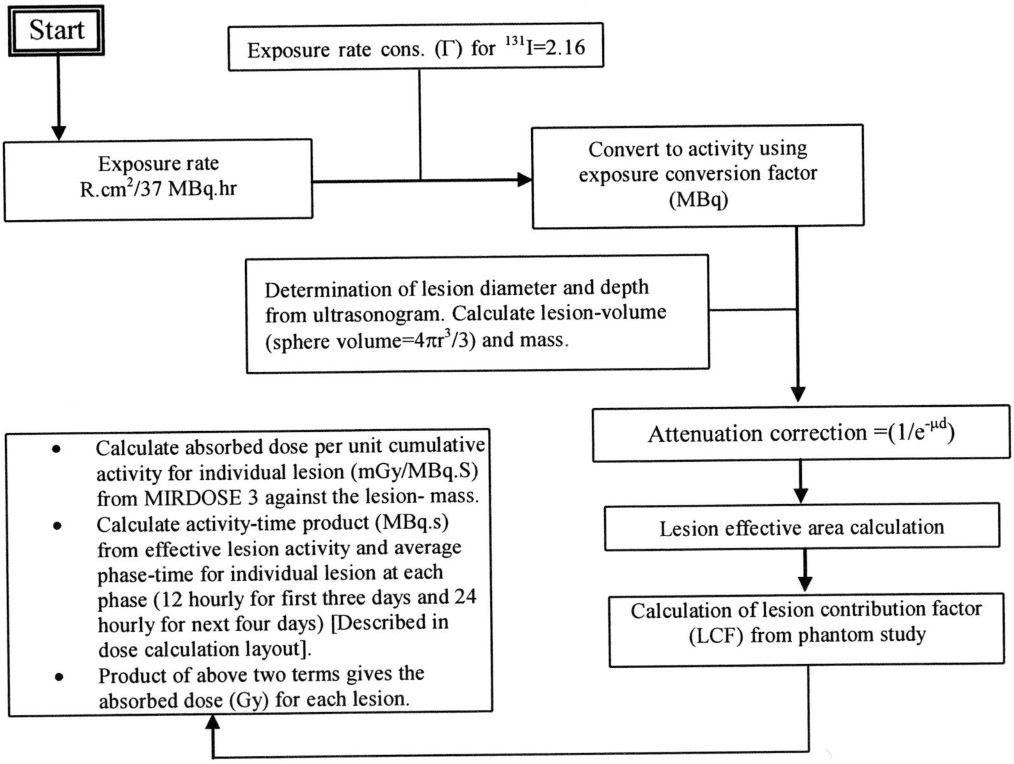

3. Results

Figure-3.1 shows the effective decay-curves for different organs plotted in terms of exposure rates measured at different time intervals. The exponential nature of the decay curves shows a symmetric approach with different effective half lives for different organs.

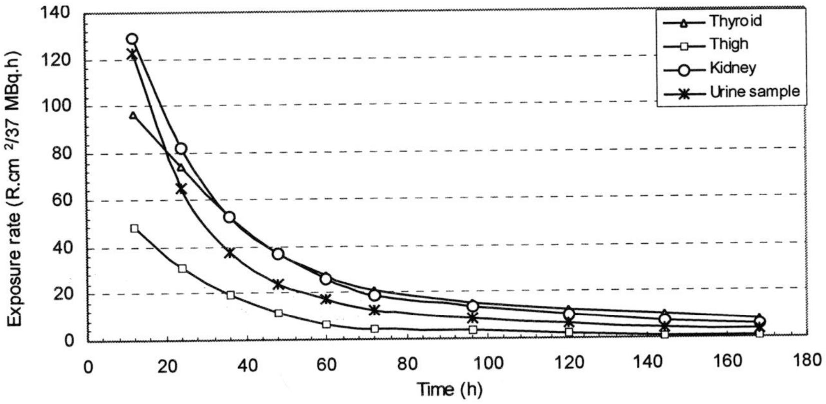

Figure 3.1: Effective decay curves for different organs

The long-term post therapeutic observation was especially designed to quantify the flow of radioisotope through urinary tract and to calculate the effective and biologic half lives for the entire period of observation considering the physical half life (8 days) of iodine. As the flow of iodine was more intense for the first few days than for the rest of the period, so the effective half lives were calculated in two phases for the urine sample and it was found to be 24.81±0.74 h for the first 72 h and 73.25±0.64 h for the next 96 h. The effective and biologic half-lives with corresponding residence-times (required for MIRDOSE 3) for all the organs are summarized in table-1. Figure-3.2 shows about 87% excretion of the radioisotope through urinary tract in first 72 h [24]. Though it is found some noticeable standard deviation (figure-3.2) within first 60 h, but after that, it is almost flat.

Table-1: Effective and biologic half-lives for thyroid, thigh, stomach and urine with corresponding residence time.

				Urine	
	Thyroid	Thigh-muscle	Stomach	First 3 days (87%)	Next 4 days (9%)
Effective half life § (h)	39.18 ± 0.85	31.50 ± 0.40	33.11 ± 0.70	24.8 ± 0.75	73.25 ± 0.65
Biologic half life § (h)	49.22 ± 0.70	37.68 ± 0.55	40 ± 0.65	28.5 ± 0.95	118.43 ± 0.50
Residence time (h)	56.42	45.36	47.68	1.23‡	

§Average±S.D ‡Calculated using Dynamic Bladder Model of MIRDOSE3

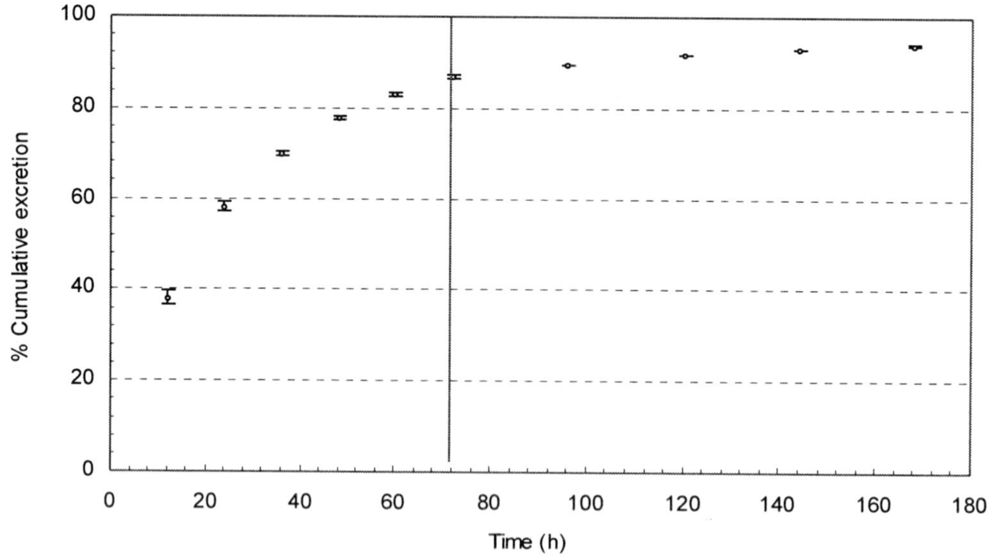

Figure 3.2: Excretion of iodine (measured from urine sample).

Table 2: Absorbed doses to different organs for four groups (classified according to given dose).

	Absorbed dose§ (mGy)		
Group dose (MBq)	Thigh-muscle	Stomach	Urine-bladder
a 3700 – 4625 (n=7)	61.30 ± 5.38	685.82 ± 13.73	2118.19 ± 454
b 4626 – 5550 (n=6)	70.62 ± 6.20	790.18 ± 15.81	2477.94 ± 569
c 5551 – 6475 (n=8)	81.28 ± 7.08	909.45 ± 18.11	2869.21 ± 646
d 6476 – 7400 (n=8)	93.50 ± 8.18	1046.19 ± 20.84	3295.11 ± 717

§Group average ± SD

Table 3: Absorbed dose to bladder at different voiding intervals for four groups (classified on given dose).

Group no. with dose limit (MBq)	Average of total activity passes urinary tract (MBq) for first 72 hrs§	Average of total activity passes urinary tract (MBq) for next 96 hrs§	Bladder voiding interval (hr)	Absorbed dose (mGy)
a (3700-4625) (n=7)	3636±160	367±18	1	687
			2	1385
			3	2077
			4	2770
b (4626-5550) (n=6)	4265±130	418±25	1	821
			2	1645
			3	2481
			4	3316
c (5551-6475) (n=8)	4936±186	487±20	1	951
			2	1905
			3	2873
			4	3840
d (6476-7400) (n=8)	5668±241	560±30	1	1092
			2	2188
			3	3299
			4	4410

§Average value ± SD

The absorbed doses due to uptake of radioiodine in different organs are shown in table-2. The thyroid-absorbed doses (target doses) were found much higher than those of others (discussed later). Among the secondary platforms of body organs, urine bladder doses are found significantly high (as low as 2118.19 ± 454mGy for Gr.a and as high as 3295.11 ± 717mGy for Gr.d). The stomach-absorbed doses (685.82 ± 13.73mGy for Gr.a and 1046.19 ± 20.84mGy for Gr.d) are found lower than urine bladder but higher than that of thigh-muscle.

The absorbed doses in thigh-muscle are found within a range of 61.30±5.38mGy (Gr.a) to 93.50±8.18mGy (Gr.d) [25].

The absorbed doses to urine bladder for different voiding intervals are summarized in table-3 for four groups divided on given radioiodine dose. The absorbed dose increases around 100% if the voiding interval increases from 1 h to 2 h. This dose increases by 50% for the next hour and 33% for one more hour consecutively [24]. The absorbed dose between two consecutive groups (dose difference 925 MBq) for same voiding interval differs as follows (approximately):

Gr.a–Gr.b: + 19%, Gr.b–Gr.c: +16%, and Gr.c–Gr.d: + 15%.

Figure-3.3 shows the absorbed doses with corresponding standard deviation (SD) (calculated with urine bladder model of MORDOSE 3) in urine bladder per liter of water drunk for four groups (classified on drinking water). Average biologic half-lives and fractions of total doses passing through urinary tract for four groups were considered same; 85% excretion with half life (28.5±0.64) h and 9% with half-life (118.43±0.53) h. The absorbed dose was calculated for each patient individually depending on one's voiding interval. Then the ratio of absorbed dose and water drunk was calculated for each patient and was averaged over group. Between the two columns (one for first 3 days and one for next 4 days) for each group of figure-3.3, the second one looks almost flat and hence indicates minimum level of absorbed dose to bladder during the next 4 days.

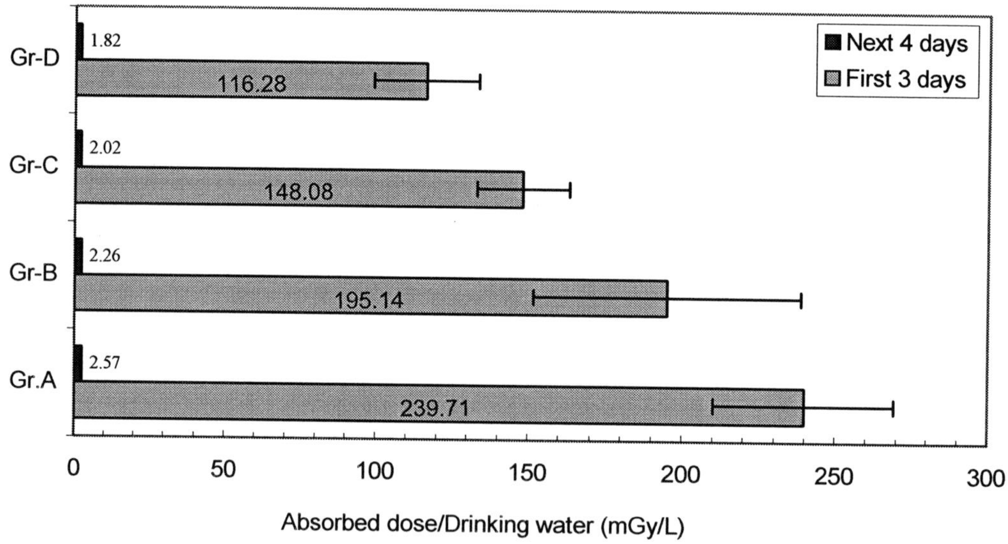

Figure 3.3: Absorbed dose and water intake ratio for four groups (classified on drinking water).

From statistical analysis, the correlation coefficient (r) among the measured uptakes was found very significant ($p<0.001$) for thyroid-thigh and stomach-urine (table-4). This was found fairly significant ($p<0.01$) for thigh-stomach but non-significant for thyroid-stomach and thyroid-urine ($p<0.1$).

Effective dose equivalent (EDEs) were calculated individually considering three source organs,- thyroid, stomach and bladder (act as platform in excretion process), for all the target organs (except thyroid) assigned as sensitive tissues for fatal occurrences described by ICRP 60 [10,25]. Therapeutic doses (thyroid doses) were not taken into account in calculating the total effective dose equivalent. Figure-3.4 shows the effective dose equivalent calculated individually for three source organs and the doses for stomach were found remarkably highest among the three source organs.

Table 4: Correlation coefficient and the level of significance between different organ pair

Organ pair	Correlation Coefficient (r)	Level of significance (df = 27)
Thyroid -Thigh	0.61	$p<0.001$
Stomach-Urine	0.64	$p<0.001$
Thigh-Stomach	0.51	$p<0.01$
Thyroid-Stomach	0.33	$p<0.1$
Thyroid-Urine	0.34	$p<0.1$

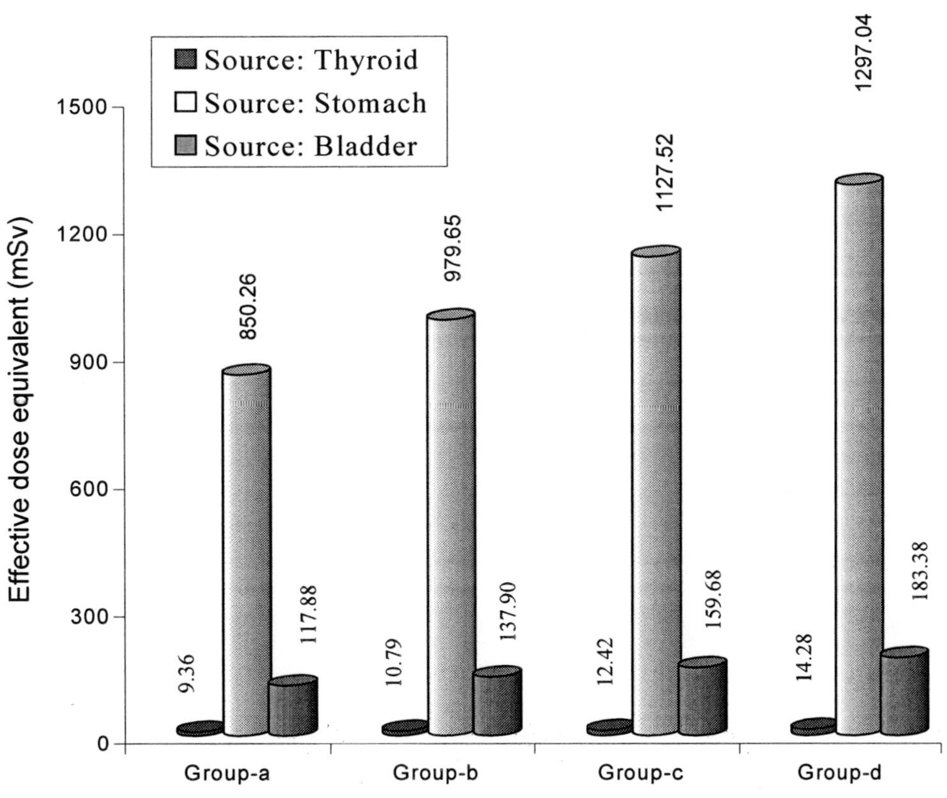

Figure 3.4: Effective dose equivalent for 4 groups (classified on given activity).

Figure-3.5 (log-log graph) was drawn from the nodule-module model of MIRDOSE 3 to calculate the absorbed dose per unit-cumulated activity for thyroid remnant tissue. Individual specifications and all the parameters relevant to remnant-tissue dose measurement are summarized in table-5.

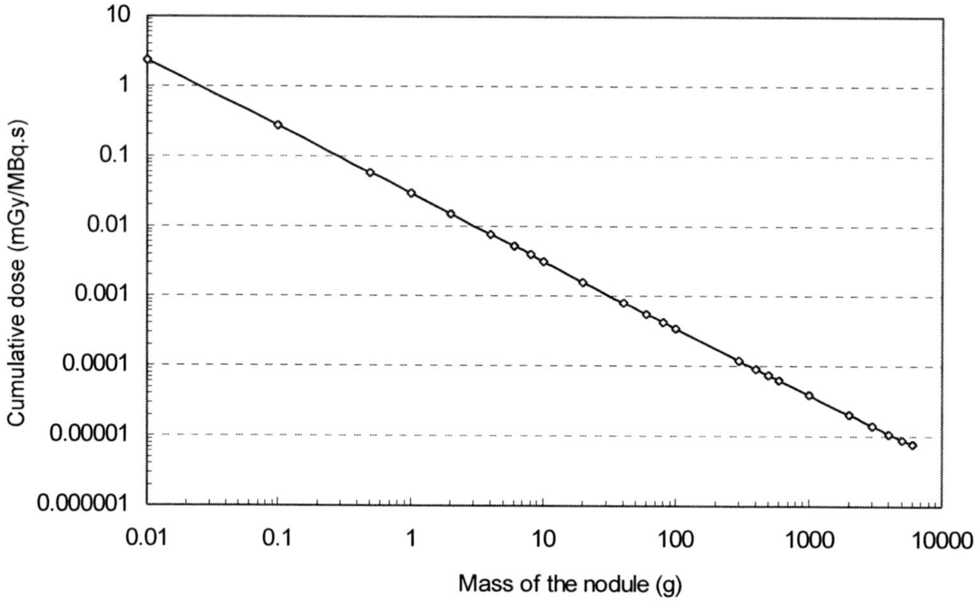

Figure 3.5: Nodule mass - Absorbed dose curve (MIRDOSE 3 table)

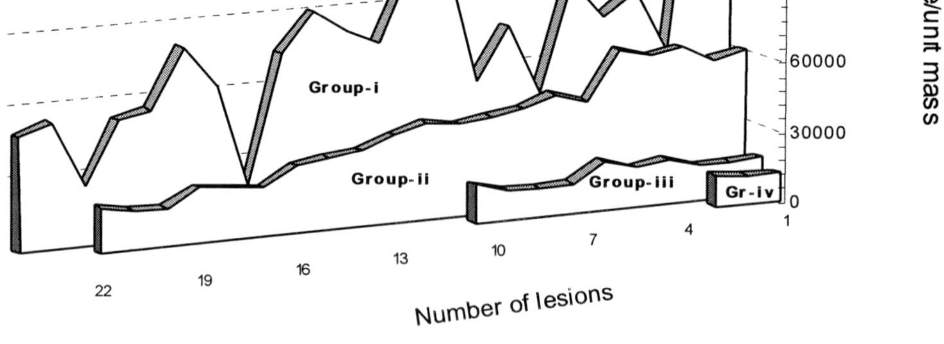

Figure 3.6: Lesion-absorbed dose per unit mass for 4 groups (classified on lesion-size).

Figure-3.6 shows 3d view of absorbed dose per unit mass of remnant tissues for four groups (classified depending on the size of the remnant-tissue spot). The length of each graph indicates the number of lesions belong to that group. Graph for group-i (radius<0.75 cm) shows extreme zigzag pattern and hence exhibits large uncertainties associated with target dose calculation (ablation dose) for very small spot. Minimum uncertainties are observed with bigger (1.00<radius<1.7 cm) tissue spots. Figure-3.7 shows the average absorbed dose along with standard deviation (SD) for each group (classified depending on the size of the remnant-tissue spot) and satisfies the results of figure-3.6.

Table 5: Calculation of parameters for target dose measurement of remnana tissues

Group	Patient's No.	Lesion No.	Radius of fic-sphere cm	Tiss-vol = $4/3\pi r^3$ cm^3	Tiss-mass [ρ=1.03 g/cc] g	Cumula - activity [Fig. 3.5]	Lesion effective area to GM head = $\pi r^2/\pi r_d^2$ [r_d=1.6cm]	Lesion depth cm	Attenuatn $1/e^{-\mu d}$ [μ=0.110 cm^{-1}]
Gr. i	1	1	0.56	0.74	0.76	-0.100	0.12	6.25	1.99
Radius<		2	0.625	1.02	1.05	0.550	0.15	7.50	2.28
0.75cm	7	1	0.605	0.93	0.95	-0.550	0.14	6.50	2.04
		2	0.585	0.84	0.86	-0.200	0.13	8.25	2.48
	10	1	0.59	0.86	0.89	-0.220	0.14	9.00	2.69
		2	0.675	1.29	1.33	0.100	0.18	6.00	1.93
	21	1	0.595	0.88	0.91	-0.280	0.14	8.50	2.55
		2	0.635	1.07	1.10	0.280	0.16	5.50	1.83
		3	0.71	1.50	1.54	0.070	0.20	6.00	1.93
	3	1	0.645	1.12	1.16	0.200	0.16	4.00	1.55
		2	0.655	1.18	1.21	0.150	0.17	4.50	1.64
	6	1	0.565	0.76	0.78	-0.130	0.12	4.75	1.69
		2	0.55	0.70	0.72	-0.080	0.12	4.00	1.55
		3	0.645	1.12	1.16	0.200	0.16	6.25	1.99
	17	1	0.65	1.15	1.18	0.170	0.17	5.25	1.78
		2	0.61	0.95	0.98	-1.250	0.15	5.50	1.83
		3	0.7	1.44	1.48	0.070	0.19	5.75	1.88
	5	1	0.69	1.38	1.42	0.080	0.19	4.25	1.60
	9	1	0.705	1.47	1.51	0.073	0.19	4.50	1.64
		2	0.73	1.63	1.68	0.058	0.21	3.75	1.51
	11	1	0.615	0.97	0.97	-0.900	0.15	5.00	1.73
		2	0.73	1.63	1.68	0.058	0.21	5.25	1.78
	12	1	0.715	1.53	1.58	0.067	0.20	4.00	1.55
Gr. ii	4	1	0.77	1.91	1.97	0.040	0.23	5.25	1.78
0.75 <		2	0.805	2.18	2.25	0.032	0.25	6.00	1.93
Radius <	2	1	0.775	1.95	2.01	0.040	0.23	3.50	1.47
1.00 cm		2	0.805	2.18	2.25	0.035	0.25	4.00	1.55
	5	2	0.81	2.22	2.29	0.035	0.26	4.00	1.55
	9	3	0.84	2.48	2.56	0.032	0.28	4.00	1.55
	11	3	0.79	2.06	2.13	0.040	0.24	5.50	1.83
	12	2	0.78	1.99	2.05	0.040	0.24	5.25	1.78
		3	0.815	2.27	2.33	0.035	0.26	5.00	1.73
	13	1	0.81	2.22	2.29	0.035	0.26	3.00	1.39
		2	0.785	2.03	2.09	0.040	0.24	3.75	1.51
		3	0.85	2.57	2.65	0.030	0.28	4.25	1.60
	8	1	0.86	2.66	2.74	0.032	0.29	3.75	1.51
		2	0.915	3.21	3.30	0.030	0.33	4.00	1.55
		3	0.965	3.76	3.88	0.022	0.36	5.50	1.83
	15	2	0.98	3.94	4.06	0.025	0.38	3.50	1.47
	16	1	0.995	4.12	4.25	0.022	0.39	4.50	1.64
		2	0.93	3.37	3.47	0.023	0.34	4.25	1.60
	18	3	0.96	3.70	3.82	0.022	0.36	3.75	1.51
		4	0.935	3.42	3.52	0.022	0.34	4.25	1.60
	20	1	0.945	3.53	3.64	0.027	0.35	5.50	1.83

Table 5: Continued

Group	Patient's No.	Lesion No.	Radius of fic-sphere cm	Tiss-vol $= 4/3\pi r^3$ cm^3	Tiss-mass [ρ=1.03 g/cc] g	Cumula - activity [Fig. 3.5]	Lesion effective area to GM head $= \pi r^2/\pi r_d^2$ [r_d=1.6cm]	Lesion depth cm	Attenuatn $1/e^{-\mu d}$ [μ=0.110 cm^{-1}]
Gr. iii 1.00 < Radius< 1.25 cm	14	1	1.12	5.88	6.06	0.018	0.49	6.00	1.93
		2	1.175	6.79	7.00	0.015	0.54	5.75	1.88
		3	1.2	7.23	7.45	0.018	0.56	4.75	1.69
	15	1	1.06	4.99	5.14	0.020	0.44	4.00	1.55
		3	1.16	6.53	6.73	0.015	0.53	4.00	1.55
	16	3	1.05	4.85	4.99	0.020	0.43	5.75	1.88
	18	1	1.21	7.42	7.64	0.018	0.57	5.00	1.73
	19	1	1.23	7.79	8.02	0.018	0.59	5.00	1.73
		3	1.19	7.06	7.27	0.014	0.55	5.00	1.73
	20	3	1.05	4.85	4.99	0.020	0.43	5.00	1.73
Gr. iv Radius> 1.25 cm	18	2	1.26	8.37	8.63	0.016	0.62	4.75	1.69
	19	2	1.26	8.37	8.63	0.016	0.62	5.25	1.78
	20	2	1.29	8.99	9.26	0.015	0.65	4.50	1.64

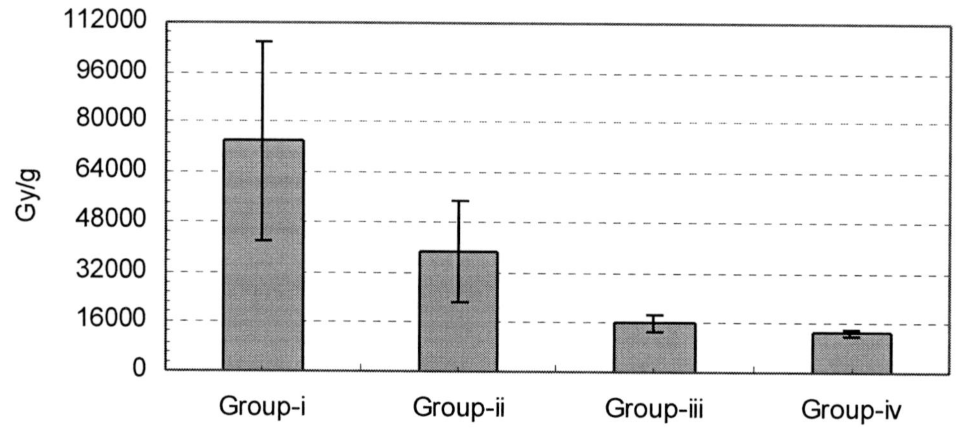

Figure 3.7: Group-average for absorbed dose per unit mass with corresponding SD.

4. Discussion

Optimization of the target dose is essential for proper ablation of the remnant thyroid tissues after thyroidectomy of the thyroid cancer patients. During dose calculation, it is important to differentiate projected doses from that what is really obtained to the target organ. These two doses differ considerably because of the irradiation from surrounding parts of the body [26]. Some studies showed that ^{131}I uptake and therapeutic outcome might not be closely related [13]. For a specific level of radiation, percent uptake per g was found inversely related to effective half life [13].

The handling of patients and data collection after giving high doses of activity, need great precautionary measures against contamination, hazard and taking of over doses by the radiation personnel. Patients-monitoring in first twenty-four hours after administered radioiodine, are very important, because most of radioiodine excretes within this period.

To investigate the influence of the diagnostic administration of low dose ^{131}I on subsequent uptake of therapeutic radiation in cases of thyroid cancer patients, Huic et al. found an effective half-life 40.3±23.0 h of the diagnostic dose in thyroid remnants [27], what satisfies the present results. From an extensive dosimetric study among thyroid cancer patients after oral administration of radioactive ^{131}I, it was found a medium effective half-life of at least 14h, with substantial variation by North et al. [15]. Normally the external radiation hazard from the radioiodide-treated thyroid cancer patients is found lesser in comparison to that of the hyperthyroid patients because of low uptake (typically <2%) and short biologic and effective half-life (typically 24 h). Zanzonico [17] found remarkably high- absorbed dose to the relevant organs among the patients treated with ^{131}I after thyroidectomy. For 7400 MBq (200 mCi) radioiodide dose to a typical 1g thyroid cancer-tissue, the absorbed dose to urinary bladder (considering 4-h voiding interval) was 300 rad considering 0.1% uptake with 2 days effective half-life [17].

Five more male patients were studied (but their data haven't included in analysis) for comparison of the results obtained in this study from female patients and with adult female phantom of MIRDOSE 3. The average effective half life for the male patients was found about 15% less than that of the present result. Four among five of the male patients (80%) comprised to Gr-D: 19-21 L (first 3 days) and 21-23 L (next 4 days). So their bladder absorbed-dose and water-intake ratio was found in the minimum level.

According to ICRP 60 [10], an annual limit of effective dose equivalent should be maintained as 20 mSv for a particular organ in case of internal exposure, so that the lifetime dose equivalent must not exceed 20 Sv for an organ, which is sufficient to avoid deterministic effects in unspecified tissues and organs. From the distribution of probabilities of fatal sites specific cancers among male and female over age 0-90 y in four countries (Japan, US, UK and Puerto Rico), an average factor was found maximum for stomach (0.225) over other organs [10]. For urine bladder, the factor was 0.044.

The absorbed doses in the urine bladder were found three times more (table-2) than that of stomach for all the groups. But, the higher tissue-weighting factor of stomach (0.16) in comparison to bladder (0.04) produces higher risks of fatal occurrences (fig-3.4) and need intense care in post therapeutic period [10].

The protocol described for target dose measurement in this study allowed dose calculation by phases rather than using a common decay constant. It seems not realistic to consider a single decay constant for a long-term observation. The excretion of iodine is much more intense for first few hours than rest of the period in general and also depend on the amount of water by the patients. So it is most likely that a significant error should propagate in dose calculation when a constant decay factor is used for entire period of dose calculation.

The nodule-module protocol of MIRDOSE 3 shows that absorbed dose to soft tissue strongly depends on the mass/volume of the target organ. The absorbed dose per unit cumulated activity (mGy/MBq.s) increases very sharply as mass of the target tissue decreases. In the present study, the absorbed dose/g is found as high as 1.72E+05 Gy (Gr-i; radius<0.75) and as low as 1.22E+04 Gy (Gr-iv; radius>1.25 cm). This figure is significantly higher than some previous results [28].

It was not possible to monitor the progression of ablation frequently for entire period. The patients were monitored in six months interval after hospital discharge and most of the spots (r<1.0 cm) were found properly ablated in first six-month period. Some of the larger spots (radius>1.25 cm) took longer time (up to 3 follow-up cycle; 6 months×3) for full ablation.

REFERENCES

[1] Early, P.J & Sodee, B. Principles and practice of Nuclear Medicine, 2nd ed. St. Louis, Missouri: Mosby-year book, Inc, 1995, 752-756

[2] Loevinger, R; Budinger, T.F & Watson, E.E. MIRD primer for absorbed dose calculations. Revised ed. New York: Society of Nuclear Medicine, 1991.

[3] Snyder, W; Ford, M; Warner, G & Fisher, H. Jr. Estimates of absorbed fractions for monoenergetic photon sources uniformly distributed in various organs of a heterogeneous phantom. MIRD pamphlet 5, *J Nucl Med* (Suppl 3), 1969, 5: 6-52.

[4] Snyder, W; Ford, M; Warner, G & Watson, S. "S" absorbed dose per unit cumulated activity for selected radionuclides and organs. MIRD pamphlet 11. New York: Society of Nuclear Medicine, 1975.

[5] Smith, E.M & Warner, G.G. Estimate of radiation dose to the embryo from nuclear medicine procedures, *J Nucl Med*, 1976, 17:836-839.

[6] Stabin, M. M I R D O S E 3, Documentation Package. Oak Ridge, USA: Radiation Internal Dose Information Center, 1994.

[7] Cloutier, R; Smith, S; Watson, E; Snyder, W & Warner, G. Dose to the fetus from radionuclides in the bladder. *Health Phys*, 1973, 25:147-161.

[8] Whitwell J.R, Spiers F.W. Calculated beta-ray dose factors for trabecular bone, *Phys Med Biol*, 1976, 21:16-38.

[9] International Commission on Radiological Protection. Limits for intakes of radionuclides by workers. ICRP Publication 30, New York: Pergamon press, 1979.

[10] International Commission on Radiological Protection.1990 Recommendations of the International Commission on Radiological Protection. ICRP Publication 60, *Ann ICRP* 21(1-3), Oxford, England: Pergamon press, 1991.

[11] Stabin, M; Stubbs, J. Radiation dose to the walls of hollow organs. *J Nucl Med*, 1994, 35(5): 788.

[12] Freitas, J.E; Gross, M.D; Ripley, S & Shapiro, B. Radionuclide diagnosis and therapy of thyroid cancer: Current status report. *Semin Nucl Med*, 1985, 15: 106-131.

[13] Reynolds, J. C. Percent ^{131}I uptake and post-therapy in ^{131}I scan: Their role in the management of thyroid cancer. *Thyroid*, 1997, 7(2): 281-284.

[14] M'Kacher, R; Schlumberger, M; Legal J.D. et al. Biologic dosimetry in thyroid cancer patients after repeated treatments with ^{131}I. *J Nucl Med*, 1998, 39: 825-829.

[15] North, D.L; Shearer, D.R; Hessessey, J.V. & Donovan G. L. Effective half-life of ^{131}I in thyroid cancer patients. *Health Phys*, 2002, 81(3): 325-329.

[16] Maxon, H.R; Thomas, S.R; Samaratunga, R.C. Dosimetric considerations in the radioiodine treatment of macrometastases and micrometastases from different thyroid cancer. *Thyroid*, 1997, 7(2): 183-187.

[17] Zanzonico, P.B. Radiation dose to patients and relatives incident to ^{131}I therapy. *Thyroid*, 1997, 7(2): 199-204.

[18] Hall, P; Holm, L.E; Lundell, G; Ruden, B.I. Tumors after radiotherapy for thyroid cancer. A case-control study within a cohort of thyroid cancer patients. *Acta Oncol*, 1992, 31(4): 403-7.

[19] Culver, C.M; Dworkin, H.J. Radiation safety considerations for post ^{131}I hyperthyroid therapy. *J Nucl Med*, 1991, 32: 169-173.

[20] Culver, C.M; Dworkin, H.J. Radiation safety considerations for post ^{131}I thyroid cancer therapy. *J Nucl Med*, 1992, 33:1402-1405.

[21] Sorenson, J.A & Phelps, M.E. Physics in Nuclear Medicine. Orlando, Florida: Grune & Stratton, Inc. 1987.

[22] Henkin, R.E. et al. Nuclear Medicine. Vol- I, St. Louis, Missouri: Mosby-year book, 1996, pp316-333.

[23] Mould, R.F. Introductory Medical Statistics. 3rd ed. Bristol, UK: IOP Publishing Ltd, 1998, pp178-195.

[24] Ahmed, Sabbir A.S.M; Demir, M; Yasar, D & Uslu, I. Quantification of absorbed dose to urine bladder depending on drinking water during radioiodine therapy to thyroid cancer patients: a clinical study using MIRDOSE 3. *Nucl Med Commun*, 2003, 24(7), 749-54.

[25] Ahmed, S; Jahan Q.M; Demir, M; Zakaria, G.A. Study in radioiodine distribution over several organs of the thyroid cancer patients to determine the effective dose equivalent that relates to fatal occurrences: A clinical perspective. *World J Nucl Med*, 2004, **3**(2), 131-136.

[26] Fueger, G.F. Dosimetry and dose-schedule of radioiodine therapy with ^{131}I. *Acta Med Austriaca*, 1987, 14(3-4): 87-8.

[27] Huic, D; Medvedec, M; Dodig, D; Popovic, S; Ivancevic, D; Pavlinovic, Z & Zuvic, M. Radioiodine uptake in thyroid cancer patients after diagnostic application of low dose ^{131}I. *Nucl Med Commun*, 1996, 17(10): 839-42.

[28] Kenneth, F. K; Ronald, S. A; Carey, J.E & Beierwaltes W. H. Iodine-131 treatment of thyroid cancer: Absorbed dose calculated from post-therapy scans. *J Nucl Med*, 1986, 27:1207-1211.

In: Trends in Thyroid Cancer Research
Editor: Carl A. Milton, pp. 183-201
ISBN 1-59454-627-4

Chapter IX

An Update and Review of Oncogenes, Tumor Suppressor Genes, and Other Tumor Markers in Thyroid Carcinomas

Salwa S. Sheikh*
Pathology Services Division, Dhahran Health Center,
Saudi Aramco, Saudi Arabia

Abstract

Cancer of thyroid gland is an uncommon tumor that predominantly affects women most often in 3rd-5th decade. Thyroid tumors develop when the growth of a single thyroid epithelial cell escapes from the normal mechanisms regulating cell divisions and gains a selective growth advantage. Unregulated cell division can result from mutations in both oncogenes and tumor suppressor genes. An understanding of mutations of the proto-oncogenes and tumor suppressor genes that occur in these tumors should eventually explain the diverse clinical characteristics of thyroid tumors and also direct therapy. These genetic abnormalities usually represent somatic / acquired mutations as opposed to germline / inherited mutations because most thyroid tumors are sporadic and not familial. This review will discuss the tumorigenic changes found in thyroid epithelial (non-medullary) cancers.

Papillary thyroid carcinomas (PTC), representing most common malignant tumor of thyroid, are associated with rearrangements of 2 different transmembrane tyrosine kinase genes—RET and NTRK1 resulting in production of chimeric proteins (RET/PTC and TRK) that contribute to the development of malignant phenotype. Expression of wild type RET is detected in half of RET positive tumors and is an independent risk factor for aggressive PTC. Mutation of BRAF gene is present in 30% of PTC. This is isoform of RAF proteins (serine-threoninekinases) that activate RAF/ MEK/ MAPK signaling pathway.

* Address for correspondence: P.O.Box: 12113, Dhahran 31311, Saudi Arabia. Fax: 00966-3-8776783 Tel: 00966-3-8776788 / 6780. E-mail: sheikhss@aramco.com.sa

A small number of PTC cases show deletions in the expressed RNA for p21/ Waf1, a cell cycle inhibitor protein. It also shows increased incidence in patients with familial adenomatous polyposis caused by germline mutations of APC gene. Familial predisposition has been linked to chromosomes 19 and 1. Follicular variant of PTC is characterized by a high frequency of ras mutations as compared to classical PTC that shows almost no ras mutations.

Recently PAX8-PPAR rearrangement has been identified in majority of follicular carcinomas (FC). A translocation has been shown in many FCs t(2,3)(q13;p25) that results in fusion of part of PAX8 gene (thyroid transcription factor) and PPAR-gamma-1 gene (transcription factor that stimulates cell differentiation and inhibits cell growth). The fusion product blocks action of PPAR-gamma-1 gene and thus most likely stimulates cell growth and inhibits cell differentiation. Mutations of K-ras, N-ras, and H-ras proto-oncogenes and over-expression of normal c-myc and c-fos genes are also found in FCs and occasionally PTCs. Hypermethylation of RASSF1A, a tumor suppressor gene, is also described in 2/3 of FC and minority of PTC. The frequency of allelic loss (FAL) using a panel of tumor suppressor genes in follicular derived neoplasms correlates with histological aggressiveness of the tumor.

Mutation of p53 tumor suppressor gene leading to production of an inactive p53 protein is seen in most anaplastic carcinomas which are the most aggressive of all thyroid carcinomas. Some cases, in particular those with areas of papillary differentiation, also show mutational activation of BRAF gene.

Immunohistochemically focal CK 19 staining may be seen in benign lesions however diffuse positivity is characteristic of PTC. HBME-1 positivity indicates malignancy but not papillary differentiation. Ret reflects RET/ PTC rearrangement and is seen in majority of classic PTCs. Only rarely all these markers are negative in PTC. Over-expression of cyclin-D1 and under-expression of p27 is also reported to predict lymph node metastasis in PTCs and thus has a role in identifying PTC with metastatic potential.

This article reviews and updates in detail, yet in a simplified manner, the tumor markers and genes involved in thyroid cancers.

Keywords: Thyroid, carcinoma, tumor, markers, genes, immunohistochemistry, molecular genetics, mutation.

WHO Classification of Thyroid Tumors [1]

Thyroid Carcinomas

1- Papillary carcinoma
2- Follicular carcinoma
3- Poorly-differentiated carcinoma
4- Undifferentiated carcinoma
5- Squamous cell carcinoma
6- Mucoepidermoid carcinoma
7- Sclerosing Mucoepidermoid carcinoma with eosinophilia
8- Mucinous carcinoma
9- Medullary carcinoma

10- Mixed medullary and follicular carcinoma
11- Spindle cell tumor with thymus-like differentiation
12- Carcinoma showing thymus-like differentiation

Thyroid Adenoma and Related Tumors

1- Follicular adenoma
2- Hyalinizing trabecular adenoma

Other Thyroid Tumors

1- Teratoma
2- Primary lymphoma and plasmacytoma
3- Ectopic thymoma
4- Angiosarcoma
5- Smooth muscle tumors
6- Peripheral nerve sheath tumors
7- Paraganglioma
8- Solitary fibrous tumor
9- Follicular dendritic cell tumor
10- Langerhans cell histiocytosis
11- Secondary tumors

INTRODUCTION

Thyroid tumors develop when growth of a single thyroid epithelial cell escapes from the normal mechanisms regulating cell divisions and gains a selective growth advantage. Unregulated cell division can result from mutations in both oncogenes and tumor suppressor genes. An understanding of mutations of the proto-oncogenes and tumor suppressor genes that occur in these tumors should eventually explain the diverse clinical characteristics of thyroid tumors and also direct therapy. These genetic abnormalities usually represent somatic / acquired mutations as opposed to germline / inherited mutations because most thyroid tumors are sporadic and not familial [2]. This review will discuss the tumorigenic changes found in thyroid epithelial follicle-cell derived (nonmedullary) cancers.

Thyroid cancer is an uncommon tumor that accounts for approximately 1% of all malignancies in developed countries. It predominantly affects women, most often between the ages of 30 to 50. Benign thyroid nodules are encountered more often. Even though thyroid malignancies are relatively rare, they represent the most common malignancies of the endocrine system. The majority of these malignancies originate from follicular cells and behave indolently with a 10 year survival of more than 90%. Other malignancies such as lymphomas and nonepithelial tumors are exceptionally rare. Thyroid carcinomas occur primarily in young to middle aged adults with mean age at diagnosis to be mid 40s to early 50s for papillary carcinoma, 50s for the follicular and medullary types, and 60s for the poorly differentiated and the undifferentiated carcinomas. It is twice to four times as common in females than males suggesting the possibility of a specific susceptibility gene with sex hormone receptor element involvement in the pathogenesis. Classification of the four major groups of papillary, follicular, medullary, and anaplastic / undifferentiated carcinomas that is based on clinical as well as morphologic features is now strongly supported by molecular studies showing distinct involvement of certain genes in these groups. Well-differentiated follicular cell-derived thyroid carcinomas are generally divided into papillary and follicular types. Well-differentiated carcinoma is relatively common but also a generally indolent cancer that is rarely fatal. Death from disease is most often due to widespread metastasis or anaplastic transformation. The rate of transformation from well-differentiated to undifferentiated carcinoma is not very well understood but has been estimated to be less than 1% [3, 4]. Both tumor groups have distinct clinical behavior, including route of metastasis and prognosis. Poorly-differentiated tumors are best treated as a separate type as they may or may not show dedifferentiation from a well-differentiated carcinoma, such as papillary or follicular types, however, they have a distinct clinical significance.

Papillay carcinoma development can be influenced by environmental, hormonal, and genetic factors. The environmental factors can be divided into genotoxic (leading to DNA damage), such as radiation and nongenotoxic, such as TSH stimulation secondary to Iodine deficiency. Follicular carcinomas can also develop secondary to radiation exposure, however they probably have a much longer latent period.

Radiation causes breaks in double stranded DNA which is a necessary precursor to RET and TRK rearrangements. This explains the high association of radiation to papillary rather than follicular carcinomas. On the other hand, follicular carcinoma is more often associated with Iodine deficiency.

Genetic susceptibility also plays a major role in particular with the medullary carcinoma. Approximately 25% of these tumors are seen in one of the recognized syndromes such as MEN 2A, MEN2B, and FMTC. Almost all these cases show germline mutation of RET oncogene. There is also a strong yet unexplained familial factor in the development of papillary carcinoma.

Significant advances have been made in the last few years in the pathogenesis of thyroid carcinoma development at the molecular level. Papillary carcinomas characteristically show RET and TRK (Tyrosine Receptor Kinase) genes rearrangements that are most likely secondary to radiation-induced DNA damage. Cases lacking these rearrangements often show BRAF mutation or rearrangements in other genes involving RET signaling pathways. Follicular carcinomas and some adenomas often show RAS mutations and PAX8/PPAR gamma rearrangements. RET mutations are causally related to development of medullary carcinomas with RET germline mutation in hereditary medullary carcinomas and somatic mutations in sporadic cases. The poorly-differentiated carcinoma may show BRAF mutations favoring the theory of their papillary origin. The anaplastic / undifferentiated carcinomas most commonly exhibit TP53 mutations.

Difficulties in diagnosing thyroid lesions even with histologic examination are well known. Many immunohistochemical markers have been used to improve the diagnosis. Two relatively new markers that look quite promising are the Galectin-3 (G-3) and thyroid peroxidase. Galectin-3 is a member of beta-galactoside family. It has antiapoptotic activity and has a role in regulation of cell-cell and cell-matrix interaction, adhesion, and migration. It is a positive marker of malignancy, meaning it is expressed in thyroid malignancies but should be negative in normal thyroid tissue or benign lesions. Thyroid peroxidase (TPO) is involved in synthesis of thyroid hormone and is a thyroid-specific enzyme. It should not be expressed in malignant lesions of thyroid as it reflects normal thyroid function. The combination of G-3 and TPO shows very high sensitivity (approximately 96%) for the detection of papillary carcinoma, however neither G-3 nor the combination showed adequate sensitivity in detecting follicular carcinoma [5]. Coexpression of fibronectin-1 and G-3 or fibronectin-1 and HBME1 is usually restricted to thyroid carcinomas, while their concurrent absence was highly specific for benign lesions [6]. In addition, the majority of follicular cell-derived malignancies including both papillary and follicular, exhibit positive staining with Lactoferrin (LF) and Ceruloplasmin (CP); whereas medullary carcinoma and most of the benign thyroid conditions show a negative immunostain reaction with these markers[7].

Papillary Carcinomas:

Papillary thyroid carcinomas (PTCs) are most commonly seen in adults 20 to 50 years of age. Even though rare, they are considered one of the most common tumors seen in the pediatric age group. The prognosis is excellent with an overall 10-year survival rate exceeding 90%. Papillary carcinoma is genetically associated with familial adenomatous polyposis coli (FAPC), Cowden syndrome, and Carney complex, and appears to have familial tendency.

PTC is characterized by distinctive nuclear features such as nuclear elongation, crowding, overlapping, nuclear irregularities, grooves, pseudoinclusions, and clearing or ground glass appearance. The tumor shows follicle cell differentiation and often exhibits papillary architecture.

A number of histologic variants of papillary carcinomas are described:

1- Follicular variant
2- Macrofollicular variant
3- Solid variant
4- Cribriform variant
5- Oncocytic variant
6- Clear cell variant
7- Columnar cell variant
8- Tall cell variant
9- Papillary carcinoma with focal insular component
10- Papillary carcinoma with fasciitis-like stroma
11- Papillary carcinoma with spindle and giant cell carcinoma

12- Papillary carcinoma with squamous cell or mucoepidermoid carcinoma
13- Combined papillary and medullary carcinoma.
14- Papillary microcarcinoma

MOLECULAR GENETICS:

RET / PTC Rearrangements

The most common genetic alteration identified in papillary carcinomas are rearrangements of transmembrane tyrosine kinase genes, RET and TRK, resulting in production of proteins with tyrosine kinase activity. Somatic mutations of RET and TRK lead to a constitutive increase in tyrosine kinase activity that activates growth pathways. This may be sufficient to cause the PTC. Tumors with TRK and RET / PTC rearrangements often behave more aggressively than those lacking the rearrangements. RET gene rearrangements produce a chimeric gene referred to as RET / PTC seen in 20 to 30% of sporadic cases, 45 to 60% in children and young adults, and 50 to 80% in those exposed to irradiation [8].

Several different types of rearrangements of RET gene, located on chromosome 10q, occur. RET fused genes may have an impact on phenotype of the tumor. RET / PTC1 is most commonly found in papillary microcarcinomas as well as tumors with classic papillary architecture. It is also considered as one of the proven specific genetic events leading to the development of PTC [9]. RET / PTC3 is more often seen in children exposed to radiation and predominates in the solid and tall cell variants of papillary carcinomas. Other RET / PTC rearrangements such as RET / PTC2 are less common.

All types of RET / PTC rearrangements, have in common replacement of extracellular ligand-binding domain of the RET gene by the RET-fused genes, leading to ligand-independent activation of RET kinase; thus causing neoplastic transformation of the follicular cells.

The solid variant of papillary carcinoma is a rare and poorly-characterized variant that is associated with a slightly higher frequency of distant metastasis and less favorable prognosis. These tumors should be distinguished from poorly-differentiated carcinomas which have a reportedly lower survival rate [10].

A study looked at the relationship between presence of RET and NTRK1 oncogenic rearrangements and age at surgery (four to 80 years). This was independent of radiation exposure. The study showed significant higher frequency of RET and NTRK1 activation in group of patients aged four to 30 years. This supports the concept that age could be contributing to this thyroid specific carcinogenic process [11].

TRK Rearrangements

10% of papillary carcinomas show TRK rearrangements. The rearrangements result from fusion of tyrosine kinase of TRK on chromosome 1q to tropomyosin (TRK), or translocated promotor region / TPR genes located on chromosome 1q (TRK1 & TRK2), or TRK-fused gene / TRF on chromosome 3. Different TRK rearrangements are seen, all occurring in similar frequency in papillary carcinomas except TRK / TPM3 that predominates in radiation associated tumors.

BRAF Mutations

The BRAF isoform of RAF has been implicated in development of papillary carcinomas. RAF proteins are serine-threonine kinases that activate RAF / MEK / MAPK signaling pathway leading to activation of MAPK cascade. Point mutation of BRAF gene occurs when thymine-to-adenine transversion occurs on nucleotide position 1796. The BRAF protein product has increased basal kinase activity. This mutation is not identified in other thyroid tumor types. A substantial proportion of tumors that are BRAF positive also show positivity for RET rearrangements suggesting the possibility that BRAF may help RET / PTC in development of papillary carcinomas. In PTCs, BRAF mutations are seen in association with older age, extrathyroidal extension, classic papillary phenotype or tall cell variant histology, and more frequent presentation at stages III and IV. An exceedingly low prevalence of BRAF mutation is noted in the follicular variant. Several studies have identified BRAF mutation to be the most common genetic event in papillary carcinoma, the prevalence varying from 36% to 69% [12]. Almost all BRAF mutation positive carcinomas (poorly-differentiated and anaplastic) contained areas of preexisting papillary carcinoma with the mutation being present in both well-differentiated and dedifferentiated components. This shows that there is distinct association between the phenotypical and biological properties of papillary carcinoma and BRAF mutation that may participate in progression to poorly-differentiated and anaplastic carcinomas.

RAS Mutations

Mutations in the RAS genes have been identified in a wide variety of human malignancies. The RAS proto-oncogenes play an important role in cellular proliferation and differentiation. There are three structurally related RAS genes (H-RAS, K-RAS, and N-RAS) that encode membrane-bound proteins (p21) which have intrinsic GTPase activity. Point mutations that block GTPase cause activation of RAS proto-oncogenes and convert them into transforming oncogenes. Less than 10% of papillary carcinomas show activating point mutations of one of three RAS proto-oncogenes with N-RAS being the most frequent one. Some studies show RAS point mutations to be seen distinctly in high frequency in the follicular variants of papillary carcinoma. The majority of mutations in papillary carcinomas reportedly occur in codon 12/13 of the K-RAS or H-RAS genes; while the majority of mutations in follicular carcinomas involve codon 61 of H-RAS or N-RAS. Thus raising the possibility that the site of mutations may serve as biological markers, reflecting an association between specific RAS mutations and the pathological type of thyroid tumor [13, 14].

Beta- Catenin

Frequent somatic mutations of the gene encoding beta-catenin are observed in the cribriform variant of papillary carcinoma.

Adenomatous Polyposis Coli (APC) Gene

Familial adenomatous polyposis is an autosomal dominant precancerous condition of the colon that is caused by germ-line mutations of the tumor suppressor gene APC located in 5q21 region. Somatic APC gene mutations have been identified in only the cribriform-morular variant of papillary carcinoma that shows an association with familial adenomatous polyposis (FAP) [15].

Patients with papillary carcinomas associated with FAP may show RET rearrangements. One report shows that the loss of function of APC coexists with the gain of function of RET in some papillary carcinomas, suggesting that RET / PTC1 oncogene activation could be a progression step in the development of FAP-associated thyroid tumors [16].

P21 / Waf1 – Cell-Cycle Inhibitor Protein

A small number of papillary carcinomas show deletions in expressed RNA, and not the gene, for P21 / Wafl protein, suggesting that splicing is probably the cause of P21 / Wafl deletion. The significance of this has yet to be established. P21 / Wafl gene is located on chromosome 6p and encodes a protein, transcription of which can be activated by the tumor suppressor gene p53. This provides a link between the tumor suppressing activity of p53 and cell cycle control [4].

Chromosome 2q21, 1 , and 19 - Susceptibility Loci for FNMTC

The familial form of nonmedullary thyroid carcinomas (FNMTC) is increasingly recognized as a distinct clinical entity characterized by multifocality and more aggressive behavior and mortality as compared to its sporadic counterparts. There is evidence in favor of existence of a susceptibility locus for FNMTC at 2q21. This locus appears particularly relevant to families with at least one case of follicular variant of PTC [17].

Although mostly seen as sporadic tumors, PTCs can occur in familial syndromes. A distinct inherited tumor syndrome has been characterized by familial association of PTC and nodular thyroid disease, and papillary renal neoplasia. The predisposing gene in a large kindred with this syndrome has been mapped to 1q21 [18].

Linkage analysis mapped a new gene TCO (thyroid tumor with cell oxyphilia) to chromosome 19p13.2 [19]. Interestingly, both malignant and benign tumors in the studied family with TCO positivity exhibited some extent of cell oxyphilia. This suggests that relatives of patients with sporadic NMTC with cell oxyphilia should be carefully investigated.

More studies to further identify any additional susceptibility genes are required.

Loss of Heterozygosity (LOH)

An analysis of LOH showed a sharp distinction between PTC and follicular carcinoma in their tendency to lose genetic material. This most likely is secondary to differences in mechanisms controlling chromosome stability in both forms of carcinomas that in turn probably have implications for tumor behavior and prognosis [20]. One study used a microdissection and genotyping assay to study the patterns of LOH of tumor suppressor genes in both microscopic (less than 1 cm) and clinical PTCs. The results indicated that all papillary carcinomas harbor mutations with similar frequencies and distribution patterns, regardless of the size of the tumor [21].

Microarray Expression Profile

An independent microarray expression analysis showed distinctive expression profiles for both PTCs and Follicular carcinomas. This suggests that either they have different molecular origin or they diverge distinctly from a common origin. The analysis performed used five genes including claudin-10 (CLDN10), CITED1, and insulin-like growth factor-binding protein 6 (IGFBP6) that were overexpressed in PTCs; follicular carcinomas, on the other hand, showed decreased expression of caveolin-1, and caveolin-2 and IGFBP6 and had no expression of CLDN10 [22].

Immunohistochemistry

Papillary carcinomas are positive for epithelial markers, thyroglobulin, and thyroid transcription factor-1 (TTF-1). High molecular weight cytokeratin (Cytokeratin 19) has been widely applied in this tumor, however it is also seen in chronic lymphocytic thyroiditis. Recognition of RET/PTC rearrangements by identifying RET staining depends on availability of antibodies with high sensitivity and specificity.

Interestingly, tumors without metastasis are positive for p27 and are negative for cyclin D1. Tumors with metastasis, show loss of p27 or cyclin D1 upregulation. Metastatic tumors are positive for thyroglobulin and TTF-1. Metastatic tumor from other sources will be negative for both. Pulmonary primaries are positive for TTF-1 but show negative staining by thyroglobulin. The combination of G-3 and TPO shows very high sensitivity (approximately 96%) for the detection of papillary carcinomas but neither G-3 nor the combination showed adequate sensitivity in detecting follicular carcinoma [23].

In a recent study, p63 was detected in approximately 80% of PTCs and Hashimoto's disease cases, which was in contrast to uncommon, or negative expression in nonpapillary thyroid neoplasms and Grave's disease [24].

FOLLICULAR CARCINOMA

Follicular carcinoma is more often seen in the 50s with the oncocytic follicular carcinoma type seen in the 60s. It is more common in females, rarely encountered in children, and accounts for 10-15% of all thyroid malignancies. The incidence is higher in Iodine deficient areas and in those exposed to radiation. Dietary Iodine has been associated with an increase in relative frequency of papillary carcinoma and decrease in follicular carcinoma.

Follicular carcinoma is invasive neoplasm that shows follicle cell differentiation and lacks the nuclear features of papillary carcinoma. Depending on the degree of invasion the tumor is divided into two categories:

A) Minimally invasive follicular carcinoma: Tumor that shows limited or focal capsular and or vascular invasion.
B) Widely invasive follicular carcinoma: Tumor exhibiting widespread invasion of capsule and or vessels. The term "Grossly encapsulated angioinvasive follicular carcinoma" is limited to cases demonstrating only vascular invasion.

Several histological variants are described:

1- Oncocytic variant
2- Clear cell variant

MOLECULAR GENETICS

PPAR-Gamma Rearrangements

Approximately 25 to 50% of follicular carcinomas show rearrangements of PPAR-gamma (peroxisome proliferator-activated receptor gamma) gene which is a transcription factor that stimulates cell differentiation and inhibits cell growth. These rearrangements produce various chimeric fusion proteins, most common one being PAX8-PPAR-gamma. This relatively new gene fusion, identified at significant frequency in follicular carcinomas with cytogenetically detected translocation t(2;3)(q13;p25), causes fusion of part of the DNA-binding segment of PAX8 gene, a thyroid transcription factor, and PPAR-gamma-1 gene. The product blocks the action of PPAR-gamma-1 leading to deregulation of ligand-inducible transcription by PPAR-gamma, apoptosis inhibition, proliferation promotion, anchorage-independent growth of follicular cells. PPAR-gamma rearrangements are most consistently identified in low stage follicular carcinomas and only some locally aggressive and metastatic tumors. The rearrangement appears to be restricted to the conventional type of follicular carcinomas and is not identified in oncocytic tumors or papillary carcinomas. Interestingly, the prevalence of PAX8-PPAR-gamma is found to be much higher in follicular tumors with history of radiation exposure as reported by some studies. This may lead to the speculation that radiation exposure may be directly responsible for the generation of PAX8-PPAR-gamma in thyroid cells as is suggested for RET / PTC rearrangements in papillary carcinomas; however larger studies are required to prove or disprove this speculation [8, 25]. Follicular carcinomas that are positive for PAX8-PPAR-gamma rearrangement are often overtly invasive, whereas tumors negative for PAX8-PPAR-gamma, in general, are minimally invasive. In addition, a few cases of follicular adenomas also show PAX8-PPAR-gamma rearrangement [26]. This suggests that these tumors most probably represent early follicular carcinomas that are removed at a preinvasive stage. There is a correlation between PAX8-PPAR-gamma rearrangement detected by RT-PCR and immunohistochemistry only when there is diffuse strong nuclear staining [8].

RAS Point Mutations

Approximately 20 to 50% of all follicular carcinomas show point mutations of the RAS proto-oncogenes. The most commonly encountered mutations are the activating mutations in codon 61 of the N-RAS and H-RAS genes [8, 27, 28]. These probably represent an early event in tumorogenesis as RAS mutations are seen in similar prevalence in benign as well as malignant thyroid tumors [29]. Some studies reported majority of mutations in PTCs to be involving a different codon of RAS genes (codon 12/13 of the K-RAS or H-RAS) as compared to follicular carcinomas that affect different codon (codon 61 of H-RAS or N-RAS).Thus suggesting that the site of mutations may reflect an association between specific RAS mutations and the pathological type of thyroid tumor [14].

RASSF1A Tumor Suppressor Gene Hypcrmcthylatio:

75% of follicular carcinomas as well as a small percentage of follicular adenomas and papillary carcinomas may show hypermethylation of RASSF1A gene that is most likely involved in early stages of thyroid epithelial tumorogenesis.

Overexpression of c-myc AND c-fos

These changes may have a growth promoting effect that is not specific to tumor type, and may act with other oncogenes or tumor suppressor genes in tumor development [2].

Chromosomal Imbalance

The involvement of several chromsomes has been suggested, such as chromosome 2, 3p, 6, 7q, 8, 9, 10q, 11, 13q, 17p, and 22. Oncocytic tumors, in general, show numerical chromosomal alteration as the predominant chromosomal alteration. In addition mutations of mitochondrial DNA are also identified. These findings are also seen in non-neoplastic thryroid tissue exhibiting oncocytic changes. This finding suggests that certain polymorphisms may predispose to oncocytic feature, whether neoplastic or not [1, 20].

Frequency of Allelic Loss (FAL) - Tumor Suppressor Genes

Follicular patterned tumors of thyroid can be challenging and controversial in diagnostic surgical pathology. Distinguishing follicular adenoma from minimally invasive or encapsulated angioinvasive carcinoma can be very difficult. The FAL in follicular-derived neoplasms correlates with the histologic aggressiveness of the tumor. Follicular adenomas have low FAL (average 9%) and low intratumoral heterogeneity (5% variability). The minimally invasive and angioinvasive carcinomas have intermediate FAL (30%) and intermediate intratumoral heterogeneity (10% variability). The widely invasive carcinomas show high FAL (average 53%) and high intratumoral heterogeneity (24% variability) [30].

Allelic loss of chromosome 11q13, a region containing several genes involved in growth control that are identified in follicular but not papillary carcinoma suggest that loss of a tumor suppressor gene at this locus will most likely lead to the follicular phenotype of the tumor. This includes the gene predisposing to development of multiple endocrine neoplasis type I (MEN-I) [29].

Microarray Expression Profile

PTCs and follicular carcinomas have distinctive microarray expression profiles, a finding that suggests either different molecular origins of both tumor types or distinct diversion from a common origin [18].

Immunohistochemistry

Follicular carcinomas are positive for thyroglobulin, TTF-1, and low-molecular weight cytokeratin. The phenotype, in general, is Bcl-2 positive, TP53 negative, low levels of cyclin D1, high levels of p27, and low proliferation rates. They usually show membranous positivity for E-cadherin and beta-Catenin, similar to the normal thyroid tissue and other benign follicular lesions, including the follicular variant of papillary carcinoma. A subgroup of widely-invasive follicular carcinomas exhibit E-cadherin downregulation. Some follicular carcinomas show focal cytokeratin 19 positivity which is in contrast with the widespread immunoreactivity seen in papillary carcinomas. Galectin-3, HBME-1, CD44v6, and CD15 are also reported in these tumors. Immunostaining with PPAR-gamma antibody can be performed as the presence of PAX8-PPAR-gamma rearrangement detected by RT-PCR correlates with immunohistochemical staining; but only when there is diffuse and strong nuclear staining [1, 8].

Poorly-Differentiated Carcinomas

These are tumors that show some follicle cell differentiation and are intermediate between the well-differentiated carcinomas including papillary and follicular carcinomas and the undifferentiated / anaplastic carcinomas. The entity remains controversial and it is difficult to say whether the wide variation in the prevalence rate in different areas is true or is related to the difference in the diagnostic criteria used. The tumor is more commonly seen in women past their 50s. Although the majority appear to arise from the differentiated carcinomas, some are known to arise de novo. The etiology is unknown and the common presentation is that of a solitary, large mass, frequently with a history of rapidly enlarging size, with or without lymph nodes.

The entities that come under this umbrella are poorly-differentiated follicular carcinoma, solid type of follicular carcinoma, poorly-differentiated papillary carcinoma, trabecular carcinoma, poorly-differentiated carcinoma with primordial cell component, and insular carcinoma. Mutations leading to downregulation of tumor suppressor genes, TP53, PTEN, and beta-Catenin genes are thought to be involved, in some instances, in the progression of well-differentiated follicular carcinoma to poorly-differentiated[1].

Molecular Genetics

Chromosomal Alterations

Specific types of chromosomal alterations such as +20q, -1p, -6q, -13q, +17q, and +1p are associated with transition from well-differentiated to poorly-differentiated carcinomas. The same findings are seen in the undifferentiated / anaplastic carcinomas.

Complex clonal alterations are also common in poorly-differentiated carcinomas. The Comparative Genomic Hybridization (CGH) shows the DNA profile to be 80%, which is similar to that seen in anaplastic carcinoma.,The number of gains or losses is intermediate between the differentiated carcinomas and the anaplastic ones [1].

TP53 Mutations

Approximately 20 to 30% of poorly-differentiated carcinomas show TP53 mutations. P53 is a nuclear protein which has a role in regulation of normal cellular proliferation. It acts as a tumor suppressor gene. Mutations of p53 are highly prevalent in several malignancies including colon cancer, lymphoma, leukemia, and cancer of other organs such as liver, breast, lung, ovary, bladder, esophagus, and brain. Allelic deletions of the locus on chromosome 17p are highly prevalent in colon cancers whereas other p53 alleles often exhibits point mutations. Mutational activation of p53 is most likely responsible for the progression to the most malignant poorly-differentiated and undifferentiated forms of these tumors [29, 31, 32].

RAS Mutations

In contrast to the differentiated carcinomas, poorly-differentiated carcinomas show multiple activating mutations. Mutations of H, K and N-RAS account for approximately 50% of these poorly-differentiated tumors.

WNT Activation / Beta-Catenin

WNT activation as indicated by mutations and or aberrant nuclear localization of beta-Catenin is also recently recognized in poorly-differentiated carcinoma.

Tyrosine Kinase Genes Rearrangements

A small number of poorly-differentiated carcinomas show rearrangements of tyrosine kinase genes such as RET / PTC or NKTRK1.

BRAF Mutations

Almost all BRAF mutation-positive poorly-differentiated and anaplastic carcinomas contained areas of preexisting papillary carcinoma with the mutation being present in both well-differentiated and dedifferentiated components [1].

There is a distinct association between BRAF mutation and the phenotypical and biological properties of papillary carcinoma that may participate in progression to poorly-differentiated and anaplastic carcinomas.

Immunohistochemistry

Poorly-differentiated carcinomas are thyroglobulin and TTF-1 positive. The tumor shows focal TP53 nuclear staining with aberrant TP53 immunoreactivity detected in 40-50% of cases. There is increased Ki-67 / MIB-1 index usually exhibiting 10-30% positive cells. The tumor cells are usually positive for Bcl-2. In addition most tumors show absence of E-cadherin membranous expression which is in contrast to that seen in differentiated carcinomas [1].

UNDIFFERENTIATED / ANAPLASTIC CARCINOMA

Undifferentiated or anaplastic carcinomas are highly aggressive malignant tumors that are widely invasive and account for less than 5% of all thyroid carcinomas. Although rare these tumors are universally fatal. Histologically, there is predominant or sole composition of the tumor by undifferentiated cells that show epithelial differentiation immunohistochemically or ultrastucturally. It is more predominant in women and is commonly seen in 60s and above. Patients present with a rapidly enlarging neck mass that is often associated with hoarseness, dysphagia, vocal cord paralysis, and pain. Approximately 40% of these patients have widespread metastasis at the time of presentation. The overall five-year survival ranges from 0-14%. Most cases, when sampled enough, show a preexisting differentiated or poorly-differentiated carcinoma suggesting that these tumors originate from follicular cells. Histologically the tumor is composed of a variable admixture of spindle cells, pleomorphic giant cells, and epithelioid cells.

EBV expression has been detected in almost all cases of thyroid cancers, however the strength of signal is stronger in the undifferentiated ones, suggestive of dedifferentiation or progression from well-differentiated carcinoma to undifferentiated carcinoma [33]. The factors that lead to anaplastic transformation are thought to be related to tumor suppressor genes accounting for the tumor's recessive phenotype. This is in sharp contrast to the typical dominant oncogene mutation. The tumor suppressor genes that have been implicated include p53, PTEN, and other tumor suppressor genes localized in 5q11-31 region [3]. In general, anaplastic carcinomas and coexistent well-differentiated carcinomas share a common core of genetic loci with identical allelic imbalance. The anaplastic component shows additional loci with allelic loss, consistent with the theory of multistep carcinogenesis with acquired mutational damage.

Several histological variants are described that are only rarely encountered:

1- Osteoclastic variant
2- Carcinosarcoma variant
3- Paucicellular variant
4- lymphoepithelioma-like variant

MOLECULAR GENETICS

Chromosomal Alterations

Complex chromosomal alterations with DNA imbalance are characteristically seen in anaplastic carcinomas. The median chromosomal loss or gain is higher than that seen in differentiated carcinomas and the poorly-differentiated carcinomas. The undifferentiated carcinoma usually show increased rates of mutations as compared to the differentiated ones that may be present in different areas of the same tumor. This is consistent with the multistep carcinogenesis.

Allelic losses of chromosomes such as 1q, 1p, 5, 8, 9p, 11, 17p, 19p, 22q, 16p, and 18q are described in association with anaplastic carcinomas.

The average frequency of allelic (FAL) loss in anaplastic carcinoma is about 71% which is much higher than differentiated carcinomas such as papillary carcinoma that has an average FAL 25% and Hurthle cell tumors with FAL of 45%. Hurthle cell tumors with higher rate of allelic imbalance are possibly at higher risk of anaplastic transformation.

Specific loss or gain of certain chromosomal material is associated with progression from poorly-differentiated to undifferentiated carcinoma. Examples include 3p+, 5q-, 11q+, and losses and gains of 8p and 8q regions [1, 3].

Mutations of p53 Gene

The normal p53 protein is a transcription factor that regulates apoptosis and cell cycle. P53 mutation is consistently identified in most undifferentiated / anaplastic carcinomas. Mutation of this tumor suppressor gene leads to synthesis of inactive p53 protein. Inactivation of p53 confers thyroid tumors with aggressive properties [29].

Mutations of BRAF Gene

Activating point mutations of the BRAF oncogene can be detected in up to 50% of anaplastic carcinomas showing BRAF gene transversion of T to A at 1796 nucleotide location. Many of these tumors show areas of differentiated carcinomas, such as papillary carcinomas, that are often positive for the same mutation. This supports the notion that many anaplastic carcinomas actually represent progressive malignant degeneration of a preexisting well-differentiated / papillary carcinoma. The high frequency of BRAF mutations in a tumor that is regarded as uniformly fatal justifies evaluation of potential benefits of anti-BRAF-therapy for these patients with anaplastic carcinoma. This is contrary to papillary carcinoma patients who harbor the same mutation, but have little to benefit from anti-BRAF therapy as these patients have an excellent prognosis and respond well to current therapies [34].

Beta-Catenin

Beta-Catenin / CTNNB1 mutations have been described in anaplastic carcinomas of thyroid.

Alterations in Components of Cell Cycle Control

The increased replicative potential is reflected by alterations in components involved in cell-cycle control mechanisms. The reported changes in literature include overexpression of cyclin D1, decreased expression of p27, and inactivation of p16 and PTEN [1, 2].

IMMUNOHISTOCHEMISTRY

The tumor is negative for thyroglobulin and only rarely shows positivity for TTF-1. Majority of cases show immunoreactivity for cytokeratin. Epithelial membrane antigen is seen only in 30 to 50% of cases with only less than 10% of tumors exhibiting CEA positivity, mostly in cases with squamoid features [1].

REFERENCES

[1] Delellis R, Lloyd R, Heitz P, and Eng C. Tumors of Thyroid and Parathyroid. *In:* WHO Classification of Tumors. Pathology & Genetics. *Tumors of Endocrine Organs*. IARC Press; Lyon, 2004.

[2] Malchoff C. Oncogenes and tumor suppressor genes in thyroid nodules and thyroid cancer. UpToDate online 12.3, 2004.

[3] founded by Burton D. Rose, MD & Joseph M. Rush, MD, www.uptodate.com

[4] Hunt J, Tometsko M, LiVolsi V, Swalsky P, Finkelstein S, and Barnes L. Molecular evidence of anaplastic transformation in coexisting well-differentiated and anaplastic carcinomas of the thyroid. *Am J Surg Pathol 2003*; 27 (12): 1559-1564.

[5] Shi Y, Farid N, and Al-Sedairy S. Evidence of gene deletion of p21 (WAF1 / CIP1), a cyclin-dependant protein kinase inhibitor, in thyroid carcinomas. *Br J Cancer 1996*; 74: 1336-1341.

[6] Weber K, Shroyer K, Heinz D, Nawaz S, Said M, and Haugen B. The use of a combination of Galectin-3 and Thyroid peroxidase for the diagnosis and prognosis of thyroid cancer. *Am J Clin Pathol 2004*;122: 524-531.

[7] Prasad M, Pellegata N, Huang Y, Nagaraja H, de la Chapelle A, and Kloos R. Galectin-3, fibronectin-1, CITED-1, HBME1, and cytokeratin-19 immunohistochemistry is useful for the differential diagnosis of thyeoid tumors. *Modern Pathol 2005;* 18: 48-57.

[8] Kondi-Pafiti A, Smyrniotis V, Frangou M, Papayanopoulo A, Englezou M, and Deligeorgi H. Immunohistochemical study of Ceruloplasmin, Lactoferrin, and Secretory Component Expression in neoplastic and non-neoplastic thyroid gland diseases. *Acta Oncologica 2000*; 39 (6): 753-756.

[9] Nikiforova M, Biddinger P, Caudill C, Kroll T, and Nikiforova Y. PAX8-PPAR γ rearrangement in thyroid tumors. RT-PCR and Immunohistochemical analysis. *Am J Surg Pathol 2002;* 26 (8): 1016-1023.

[10] Jhiang S, Sagartz J, Tong Q, Parker-Thornburg J, Capen C, Cho J, Xing S, and Ledent C. Targeted expression of the ret/PTC1 oncogene induces papillary thyroid carcinomas. *Endocrinol 1996*; 137 (1): 375-378.

[11] Nikiforova Y, Erickson L, Nikiforova M, Caudill C, and Lloyd R. Solid variant odf papillary thyroid carcinoma. *Am J Surg Pathol 2001*; 25 (12): 1478-1484.

[12] Bongarzone I, Fugazzola L, Vigneri P, Mariani L, Mondellini P, Pacini F, Basolo F, Pinchera A, Pilotti S, and Pierotti M. Age-related activation of the tyrosine kinase

receptor protooncogenes RET and NTRK1 in papillary thyroid carcinoma. *J Clin Endocrinol Metab 1996*; 81 (5): 2006-2009.

[13] Nikiforova M, Kimura E, Gandhi M, Biddinger P, Knauf J, Basolo F, Zhu Z, Giannini R, Salvatore G, Fusco A, Santoro M, Fagin J, and Nikiforova Y. BRAF mutationsin thyroid tumors are restricted to papillary carcinomas and anaplastic or poorly differentiated carcinomas arising from papillary carcinomas. *J Clin Endocrinol Metab 2003*: 88 (11): 5399-5404.

[14] Zhu Z, Gandhi M, Nikiforova M, Fischer A, and Nikiforova Y. Molecular profile and clinical-pathological features of the follicular variant od papillary thyroid carcinoma. *Am J Clin Pathol 2003*; 120: 71-77.

[15] Karga H, Lee J, Vickery,Jr., A, Thor A, Gaz R, and Jameson L. Ras oncogene mutations in benign and malignant thyroid neoplasms. *J Clin Endocrinol Metab 1991*; 73 (4): 832-836.

[16] Cameselle-Teijeiro J, Ruiz-Ponte C, Loidi L, Suarez-Penarande J, Baltar J, and Sobrinho-Simoes M. Somatic but not germline mutation of the APC gene in a case of cribriform-morular variant of papillary thyroid carcinoma. *Am J Clin Pathol 2001*; 115: 486-493.

[17] Cetta F, Chiappetta G, Melillo R, Petracci M, Montalto G, Santoro M, and Fusco A. The ret/ptc1 is activated in familial adenomatous polyposis-associated thyroid papillary carcinomas. *J Clin Endocrinol Metab 1998*; 83 (3): 1003-1006.

[18] McKay J, Lesueur F, Jonard L, Pastore A, Williamson J, Hoffman L, Burgess J, Duffield A, Papotti M, Stark M, Sobol H, Maes B, Murat A, Kaariainen H, Bertholon-Gregoire M, Zini M, Rossing M, Toubert M, Bonichon F, Cavarec M, Bernard A, Boneu A, Leprat F, Haas O, Lasset C, Schlumberger M, Canzian F, Goldgar D, and Romeo G. Localization of a susceptibility gene for familial nonmedullary thyroid carcinoma to chromosome 2q21. *Am J Hum Genet 2001*; 69: 440-446.

[19] Malchoff C, Sarfarzi M, Tendler B, Forouhar F, Whalen G, Joshi V, Arnold A, and Malchoff D. Papillary thyroid carcinoma associated with papillary renal neoplasia: Genetic linkage analysis of a distinct heritable tumor syndrome. *J Clin Endocrinol Metab 2000;* 85 (5): 1758-1764.

[20] Canzian F, Amati P, Harach R, Kraimps J, Lesueur F, Barbier J, Levillain P, Romeo G, and Bonneau D. A gene predisposing to familial thyroid tumors with cell oxyphilia maps to chromosome 19p13.2. *Am J Hum Genet 1998*; 63: 1743-1748.

[21] Ward L, Brenta G, Medvedovic M, and Fagin J. Studies of allelic loss in thyroid tumors reveal major differences in chromosomal instability between papillary and follicular carcinomas. *J Clin Endocrinol Metab 1998*; 83 (2): 525-530.

[22] Hunt J, LiVolsi V, Baloch Z, Barnes L, Swalsky P, Niehouse L, and Finkelstein S. Microscopic papillary thyroid carcinoma compared with clinical carcinomas by heterozygosity mutational profile. *Am J Surg Pathol 2003*; 27 (2): 159-166.

[23] Aldred M, Huang Y, Liyanarachchi S, Pellegata N, Gimm O, Jhiang S, Davuluri R, de la Chapelle A, and Eng C. Papillary and follicular thyroid carcinomas show distinctly different microarray expression profiles and can be distinguished by a minimum of five genes. *J Clin Oncol 2004*; 22: 3531-3539.

[24] Namba H, Matsuo K, and Fagin J. Clonal composition of benign and malignant human thyroid tumors. *J Clin Invest 1990*; 86: 120-125.

[25] Burstein D, Nagi C, Wang B, and Unger P. Immunohistochemical detection of p53 homolog p63 in solid cell nests, papillary thyroid carcinoma, and Hashimoto's thyroiditis: A stem cell hypothesis of papillary carcinoma oncogenesis. *Hum Pathol 2004*; 35: 465-473.

[26] Nikiforova M, Stringer J, Blough R, Medvedovic M, Fagin J, Nikiforova Y. Proximity of chromosomal loci that participate in radiation-induced rearrangements in human cells. *Science 2000*; 290: 138-141.

[27] Marquis A, Espadinha C, Catarino A, Moniz S, Pereira T, Sobrinho L, and Leite V. Expression of PAX8-PPARγ1 rearrangements in both follicular thyroid carcinomas and adenomas. *J Clin Endocrinol Metab 2002*; 87 (8): 3947-3952.

[28] Esapa C, Johnson S, Kendall-Taylor P, Lennard T, and Harris P. Prevalence of RAS mutations in thyroid neoplasia. *Clin Endocrinol 1999*; 50: 529-535.

[29] Lemoine N, Mayall E, Wyllie F, Williams E, Goynes M, and Wynford –thomas D. High frequency of ras oncogene activation in all stages of human thyroid tumorigenesis. *Oncogene 1989*; 4: 159-164.

[30] Fagin J, Matsuo K, Karmakar A, Chen D, Tang S, and Koeffler P. High prevalence of mutations of the p53 gene in poorly differentiated human thyroid carcinomas. *J Clin Invest 1993;* 91: 179-184.

[31] Hunt J, LiVolsi V, Baloch Z, Swalsky P, Bakker A, Sasatomi E, Finkelstein S, and Barnes L. A novel microdissection and genotyping of follicular-derived thyroid tumors to predict aggressiveness. *Hum Pathol 2003*; 34: 375-380.

[32] Gaidano G, Ballerini P, Gong J, InghiramiG, Neri A, Newcomb E, Magrath I, Knowles D, and Dallafavera R. p53 mutations in human lymphoid malignancies associated with Burkitt lymphoma and chronic lymphocytic leukemia. *Proc Natl Acad Sci 1991*; 88: 5413-5417.

[33] Nigro J, Baker S, Preisinger A, Jessup J, Hostetter R, Cleary K, Bigner S, Davidson N, Baylin S, Davilee P, Glover T, Collins F, Weston A, Modali R, Harris C, and Vogelstein B. Mutations in the p53 gene occur in diverse human tumour types. *Nature 1989*; 342: 705-708.

[34] Shimkage M, Kawahara K, Sasagawa T, Inoue H, YutsudoM, Yoshida A, and Yanoma S. Expression of Epstein-Barr virus in thyroid carcinoma correlates with tumor progression. *Hum Pathol 2003*; 34: 1170-1177.

[35] Begum S, Rosenbaum E, Henrique R, Cohen Y, Sidransky D, and Westra W. BRAF mutations in anaplastic thyroid carcinoma: implications for tumor origin, diagnosis and treatment. *Modern Pathol 2004*; 17: 1359-1363.

In: Trends in Thyroid Cancer Research
Editor: Carl A. Milton, pp. 203-220
ISBN 1-59454-627-4

Chapter X

Recent Advances in the Clinical Management of Thyroid Cancers

Stephen L. Hyer and Clive Harmer
Thyroid Unit, Royal Marsden Hospital, UK

Abstract

Thyroid cancer is increasingly being diagnosed at an earlier stage and treatment is now usually associated with a long life expectancy. New information from large retrospective series has helped identify prognostic factors more accurately so that management can be adapted appropriately.

Results from recent studies show that differentiated carcinoma in the elderly behaves more aggressively and has a less favourable prognosis compared with younger patients. In a series of 111 patients aged 70 years or older at the time of initial diagnosis, 70% of tumours at presentation were pathological stage T3 or over, 44% demonstrated lymphatic spread and 23% had evidence of distant metastases. Cause specific survival was only 50% at 5 years. By contrast, thyroid cancer discovered incidentally at surgery for benign thyroid disease, or presenting in pregnancy has an excellent prognosis.

The use of diagnostic radioiodine scanning is declining both for initial diagnosis in a thyroid nodule and in the detection of recurrence. There is new evidence that it adds little additional information to influence clinical management.

In a retrospective analysis of 153 consecutive patients treated between 1990 and 2000, no patient with a positive diagnostic scan received radioiodine therapy which would not otherwise have been given based on clinical findings and serum thyroglobulin. Thyroglobulin estimation following rhTSH stimulation is rapidly gaining acceptance as the preferred way for detecting persistent or recurrent disease.

As the majority of patients with differentiated carcinoma are young with a good prognosis, the effect of treatment on reproductive function is an important area of concern. In 122 young men treated for differentiated thyroid cancer with a median follow-up of 21 years, no effect was observed on long term fertility even after multiple administrations. Similarly, no case of permanent ovarian failure was seen in 409 young women with a median follow-up of 18 years.

Prognostic factors for medullary thyroid cancer (MTC) have recently been clarified and include age at diagnosis, lymph node involvement and completeness of initial surgical resection. Prognosis for MTC when part of multiple endocrine neoplasia (MEN) 2A is excellent and is mainly accounted for by the earlier stage at which disease is diagnosed, thus emphasizing the need for early detection.
There is now general agreement that management of patients with thyroid cancer should be within a multidisciplinary team, working in specialised units and following evidence-based guidelines.

INTRODUCTION

This chapter will focus on recent developments regarding thyroid cancer in the elderly, diagnostic strategies, surveillance and detection of recurrence, thyroid cancer found incidentally at surgery, thyroid cancer in pregnancy, the long term consequences of thyroid cancer treatment for reproductive health, and prognostic factors for medullary carcinoma. More comprehensive reviews have recently been published (Vini & Harmer, 2002; Sherman, 2003).

Cancer of the thyroid gland represents less than 0.5% of all malignancies in England and Wales (Coleman et al. 1999). Annually in the UK there are approximately 1400 new cases and about 300 deaths from thyroid cancer. The greatest incidence is seen in North and Mid Wales where levels of radiation are highest.

Differentiated thyroid carcinomas derive from the follicular epithelial cells and are either of papillary or follicular subtype. They constitute about 90% of all thyroid cancers. The remainder include medullary carcinoma derived from the neuroendocrine C cells of the thyroid (about 6%) and anaplastic carcinomas (2%). Hurthle-cell carcinoma, previously considered a variant of follicular carcinoma, is now recognised as a distinct clinico-pathological entity (Stojadinovic, 2001). Rare tumour types include sarcomas and primary thyroid lymphoma.

Differentiated thyroid carcinoma predominately affects young adults with the highest incidence occurring between 25 and 54 years of age (SEER, 1997). The median age at diagnosis for papillary carcinoma is 40 years for females and 44 years for males, while for follicular cancer the median age is 48 years for females and 53 years for males (Corea et al. 1995). However, thyroid cancer affects all age groups including the very young and the elderly. Between 2.5 and 12% of differentiated carcinomas occur in individuals over the age of 65 years and the incidence in this age group appears to be rising in recent series (Girelli et al, 1999; Lin et al, 2000).

THYROID CANCER IN THE ELDERLY

We recently reported a study of 111 patients who were aged 70 years or over at the time of diagnosis for differentiated thyroid cancer (Vini et al. 2003). Their records were reviewed in respect of clinical presentation, pathological features, treatment, pattern of recurrence, and survival. There were 83 females and 28 males giving a female to male ratio of 3:1. The median follow-up period was 9 years. The oldest patient was 93 years old and the median age was 75 years.

Older patients were found to have more locally aggressive tumours and a higher incidence of distant metastases at diagnosis. Enlarged lymph nodes in the neck was the presenting symptom in 17 cases and bone pain in 6, including 2 with pathological fracture.

The majority of tumours were locally advanced, 78 (70%) being more than 4 cm or infiltrating beyond the thyroid capsule (pT3 or T4). At diagnosis, lymph nodes were involved in 49 patients (44%) while distant metastases were documented in 26 (23%). Sites of distant spread included the skeleton (12), lung (7), lung and bone (6) and soft tissue (1). Asymptomatic metastatic disease was discovered on the post-ablation 1-131 scan in 7 patients.

Older patients developed clinical recurrence rapidly after initial treatment with a median time of 9 months (range 2-32 months). Local relapse frequently preceded the appearance of distant metastases.

Overall cause-specific survival at 5, 10 and 15 years was 75%, 50% and 50% respectively. In multivariate analysis, the only two factors that emerged with adverse statistical significance for cause specific survival were metastatic spread and use of external beam radiotherapy. The outcome for patients treated with total thyroidectomy was much improved compared to those receiving biopsy alone but at multivariate analysis, the independent effect of surgery did not achieve statistical significance ($p = 0.07$). No significant benefit of ablative radioiodine on cause-specific survival was evident in this study (Hazard Ratio for ablation versus none 0.98; 95% CI: 0.53 – 1.81).

Older age emerged as an important risk factor for overall survival on both univariate and multivariate analysis, with patients over 80 years having a 3-fold increased adverse risk (95% CI: 2.16-4.12) compared to under 75 year-olds. Probability of survival improved significantly according to decade of treatment ($p=0.03$; χ^2 test;). The most marked improvement was seen in patients treated since 1990 when total thyroidectomy followed by ablative radioiodine became routine. Median survival improved from 4.7 years pre 1970, 6.0 years pre 1980, 8.8 years pre 1990 and is now greater than 10 years.

In keeping with previous studies (Tubliana, 1985; Schlumberger, 1996), thyroid tumours in older patients appear to have a shorter doubling time, are less well-differentiated, and take up ^{131}I less avidly when compared to younger subjects. Girelli and colleagues (1999) reported similar observations in the only other large published series of elderly patients.

Candy (1998) has suggested that, on the basis of the unique aspects of their biological behaviour, differentiated thyroid cancer of the elderly is a different disease to that in the young, not merely a different stage of the same disease.

In children and adolescents, extensive disease including distant metastases at presentation, is compatible with long-term survival (Zimmerman et al. 1988; Newman et al. 1998; Furmanchuk et al. 1992).

However, children under the age of 10 years have a higher risk of death although only 5-14% die of the disease (Newman et al. 1998; Landau et al. 2000). Exposure to radioiodine following the Chernobyl nuclear accident has led to a 3 –75 fold increased incidence of papillary carcinoma, especially in young children in whom it typically presents with aggressive tumours (Pacini, 1997). Thus extremes of age appear to have an adverse effect on prognosis, independent of the extent of disease at presentation.

Diagnostic Strategy

In recent years the diagnostic approach has been modified and now includes widespread use of fine-needle aspiration cytology, ultrasonography, and calcitonin measurement, with a decline in use of diagnostic thyroid isotope imaging (Sherman, 2003; Schlumberger & Pacini., 2003).

Typical presentation of thyroid cancer is with a symptomless solitary thyroid nodule or neck node enlargement. Fine needle aspiration cytology is the single most informative investigation and a diagnosis of papillary carcinoma can be made reliably provided an adequate specimen has been obtained (Ravetto et al. 2000).

Cytology cannot differentiate follicular thyroid adenoma from carcinoma since this distinction is based on capsular or vascular invasion which demands excision with formal histology. It is also less reliable in thyroid lymphoma, where a core biopsy or lymph node excision permits immunohistochemical typing (Vini & Harmer, 2002). Repeat fine needle aspiration is recommended when initial aspiration yields inadequate material. This may preferably be performed under ultrasound guidance (Cramer, 2000).

High resolution ultrasonography is increasingly being used as part of the initial investigation of a thyroid nodule. It provides useful information on the number, size and nature of nodules (cystic, solid or mixed) and detects lymph node enlargement. Certain ultrasound appearances such as the absence of a peripheral halo, microcalcifications and increased vascularity on Doppler studies, have been identified as more common in malignancy but their predictive value is low and fine needle aspiration is still required (Schlumberger & Pacini, 2003).

The routine measurement of circulating serum calcitonin concentration in patients with thyroid nodules is controversial. In a study from Pisa, routine calcitonin measurements in approximately 10, 000 patients with thyroid nodules screened over 10 years, detected one medullary thyroid cancer in every 200 patients (Elisei et al. 2004). Patient survival at 10 years was better in this group of patients compared to historical controls not screened in this way. Routine calcitonin screening of thyroid nodules was more accurate than fine-needle aspiration. If the prevalence of medullary thyroid cancer is similar elsewhere, routine calcitonin measurements should be cost-effective and part of the initial diagnostic strategy.

Thyroid scintigraphy with technetium (^{99m}Tc) can distinguish between functioning (hot) and non-functioning (cold) nodules. A cold nodule may be solid or cystic and scanning will not be able to differentiate between these. Hence the finding of a cold nodule is non-specific and non-diagnostic. Radionuclide scanning remains valuable in detecting functioning thyroid adenomas (autonomous nodules) in patients with thyrotoxicosis (Cases & Surks, 2000), but use in the diagnosis of malignancy has declined with the advent of fine-needle aspiration and high resolution ultrasonography.

DETECTION OF RECURRENT DISEASE

Management of differentiated thyroid carcinoma is usually with total or near-total thyroidectomy followed by ^{131}I ablation of remnant thyroid tissue. Before the widespread availability of serum thyroglobulin (Tg) measurement, follow-up consisted of repeat clinical examination and ^{131}I whole body scans.

Recognition of the importance of serum Tg has changed follow-up strategies. Since Tg is derived exclusively from thyroid follicular cells; it should be undetectable after successful surgery and remnant thyroid ablation. Detectable and particularly rising concentrations of Tg following ablative therapy indicates persistent or recurrent disease (Spencer et al. 1999). In recent years serum Tg measurements have become more sensitive and more reliable.

The sensitivity of Tg concentrations to detect disease is enhanced by TSH stimulation, either in the hypothyroid state following hormone withdrawal or after recombinant thyroid stimulating hormone (rhTSH) administration. The latter is becoming increasingly popular as it avoids the unpleasant and debilitating symptoms of hypothyroidism (Haugen et al. 1999). In the presence of TSH suppression, the sensitivity of Tg in detecting small volume residual or recurrent disease may be as low as 50%. Schlumberger and Pacini (2003) summarising studies performed on more than 2000 patients conclude that serum Tg measured 3 days after the second injection of rhTSH is highly sensitive for detection of persistent or recurrent disease.

One limitation to use of serum thyroglobulin in the surveillance of thyroid carcinoma is the presence of antibodies to thyroglobulin which can spuriously lower Tg levels and interfere with the Tg assay.

Such antibodies may be present in up to 25% of patients with thyroid cancer and, in these patients, monitoring of Tg is unreliable (Hollowell et al. 2002).

In patients with suspected recurrence, both high resolution ultrasonography of the neck and ^{131}I diagnostic scanning have been advocated. Ultrasound can accurately identify locoregional disease, with diagnosis confirmed by fine-needle aspiration (Antonelli et al. 1995; Krishnamourthy et al. 2001).

Newer scanning modalities including CT, MRI, and FDG-PET imaging are not required for routine surveillance but may be helpful in patients with a rising Tg to identify a potentially resectable recurrence. CT appears less sensitive than ultrasound in detecting small lesions and use of contrast is preferably avoided as ^{131}I therapy may be required. Interpretation of CT and especially MRI in the neck may be difficult after surgery. PET scanning is a promising technique which may be particularly useful for detecting mediastinal lymph node metastases; rhTSH stimulation may increase both specificity and sensitivity.

The value of ^{131}I diagnostic imaging after thyroid ablation was questioned by Cailleux *et al.* (2000) who suggested that measurement of serum Tg after thyroxine withdrawal was a sufficiently sensitive marker of residual or metastatic disease by itself and that a diagnostic whole body scan yielded no additional information of clinical value. Similar conclusions were reached by Pacini *et al.* (2002) in a study of patients with undetectable serum Tg after thyroid ablation .

We recently reported our experience in 153 consecutive patients undergoing initial ^{131}I diagnostic whole body scan 4 - 6 months following total thyroidectomy and ablative ^{131}I treatment for thyroid cancer (Taylor et al, 2004).

The diagnostic scan was positive in 20 patients (13%) and faintly positive in 16 (11%). The majority (117) had negative scans. Of the 20 patients with a positive scan, 4 received no further treatment, 9 showed no abnormal uptake following a second ablative ^{131}I dose, and 7 had uptake in the thyroid bed (6) or in neck nodes (1) after repeat ablation. In the group of 20 patients with positive scans, the 4 who received no further treatment and the 9 with a negative second ablation scan remained disease-free during follow-up of at least 4 years. No patient with a positive diagnostic scan received additional ^{131}I therapy which would not otherwise have been given based on clinical findings, serum Tg, or the presence of anti-Tg antibodies. Ten of the 117 patients with negative scans developed recurrent disease which was always detected clinically or by a rising serum Tg.

Thus routine diagnostic whole body ^{131}I scanning adds little extra information and in our experience, does not influence patient management. We now reserve these scans for patients in whom serum Tg levels are unreliable because of the presence of antibodies or when there is clinical suspicion of tumour.

Thyroid Cancer in Pregnancy

Management of the pregnant woman with cancer is inevitably associated with considerable anxiety in both patient and clinician, mainly regarding the timing of any recommended treatment. In the case of thyroid cancer, this anxiety is compounded by reports that pregnancy may accelerate the course of the disease (Kobayashi et al. 1994; Rosen et al. 1986). Recent evidence suggests that the prognosis of differentiated thyroid cancer in pregnancy is similar to that occurring in non-pregnant women of similar age with similar rates of recurrence, distant metastases and cause-specific mortality (Moosa & Mazzaferri, 1997).

However, pregnancy complicates management of thyroid cancer as isotope and radiological investigations and treatment may be harmful to the developing fetus and there are concerns regarding surgery and anaesthesia. If treatment is delayed until after delivery and after the mother has stopped breast-feeding to avoid the risk of infant exposure to radioiodine, then patients with a malignant thyroid nodule discovered early in pregnancy are likely to wait for a year or more.

Our reported experience of thyroid cancer diagnosed during pregnancy (Vini et al. 1999) described 9 women with a median age of 28 years, representing 0.64% of all differentiated thyroid cancers on our database of 1398 patients. A thyroid nodule was discovered by the clinician during routine antenatal examination in 4 cases; the remainder had noted a lump in the neck which had increased in size. Iin 2 cases the tumour measured >4 cm and one patient had local spread to cervical lymph nodes.

Only one of our patients underwent thyroidectomy during pregnancy; the others were operated on less than a year after delivery. All tumours were well differentiated carcinoma and ranged in size from 1 - 6 cm. The median follow-up was 14 years (5 - 31 years). Outcome was good in all patients except one whose treatment was delayed over 2 years from initial presentation because of a further pregnancy. She died with metastatic disease but the other 8 of the original cohort of patients are currently disease free. The poor outcome in the patient who developed metastatic disease was likely due to delay in treatment.

We recommend thyroidectomy in the mid-trimester for thyroid cancer found early in pregnancy; those found later in pregnancy can safely be left until after delivery. Thyroid surgery in pregnancy is reported to be safe (Hamilton et al. 1968) although it is associated with increased fetal loss if more extensive surgery including neck dissection is performed (Cunningham & Slaughter, 1970). In all cases further investigation, including whole body radioiodine scan and ablation, can be deferred until after the pregnancy and breast-feeding have been completed.

THYROID CANCER IN GRAVES' DISEASE

The co-existence of Graves' disease and differentiated thyroid cancer is rare. The reported incidence of thyroid carcinoma found at surgery in hyperthyroid patients ranges from 0.21% to 8.7% depending on the criteria used to select patients for surgery, patient characteristics and history of previous neck irradiation.

It has been suggested that thyroid cancer associated with Graves' disease is aggressive because of stimulation of thyroid cancer cells by TSH-receptor antibodies and should therefore be treated vigorously (Belfiore et al. 1990). Other investigators (Hales et al. 1992) have not confirmed this finding. The issue remains controversial as the influence of thyroid autoimmunity on the natural history of thyroid cancer is poorly understood.

Previous studies have suggested that thyroid cancer occurs more frequently in patients operated for hyperthyroidism compared with euthyroid patients (Sokal, 1954; Shapiro et al. 1970; Farbota et al. 1985; Pacini et al. 1988). We examined the outcome of patients found to have differentiated cancer incidentally at the time of surgery for hyperthyroidism (Vini et al. 1999).

Among 986 patients with differentiated thyroid cancer, 23 (2.3%) had presented with symptoms and signs of hyperthyroidism. Graves' disease was diagnosed in 11, multinodular goitre in 8 and toxic adenoma in 4. Following thyroidectomy, histology revealed papillary (18), follicular (4) and Hurthle cell (1) carcinoma. Tumour size ranged from 4 mm to 5.5 cm, multifocality was detected in 3 patients, and lymph node involvement in one.

In this series of patients with occult thyroid malignancy and hyperthyroidism, there was no evidence of increased tumour aggressiveness over a median of 16 years follow-up. Only two patients recurred locally and only one developed distant metastases.

These results contrast with those of Belfiore et al. (1990) who reported a high incidence of local invasiveness, lymph node involvement and distant metastases in their patients with Graves' disease and thyroid cancer. However, all but 2 of their patients had palpable nodules, in contrast to our series in which none had clinically apparent nodules, which suggests that tumours in the Belfiore study were more advanced and detected later. In our experience, differentiated thyroid cancer found incidentally at surgery for hyperthyroidism has a good prognosis.

Reproductive Health after Thyroid Cancer Treatment

Treatment of differentiated thyroid cancer in young adults is frequently associated with normal life expectancy and hence the potential effect on reproductive function is a source of concern. Following ^{131}I administration, the gonads will be exposed to radiation derived from isotope in blood, bladder, bowels and any functioning metastases closeby. More prolonged irradiation lasting for several weeks results from organified ^{131}I incorporated into circulating iodoproteins with long half-lives (Jeevanram *et al.* 1982).

Males

In men treated with radioiodine, transient increases in serum FSH were reported by Wichers *et al.* (2000). Previously, Pacini *et al.* (1994) found that levels returned to normal in the majority of patients within 12 months after treatment, although persistent elevation of FSH levels occurred in 4 patients who had received large cumulative doses. During the hypothyroid state, the renal clearance of iodine is reduced, which may result in a higher testicular dose (Maxon *et al.* 1990). Handelsman *et al.* (1983) suggested a threshold dose for testicular damage of 3.7 GBq radioiodine since no elevation of serum FSH was seen in men treated with doses below this value in their study.

The administration of radionuclides also raises concern because of their appearance in ejaculate. Sexually active males who have been treated with radioiodine are usually recommended to use contraception for 4 months, as this period is greater than the life of a spermatozoon (ARSAC, 1998).

We examined the records of all males under the age of 40 years at the time of treatment with a minimum of 3 years follow-up. In addition, we prospectively measured radiation dose to the testes in 14 consecutive patients admitted for ^{131}I therapy (Hyer et al. 2002).

Fertility was assessed in 122 men with a median follow-up of 21 years (range 3-39) of whom 93 were under active follow-up. Altogether 106 children were fathered by 59 patients; the remainder had no wish to have children. No major malformations were reported. Of these 59 patients, 12 had received a single 3GBq ablation dose, 19 had been treated with up to 14 GBq radioiodine and 28 had received 14 to 44 GBq. In 14 patients studied prospectively, the median estimated radiation dose to each testis was 6.4 cGy following 3 GBq, 14.1 cGy after 5.5 GBq and 21.2 cGy following 9.2 GBq ^{131}I. There was a transient elevation in serum FSH after radioiodine which normalised within 9 months from the last administration.

Consistent with other investigators, we noted a transient impairment of gonadal function. The radiation dose absorbed by the testis after a single ablative dose of radioiodine was well below that associated with permanent damage to germinal epithelium and the risk of infertility in these patients was found to be minimal. However, patients requiring multiple administrations for persistent or metastatic thyroid cancer should be offered sperm banking as they are at greater risk of gonadal damage, although even in this group we found no evidence of infertility.

Females

A similar low risk of permanent gonadal damage appears to apply to women receiving ablative radioiodine. Menstrual irregularities have been reported in about one third of young female patients following administration of high activities of ^{131}I and a smaller number of women experience amenorrhoea, usually lasting less than six months (Raymond et al. 1989). The effect does not appear to be related to the activity of ^{131}I administered and is more common in older women. An increased incidence of miscarriage has also been reported within one year of radioiodine administration (Dottorini et al. 1995). Nevertheless, radioiodine treatment does not appear to affect the outcome of any subsequent pregnancy (Schlumberger et al. 1996).

To confirm these findings, we also reviewed outcome on ovarian function following therapy in young female patients treated for differentiated thyroid carcinoma (Vini et al. 2002). Of 1398 patients on our database, 496 were females under the age of 40 at the time of diagnosis who had received radioiodine. Of these, 322 received a single 3 GBq ablation dose, whilst the remainder received subsequent therapy ^{131}I to a cumulative activity of 8.5 – 59 GBq for residual, recurrent or metastatic disease. We observed transient amenorrhoea in 34 patients (8%) and lesser degrees of menstrual disturbance in a further 49 patients (12%), lasting up to 10 months. No case of permanent ovarian failure was recorded.

There were 427 children born to 276 women; only one patient wishing to achieve a successful pregnancy outcome had been unsuccessful. Four premature births and 14 miscarriages occurred but no congenital abnormalities were reported.

We selected women under the age of 40 years because these patients have the best prognosis from their thyroid cancer. The risk of permanent damage to the ovaries following radioiodine treatment appears to be low in these young patients and they can be reassured that they should experience a normal pregnancy. We did not investigate older women in whom the risk of menstrual irregularities may be greater. A recent report indicated that the age at menopause may be slightly younger following radioiodine but no correlation was observed with the cumulative dose of radioiodine received (Ceccarelli et al. 2001).

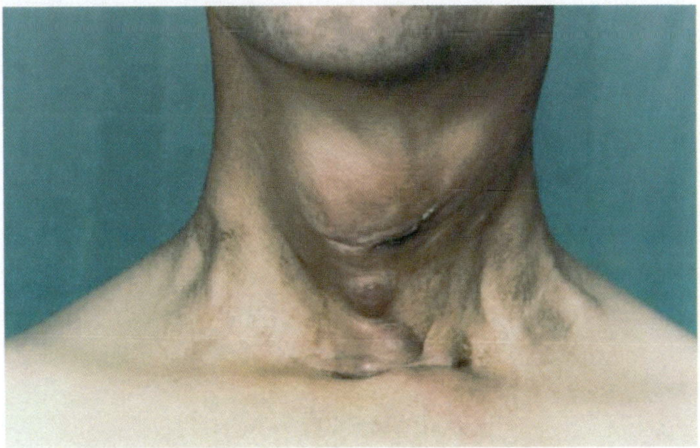

Figure 1: Early recurrent follicular thyroid carcinoma. Note scar of previous thyroidectomy and local recurrence.

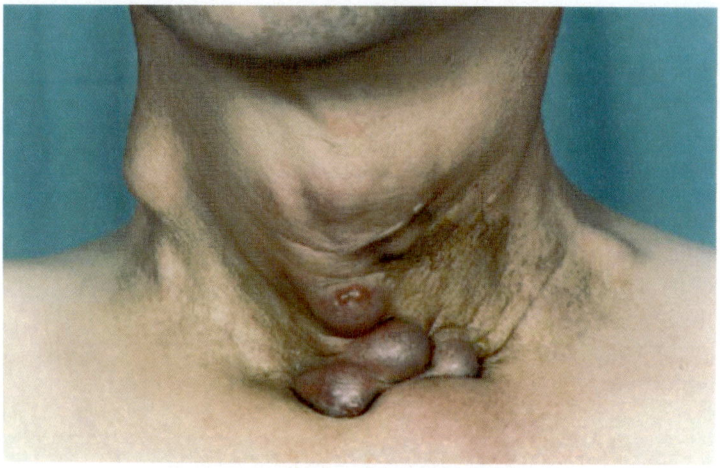

Figure 2: Late aggressive recurrent follicular thyroid carcinoma.

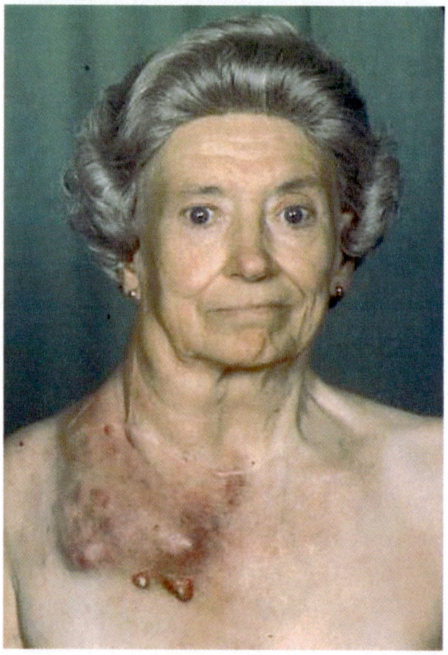

Figure 3: Recurrent medullary thyroid carcinoma. Note scar from previous thyroidectomy and post-radiotherapy skin change.

Prognosis in Medullary Thyroid Cancer

Medullary thyroid carcinoma (MTC) is a rare tumour derived from the parafollicular or C cells of the thyroid, accounting for 5-10% of all thyroid malignancies (Chong et al. 1975; Nguyen et al. 1992). It occurs in sporadic and familial forms, either alone or as part of a multiple endocrine neoplastic syndrome (MEN type IIA or type IIB). As many as 20-25% of all cases are inherited (Raue et al. 1993; Saad et al. 1984). Detection of mutations in the *ret* oncogene have been introduced for family screening (Ponder et al. 1988).

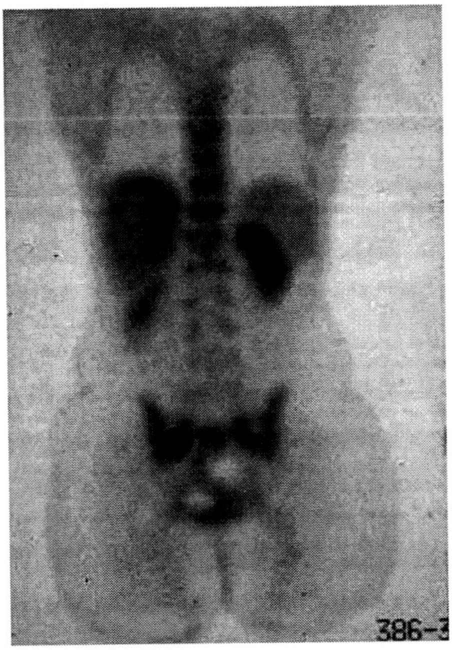

Figure 4: Metastatic medullary thyroid carcinoma (PET scan). Note recurrence in sacrum.

The initial, potentially curative treatment for MTC is surgical consisting of total thyroidectomy plus dissection of lymph nodes in the central compartment of the neck. In addition, patients with cervical lymph node spread require selective neck dissection. External beam radiation following surgery may help in the control of local disease (Fife et al. 1996).

The prognosis of MTC is intermediate between anaplastic and differentiated thyroid cancer, although duration of survival is very variable. A number of factors influencing prognosis have been documented including age and gender, sporadic versus familial disease, and the extent of the tumour at presentation but their relative importance is not clear.

We reviewed all 162 patients with MTC treated in our unit between 1949-1998 to investigate the prognostic value of various clinical parameters (Hyer et al. 2000). We also examined local tumour control and survival in patients treated with external beam radiation.

The overall survival was 72% (95% CI: 64 -78) at 5 years, 56% (95% CI: 47 - 64) at 10 years, 40% (95%CI: 31-49) at 15 years and 30% (95% CI: 20 - 40) at 20 years. Cause specific survival and overall survival (at 5 and 10 years) were very similar. Patients diagnosed before the age of 50 years had a significantly longer survival rate than those diagnosed when older ($p<0.001$). Women had a significantly better prognosis than men ($p<0.01$). The survival of patients with a family history of MTC (52 patients) was not significantly different from those with sporadic disease.

In univariate analysis, the following factors were found to be significant predictors of survival: age at diagnosis, gender, tumour size, lymph node disease, metastases at presentation, and extent of surgery. These six variables were then entered into multivariate analysis and four significant variables remained: age at diagnosis, lymph node disease, metastases at presentation, and extent of surgery. The presence of a positive family history did not predict survival.

Overall survival was similar in patients receiving external beam radiotherapy compared with those treated with surgery alone, despite irradiated patients having more advanced disease. Local recurrence rates were significantly reduced by radiotherapy only in the group of patients with ipsilateral nodal disease (N1a). The reduction in local relapse rates in the N1b group did not quite reach statistical significance (p=0.06). The median time to relapse in N1a patients was 894 days following surgery alone but 3317 days when post-operative irradiation was added (p<0.05).

The difference in local relapse rates in patients with N1a and N1b disease after radiotherapy was not due to differences in the extent of surgical resection of nodes as completeness of surgery was similar in both groups.

When the effect of irradiation on local recurrence rates was compared within patient groups stratified according to tumour size or presence/ absence of metastases, no significant differences were found.

Data on serum calcitonin levels are incomplete due in part to changes in methods of assessment over the long period of this study. Hence we were unable to evaluate the value of calcitonin measurements as a prognostic indicator. They are certainly useful in following the course of disease to document residual tumour and relapse. Carcino-embryonic antigen (CEA) was also used as a complementary tumour marker (Palmer et al. 1984).

The overall 5- and 10- year survival rates were 72% and 56% respectively, similar to those reported by other investigators (Brierley et al. 1996; Gharib et al. 1970). We have used overall survival rather than cause specific survival since it was difficult to determine accurately to what extent cause of death was related to tumour which was present in 81 of the 87 patients who died. In contrast to some previous reports (Samaan et al. 1988) but in keeping with others (Gharib et al. 1992) we found no significant difference in survival between patients with and without a family history of MTC. The more favorable prognosis in familial MTC found in earlier studies probably relates to their younger age and earlier stage when disease was first detected, rather than to any inherent difference in progression of disease (Russell et al. 1983).

The most important factors influencing the prognosis in our series were age at diagnosis, lymph node involvement, distant metastases at presentation, and extent of surgery.

Increasing age at diagnosis was an important prognostic factor on multivariate analysis, after allowing for other factors such as differences in tumour stage or extent of surgery. Patients aged less than 50 years at diagnosis survived significantly longer than those diagnosed when older. The relative risk for dying in those over 50 years at diagnosis rises to 3.7 compared to the risk in those under 40 years. Similar results have been described by other groups suggesting that older patients have more aggressive disease.

Reduced survival with male gender has been described previously in some but not all series. Associations of gender type with age, stage of disease, or completeness of surgery could act as confounding factors. In our series, male gender ceased to be of prognostic importance in multivariate analysis when these factors were taken into account. Males were more likely to have nodal disease (80% of males had nodal disease compared with 56% of females) but were similar in age and extent of surgery to females. The association with nodal status thus appears to determine the poorer prognosis.

The presence of lymph node metastases adversely affected survival with a 2.5 - 6 fold increased risk of dying relative to patients with no nodal involvement, depending whether disease was ipsilateral or had spread to mediastinal nodes. These findings are in keeping with some but not all previous studies. Such discrepancy may relate to differing prognostic significance of mobile compared with fixed nodes (in which disease has extended into surrounding tissues).

The worst prognostic group comprised patients with distant metastases but it is important to recognise that prolonged survival is still possible with metastatic disease. Our longest survivor with metastases lived for 16 years.

Pathological stage at diagnosis rather than tumour size was a strong determinant of survival. Patients with larger tumours had poorer survival on univariate analysis but this was accounted for by a strong association of tumour size with presence of nodal disease or metastases. In multivariate analysis, tumour size was not an independent risk factor.

In our series, the extent of surgery proved to be another independent influence on survival. The extent of surgery was determined by stage of disease, availability of frozen section techniques and changing concepts of the disease over time. Since bilateral or multifocal disease was found at surgery in up to a quarter of patients, we agree with other authors in recommending total thyroidectomy as treatment of choice. Dissection of the central compartment of the neck is also recommended routinely and nearly two thirds of patients had spread of disease to cervical or mediastinal lymph nodes at presentation. Selective neck dissection is often required initially and, if extensive mediastinal disease is present, a sternal split is necessary for complete resection. Other investigators report nodal disease in 40 - 75% of patients. Radical neck dissection, however, is not recommended as a routine procedure because it carries a high morbidity and does not improve survival (Simpson et al. 1982).

In the absence of prospective randomised trials, the value of external radiotherapy (RT) in the management of MTC is uncertain, with varying claims made in the literature of the benefits or otherwise of this treatment. Samaan *et al.* (1988) noted a better overall survival in those not treated with irradiation, which persisted after matching for extent of disease.

However, in a large series from Texas (Saad et al. 1984) the lower survival in patients receiving RT could be attributed to their more advanced disease at presentation. In agreement with previous authors, we found no difference in overall survival rate after RT. Since RT was given in patients with more advanced disease, their similar survival rate could suggest a beneficial effect.

We have previously reported favourable effects of RT in patients with residual microscopic disease after surgery (Fife et al. 1996). The present data extend these observations to patients with disease spread to local lymph nodes showing significantly reduced local relapse rates. Other groups (Gharib et al. 1992; Nguyen et al. 1992) have also reported improved disease control in the thyroid bed and regional lymph nodes after RT. We do not know whether a significant benefit in reducing relapse may have been demonstrated in our study had larger numbers of patients with more extensive nodal disease received RT.

In our experience chemotherapy has not prolonged survival in patients with metastases; out of six patients treated, none has shown an objective response. Similar poor response rates have been described previously (Hoskin & Harmer, 1987), although our more recent experience has been more encouraging (Harmer, 1996) We now reserve this treatment for patients with both symptomatic and progressive disease.

In a separate analysis of 55 patients with at least two first-degree relatives affected by medullary thyroid cancer; 26 were classified as MEN 2A, one as MEN 2B and 28 as FMTC (Hyer et al. 2004). Median age at diagnosis was 35 years (MEN 2A), 25 (MEN 2B) and 47.5 (FMTC). Median follow-up was 9 years (range: 4-24).

Total or near-total thyroidectomy had been performed in all patients and 11 received adjuvant external beam radiotherapy. Cause specific survival was 89% at 10 years and 77% at 20 years for MEN patients, 51% and 32% for those with sporadic MTC, and 46% and 26% for those with FMTC. In multivariate analysis, factors predicting survival were presence of metastases, nodal status and age at diagnosis. Improved survival rates associated with familial types of MTC can be accounted for by the earlier stage at which disease is detected and the younger age at presentation (Hyer et al, 2004). These observations emphasize the need for early detection and treatment of those at risk.

Conclusions

There has been significant progress in the understanding of thyroid cancer over the past decades. Despite lack of randomised controlled trials, improvements in clinical management have come from analysis of the results of large retrospective series. Consensus guidelines have now been agreed and the importance of management by multi-disciplinary teams has been emphasised. Prospective data collection and regular audit of outcomes is expected to lead to further improvement in management of this rare but fascinating disease.

References

Administration of Radioactive Substances Advisory Committee (ARSAC). Notes for guidance on the clinical administration of radio-pharmaceuticals and use of sealed radioactive sources. 1998

Antonelli A, Miccoli P, Fedeghini M et al. Role of neck ultrasound in the follow-up of patients operated on for thyroid cancer. *Thyroid* 1995 5:25-28.

Belfiore A, Garofalo MR, Giuffrida D, *et al.* Increased aggressiveness of thyroid cancer in patients with Graves' disease. *J Clin Endocrinol Metab* 1990; 70:830-35.

Brierley J, Tsang R, Simpson WJ *et al.* Medullary thyroid cancer: analysis of survival and prognostic factors and the role of radiation therapy in local control. *Thyroid* 1996; 6: 305- 310.

Cailleux AF, Baudin E, Travagli JP, Ricard M & Schlumberger M.. Is diagnostic iodine-131 scanning useful after total thyroid ablation for differentiated thyroid cancer? *Journal of Clinical Endocrinology & Metabolism* 2000 85 175-178

Candy B, Rossi R. An expanded view of risk-group definition in differentiated thyroid cancer. *Surgery* 1988; 104:947-53.

Cases JA, Surks MI. The changing role of scintigraphy in the evaluation of thyroid nodules. *Semin Nucl Med* 2000 30:81-87.

Ceccarelli C, Bencivelli W, Morciano D et al. 131 I therapy for differentiated thyroid cancer leads to an earlier onset of menopause: results of a retrospective study. *J Clin Endocrinol Metab* 2001 86: 3512-3515

Chong GC, Beahrs OH, Sizemore GW & Woolner LH. Medullary carcinoma of the thyroid gland. *Cancer* 1975; 35:695-704.

Coleman PM, Babb P, Damiecki P et al. Cancer survival trends in England and Wales 1971-1995; deptrivation amnd NHS region (Series SMPS No 61). London:HMSO, 1999:471-78.

Corea P, Chen VW, Endocrine gland cancer. *Cancer* 1995; 75:338-352.

Cramer H. Fine needle aspiration cytology of the thyroid: an appraisal. *Cancer* 2000 90:325-29.

Cunningham MP & Slaughter DP. Surgical treatment of disease of the thyroid gland in pregnancy. *Surgery Gynaecology & Obstetrics* 1970 131 486-488.

Dottorini ME, Lomuscio G, Mazzucchelli L, Vignati A, Colombo L. Assessment of female fertility and carcinogenesis after iodine-131 therapy for differentiated thyroid carcinoma. *J Nucl Med.* 1995; 36: 21-27.

Elisei R, Bottici V, Luchetti F, et al. Impact of routine measurement of serum calcitonin on the diagnosis and outcome of medullary thyroid cancer: experience in 10,864 patients with nodular thyroid disorders. *J Clin Endocrinol Metab*. 2004 89(1):163-8.

Farbota LM, Calandra DB, Lawrence AM, Paloyan E. Thyroid carcinoma in Graves' disease. *Surgery* 1985; 98:1148-1153

Fife KM, Bower M & Harmer CL. Medullary thyroid cancer: the role of radiotherapy in local control. *European Journal of Surgical Oncology* 1996; 22:588-591

Furmanchuk AW, Averkin JI, Wegloff B, et al. Pathomorphological findings in thyroid cancer of children from the republic of Belarus. A study of 86 cases occurring between 1986 (post-Chernobyl) and 1991. *Histopathology* 1992; 21:401-8.

Gharib H, McConahey WM, Tiegs RD *et al*. Medullary thyroid carcinoma: clinicopathologic features and long term follow-up of 65 patients treated during 1946-1970. *Mayo Clinic Proceedings* 1992; 67:934-940.

Girelli ME, Casara D, Rubello R, et al. Differentiated thyroid cancer in the elderly: disease outcome, therapeutic approach, and long-term results in a group of 314 patients. *J Endocrinol Invest* 1999; 22:45-46.

Girelli ME, Casara D, Rubello R, et al. Differentiated thyroid cancer in the elderly: disease outcome, therapeutic approach, and long-term results in a group of 314 patients. *J Endocrinol Invest* 1999; 22:45-46.

Hales IB, McElduff A, Crummer P, *et al*. Does Graves' disease or thyrotoxicosis affect the prognosis of thyroid cancer? *J Clin Endocrinol Metab* 1992; 75: 886-889.

Hamilton NT, Paterson PJ & Bierdahl HD. Thyroidectomy during pregnancy. *Medical Journal of Australia* 1968 1 431-433.

Handelsman, D.J. & Turtle, J.R. (1983) Testicular damage after radioactive iodine therapy for thyroid cancer. *Clinical Endocrinology*, 18: 465-472.

Harmer CL. Radiotherapy in the management of thyroid cancer. *Annals of Academic Medicine Singapore* 1996; 25:413-419.

Haugen BR, Pacini F, Reiners C. et al. A comparison of recombinant human thyrotropin and thyroid hormone withdrawal for the detection of thyroid remnant or cancer. *J Clin Endocrinol Metab*. 1999 84: 3877-85.

Hollowell JG, Staehling NW, Flanders WD et al. Serum TSH, T4 and thyroid antibodies in the United States population (1988-1994): National Health and Nutrition Examination Survey (NHANES III) *J Clin Endocrinol Metab* 2002 87:489-99.

Hoskin PJ, Harmer CL. Chemotherapy for thyroid cancer. *Radiotherapy and Oncology* 1987; 10: 187-194.

Hyer SL, K. Newbold K, Harmer CL Familial medullary thyroid cancer: clinical aspects and prognosis. *European J Surg Oncol*. 2004 (in press).

Hyer SL, Vini L, Pratt B, Harmer C. Medullary thyroid cancer: multivariate analysis of prognostic factors influencing survival. *European Journal of Surgical Oncology* 2000 26:686-690.

Hyer SL. Vini L, O'Connell M, Pratt B., Harmer C. Testicular dose and fertility in men following I-131 therapy for thyroid cancer. *Clinical Endocrinology* 2002 56, 755-758.

Jeevanram, R.K., Shah, D.H., Sharma, S.M. & Ganatra, R.D. (1982) Disappearance rate of endogenously radio-iodinated thyroglobulin and thyroxine after radioiodine treatment. *Cancer* 49:2281-2284.

Kobayashi K, Tanaka Y, Ishiguro S & Mori T. Rapidly growing thyroid carcinoma during pregnancy. *Journal of Surgical Oncology* 1994 55 61-64.

Krishnamurthy S, Bedi DG, Carawy NP. Ultrasound-guided fine needle aspiration biopsy of the thyroid bed. *Cancer (Cytopathology)* 21001 93:199-205.

Landau D, Vini L, A'Hern R, Harmer CL. Thyroid cancer in children; the Royal Marsden experience. *Eur J Cancer* 2000; 36:214-20.

Lin JD, Chao TC, Chen ST, et al. Characteristics of thyroid carcinomas in ageing patients. *Eur J Clin Invest* 2000; 30:147-53.

Maxon, H.R. & Smith, H.S. (1990) Radioiodine-131 in diagnosis and treatment of metastatic well-differentiated thyroid cancer. *Endocrinology Metabolism Clinics of North America* 19: 685-718.

Moosa M & Mazzaferri EL. Outcome of differentiated thyroid cancer diagnosed in pregnant women. *Joutnal of Clinical Endocrinology & Metabolism* 1997 82 2862-2866.

Newman KD, Black T, Heller G, et al. Differentiated thyroid cancer: determinants of disease progression in patients <21 years of age at diagnosis. A report from the Surgical Discipline Committee of the Children's Cancer Group. *Ann Surg* 1998; 227:533-41.

Nguyen TD, Chassard JL, Lagarde P *et al*. Results of postoperative radiation therapy in medullary carcinoma of the thyroid: a retrospective study by the French Federation of Cancer Institutes. *Radiotherapie Oncologie* 1992; 23: 1-5.

Pacini F, Capezzone M, Elisei R, Ceccarelli C, Taddei D & Pinchera A. Diagnostic 131-Iodine whole body scan may be avoided in thyroid cancer patients who have undetectable stimulated serum Tg levels after initial treatment. *Journal of Clinical Endocrinology & Metabolism* 2002 87 1499 –1501

Pacini F, DiCoscio GC, Anelli S, *et al*. Thyroid carcinoma in thyrotoxicosis patients treated by surgery. *J Endocrinol Invest* 1988; 11:107-12.

Pacini F, Vorontsova T, Demidchick EP et al, Post-Chernobyl thyroid carcinoma in Belarus children and adolescents: a comparison with naturally occurring thyroid carcinoma in Italy and France. *J Clin Endocrinol Metab* 1997 82:3563-3569.

Pacini, F., Gasperi, M., Fugazzola, L. *et al*. (1994) Testicular function in patients with differentiated thyroid carcinoma treated with radioiodine. *Journal of Nuclear Med*icine, 35:1418-1422.

Palmer BV, Harmer CL, Shaw HJ. Calcitonin and carcino-embryonic antigen in the follow-up of patients with medullary carcinoma of the thyroid. *British Journal of Surgery* 1984; 71:101-104.

Ponder BAJ, Finer N, Coffey R, Harmer CL *et al*. Family screening in medullary thyroid carcinoma patients presenting without a family history. *Oncological Journal of Medicine* 1988; 67:299-308.

Raue F, Kotzerke J, Reinwein D *et al*. Prognostic factors in medullary thyroid carcinoma: evaluation of 741 patients from the German medullary thyroid carcinoma register. *The Clinical Investigator* 1993; 71:7-12.

Ravetto C, Colombo L, Dottorini ME. Usefulness of fine needle aspiration in the diagnosis of thyroid carcinoma: a retrospective study in 37, 895 patients. *Cancer* 2000 90:357-63.

Raymond JP, Izembart M, Marliac V et al. Temporary ovarian failure in thyroid cancer patients after thyroid remnant ablation with radioactive iodine. *J Clin Endocrin Metab*. 1989; 69: 186-189.

Rosen IB & Walfish PG. Pregnancy as a predisposing factor in thyroid neoplasia. *Archives of Surgery* 1986 121 1287-1290.

Rougier P, Parmentier C, Laplanche A *et al*. Medullary thyroid carcinoma: prognostic factors and treatment. *International Journal of Radiation, Oncology, Biology and Physics* 1983; 9:161-169.

Russell CF, Van Heerden JA & Sizemore GW. The surgical management of medullary thyroid carcinoma. *Annals of Surgery* 1983; 106:42-44

Saad MF, Ordonez NG, Rashid RK *et al*. Medullary carcinoma of the thyroid: a study of the clinical features and prognostic factors in 161 patients. *Medicine* 1984; 63:319-342.

Samaan NA, Schultz PN & Hickey RC. Medullary thyroid carcinoma: prognosis of familial versus sporadic disease and the role of radiotherapy. *Journal of Clinical Endocrinological Metabolism* 1988; 67:801-805.

Schlumberger M, Challeton C, De Vathaire F, et al. Radioactive iodine treatment and external radiotherapy for lung and bone metastases from thyroid carcinoma. *J Nucl Med* 1996; 37:598-605.

Schlumberger M, De Vathaire F, Ceccarelli C, Delisle MJ, Francese C, Couette JE, Pinchera A, Permentier C. Exposure to radioactive iodine-131 for scintigraphy or therapy does not preclude pregnancy in thyroid cancer patients. *J Nucl Med* 1996; 37: 606-612.

Schlumberger M, Pacini F. *Thyroid tumors*. Editions Nucleon, Paris, 2003

Shapiro SJ, Friedman NB, Perzik SI, Caty B. Incidence of thyroid carcinoma in Graves' disease. *Cancer* 1970; 26:1261-70

Sherman SI. Thyroid carcinoma *Lancet* 2003 361: 501-511.

Simpson WJ Palmer JA, Rosen IB & Mustrard RA. Management of medullary carcinoma of the thyroid. *American Journal of Surgery* 1982; 144:420-422

Sokal JE. Incidence of malignancy in toxic and nontoxic nodular goitre. *JAMA* 1954; 154:1321-25.

Spencer CA, LoPresti JS, Fatemi S, Nicoloff JT. Detection of residual and recurrent differentiated thyroid carcinoma by serum thyroglobulin measurement. *Thyroid* 1999 9:435-41.

Stojadinovic A, Ghossein RA, Hoos A et al. Hurthle cell carcinomas: a critical histopathological appraisal. *J Clin Oncol* 2001; 19:2616-25.

Surveillance, Epidemiology and end Results (SEER) programme of the National Cancer Institute. *J Natl Cancer Inst* 1997; 89:1753.

Taylor H, Hyer S, Vini L, Pratt B, Cook G, Harmer C. Diagnostic ^{131}I whole body scanning after thyroidectomy and ablation for differentiated thyroid cancer. *European Journal of Endocrinology* 2004 150 (5) 649-653

Tubliana M, Schlumberger M, Rougier P, et al. Long term results and prognostic factors in patients with differentiated thyroid carcinoma. *Cancer* 1985; 2: 794-804.

Vini L, Harmer H. Management of thyroid cancer. *The Lancet Oncology* 2002 3 407-414.

Vini L, Hyer SL, Al-Saadi A, Pratt B, Harmer C. Prognosis for fertility and ovarian function after treatment with radioiodine for thyroid cancer. *Postgraduate Medical Journal* 2002; 78 92-93.

Vini L, Hyer SL, Marshall S, A'Hern R, Harmer C. Long-term results in elderly patients with differentiated thyroid cancer. *Cancer* 2003 97 (11) 2736 – 2742.

Vini L, Hyer SL, Pratt B, Harmer C. Good prognosis in thyroid cancer found incidentally at surgery for thyrotoxicosis. *Postgraduate Med J* 1999 75: 169-170.

Vini L, Hyer SL, Pratt B, Harmer C. Management of differentiated thyroid cancer diagnosed during pregnancy. *European Journal of Endocrinology.* 1999 140:404-406.

Wichers, M., Benz, E., Palmedo, H., Biersack, H.J., Grunwald, F., Klingmuller, D. (2000) Testicular function after radioiodine therapy for thyroid carcinoma. *European Journal of Nuclear Medicine,* 27:503-507.

Zimmerman D, Hay ID, Gough IR, et al. Papillary thyroid cancer in children and adults: long term follow-up of 1039 patients conservatively treated at one institution during three decades. *Surgery* 1988; 104:1157-66.

In: Trends in Thyroid Cancer Research
Editor: Carl A. Milton, pp. 221-241
ISBN 1-59454-627-4

Chapter XI

RISK FACTORS FOR ANAPLASTIC THYROID CANCER

Vladan Zivaljevic
Center for Endocrine Surgery, Institute of Endocrinology, Clinical Center of Serbia

ABSTRACT

Aims and background: The aim of the present study was to test some hypothetical risk factors for anaplastic carcinoma, the most lethal type of thyroid cancer.
Study design: A case-control study comprised 126 histologically or cytologically verified anaplastic thyroid cancer patients and 252 controls individually matched with cases by sex, age and place of residence. In the analysis of data univariate and multivariate logistic regressions analysis were used.
Results: According to the multivariate conditional logistic regression analysis following factors were significantly and independently related to anaplastic thyroid cancer: lower education level (OR=1.42, 95%CI=1.09-1.86), history of goiter (OR=37.55, 95%CI=4.86-290.11), personal history of other non-thyroid malignant tumors (OR=2.42, 95%CI=0.99-5.95), blood group B (OR=2.41, 95%CI=1.03-5.66) and age at menarche after 15 year (OR=4.06, 95%CI=1.76-9.46).
Conclusions: The results obtained are in line with the current knowledge on factors related to thyroid cancer, except for the associations between anaplastic thyroid cancer and blood group B, which has not been reported.

Key words: anaplastic thyroid cancer, risk factors, case-control study.

INTRODUCTION

At the end of the XIXth century and during the first half of the XXth century, due to rapid development of medical sciences, for most infective diseases who were until then the commonest cause of falling ill and dying, many adequate measures of prevention and treatment were found. Due to this factor, the life span of the general population increased considerably, and so did the occurrence of malignant tumors, which today represent the second most common cause of death, right after cardiovascular diseases. Today, oncology is one of the most researched and discussed topics among experts and among the general population, and most of the research in this area of medicine is focused on unveiling the risk factors of malignant tumor development and the best way to treat them. Identifying these potential risk factors would allow carrying out adequate preventive measures against the appearance of malignant tumors, since it is easier, cheaper and much better to prevent an illness from occurring than to treat that illness.

Investigating the risk factors of thyroid malignant tumor development has one dimension more and that is that the recognized and established conditions in which the risk factors work can be used in everyday practice. The number of patients with an altered thyroid gland is very big. Clinically examined, a lump or an enlargement of the thyroid gland can be found in about 5% of the general population and more frequently in women. Using an ultrasound to examine the thyroid gland increases this percentage five times, meaning that 25% of the general population has an altered thyroid gland. (1-3) As a contrast to that, cancer of the thyroid gland is a relatively rare malignancy which covers 1% to 2% of all malignant tumors, but it is on the other hand the commonest tumor among endocrine tumors. (4) More than 90% of malignant tumors of the endocrine system are malignant tumors of the thyroid gland. (5) The incidence of carcinoma of the thyroid gland is low and ranges between 1 to 8%ooo, but in most countries, shows an increase. (6, 7) Carcinoma of the thyroid gland is diagnosed in about 20.000 patients yearly, in the USA alone. (8) To put it differently, one patient in a thousand patients with an altered thyroid gland has cancer of the thyroid gland. The problem that is presented to the doctor is how to separate, from a vast amount of patients with a solitary nodule or goiter, the patients that need to be operated. Using already standard principles, the risk factors that determine malignant tumor development could be an additional entity to take into account when deciding who should undergo surgery.

The best known risk factor for malignant tumor development is exposure to external radiation. More than 50 years ago, it was shown that external radiation is associated with cancer of the thyroid gland. (9, 10) The children's thyroid gland is particularly susceptible to the cancerous effect of radiation. (11, 12) Women have a greater risk of cancer alteration of the thyroid gland, due to radiation than do men. (13, 14) It takes typically two to three decades, after exposure, for the cancerous effect of external radiation to manifest. (13, 14) The correlation between exposure to external radiation and the development of thyroid cancer is additionally proved by the high occurrence of this cancer in people who have been exposed to therapeutical radiation usually in their childhood, because of neck haemangioma, enlarged thymus gland, lymphoma, tonsillitis, acne vulgaris, and tinea capitis. (15–19) Further proof of this is a high occurrence of thyroid gland carcinoma among persons who were exposed during the nuclear havoc in Chernobyl, or among the survivors in Hiroshima and Nagasaki after the use of the nuclear bomb, or among the inhabitants of Marshall Islands who were exposed to radioactive rain after nuclear testing nearby. (20-23)

The next factor that should be taken into account is the deficiency of iodine, which is the case with the inhabitants of endemic goiter regions where there is a low concentration of iodine. (24, 25) The risk of development of cancer increases as does the duration of life spent in these regions. (26, 27) This risk is particularly evident with persons who have spent their childhood and adolescence in such regions. (28, 29) Anaplastic and follicular carcinomas of the thyroid gland are basically extensively found in these endemic regions. (30, 31)

Another risk factor for the occurrence of cancer of the thyroid gland is long-term exposure, in the line of work, to various chemicals and metals. (32, 33)

Other malignant tumors, revealed in personal anamnesis, increase the risk of a person, with goiter or a solitary nodule in the thyroid gland, to in fact have carcinoma of the thyroid gland. Around 5% of patients with cancer of the thyroid gland were previously treated because of a primary malignant tumor of a different location. (34, 35) This is mostly evident in women who underwent treatment of breast cancer. (36) The appearance of carcinoma of the thyroid gland, among patients with multiple malignant tumors, can point towards a genetic predisposition of malignant tumor expression. Furthermore, it can be the result of exposure to joint exogenous risk factors. One should have in mind that the appearance of a secondary primary malignant tumor could be, in fact, the result of various diagnostic and therapeutic procedures associated with a previous primary malignant tumor.

Finally, one of the risk factors for carcinoma of the thyroid gland is a positive family anamnesis for malignant non-thyroid tumors. (37, 38)

Thyroid gland cancer can appear in a sporadic form or in a hereditary form. Medullar carcinoma is a very rare tumor and covers less than 10% of all thyroid carcinomas. On the other hand, the congenital form of this tumor, which appears as the result of the mutation of RET proto-oncogene on the 10th chromosome, is one of the best examined tumors in oncology. Genetic screening has made it possible to operate (prophylactic thyroidectomy) carriers of the mutated RET proto-oncogene, before medullar carcinoma can develop. (39) Today it is known, due to firstly epidemiological studies and then genetic studies, that there is, apart from the congenital form of medullar carcinoma, a congenital form of non-medullar carcinoma of the thyroid gland, which is a precisely defined clinical entity. (40-42)

Other risk factors, for the occurrence of cancer of the thyroid gland, include various controversial hormone and reproductive dependant characteristics. (43) For instance, women who were pregnant have a higher risk to have carcinoma of the thyroid gland, and the risk increases with the increased times the woman was pregnant. (44, 45) Menstrual disorders, late menarche and miscarriages are also associated with carcinoma of the thyroid gland. (46-48) Carcinoma of the thyroid gland is more frequently discovered in elder pregnant women and women who used oral contraceptives. (49, 50)

Additionally, a diet rich in sea food and goiter dependant substances can result in carcinoma of the thyroid gland. (51)

For the past couple of years, the risk factors for development of carcinoma of the thyroid gland is still an extremely studied topic, which numerous published results of many studies demonstrated from all around the world. (52-56)

Most studies aim to unveil risk factors that determine the development of certain histo-pathological types of carcinoma of the thyroid gland. The vast majority of studies concentrate on well differentiated carcinomas of the thyroid gland, such as the papillary type, which is the most common histo-pathological form of thyroid gland carcinoma. In 2002, the first "case-control" study was published on factors that determine the risk for development of medullar carcinoma of the thyroid gland, using 67 persons from a few centers around the world. (57)

Up till now, this kind of a study was not used to research anaplastic carcinoma of the thyroid gland, even though it is the most aggressive histo-pathological form for this localization of malignant tumors. The lethality rate for anaplastic carcinoma of the thyroid gland is 100%, and the survival rate is, despite the multi modular approach to therapy, only 3 to 6 months. (58-60) Due to this, anaplastic carcinoma of the thyroid gland deserves full attention, and therefore the need to establish the risk factors has been presented. The reason why a "case-control" study has not been conducted so far possibly lies in the fact that anaplastic carcinoma has a low incidence in the general population, and therefore it is difficult to obtain a relevant amount of patients which would be required for this kind of a study. The yearly incidence for anaplastic carcinoma is around 2 in a million people. (61) So far, the only "case-control" study on the risk factors for development of anaplastic carcinoma of the thyroid gland consists of the preliminary results of our research, published in 2004. (62) According to the multivariate conditional logistic regression analysis following factors were significantly and independently related to anaplastic thyroid cancer: history of goiter or thyroid nodules (Odds ratio - OR = 37.55, 95% confidence interval - 95% CI = 4.86-290.11), history of residence in endemic goiter area (OR = 2.56, 95% CI = 1.05-6.22), history of previous malignant non-thyroid tumors (OR = 5.51, 95% CI = 1.04-29.25), diabetes mellitus (OR = 4.06, 95% CI = 1.29-12.81) and lower education level (OR = 2.44, 95% CI = 1.17-5.06). (62)

Material and Method

A case-control study was performed in population of Serbia (a part of the former Yugoslavia with about ten million inhabitants) from January 1996 to December 2000.

The case group comprised 126 consecutive patients with newly diagnosed anaplastic thyroid cancer at the Center for Endocrine Surgery, Institute of Endocrinology, Clinical Center of Serbia in Belgrade. Type of tumor was determined by histological analysis in operated patients (55) or by cytology in non-operated cases (71). Histological analysis confirmed anaplastic transformation of papillary thyroid cancer in 42 (33%) cases.

The control group was recruited among patients neighbours in like manner always. None among controls had prior thyroid cancer diagnose. Cases and controls were individually matched by sex, age (± 2 years) and place of residence.

One physician interviewed all participants at hospital and home. No one among cases and controls refused participation in the study. A standardized questionnaire was used to obtain information about socio-demographic characteristics, personal habits (smoking, consumption of coffee and alcohol), residence in endemic goiter area, exposure to radiation and various chemicals, personal history (thyroid gland disease, other endocrine disease, malignant tumors, some other medical conditions, diagnostic and therapeutic procedures, operations and drug consumption) and family history (thyroid gland diseases, malignant tumors, residence in endemic goiter area). Detailed data were also obtained on menstrual, reproductive and hormonal history (age at menarche, regularity of menstrual cycle, pregnancies, outcome of first pregnancy, age at first full pregnancy, miscarriage, abortion, number of live-born children, use of oral contraceptives and estrogen use in menopause). In participants who reported relevant disease in their past histories, medical records were reviewed in order to verify diagnosis.

Patients with anaplastic thyroid cancer were significantly more frequently with lower education level than their controls (incomplete or complete primary school only).

Table 1 - Demographic characteristics of anaplastic thyroid cancer patients and their controls

	CASES		CONTROLS		p*
	No	%	No	%	
Sex					
Male	49	39.0	49	39.0	Matched
Female	77	61.0	77	61.0	
Age					
30-39	1	0.8	2	0.8	
40-49	10	8.0	16	6.4	
50-59	30	24.0	40	16.0	
60-69	65	52.0	149	59.6	Matched
70-79	19	15.2	43	17.2	
80+	1	0.8	2	0.8	
Place of residence					
RURAL AREA	39	31.0	78	31.0	
Urban area	87	69.0	174	69.0	Matched
Formal education					
None or incomplete	**38**	**30.2**	**62**	**24.6**	
Primary	**66**	**52.4**	**111**	**44.0**	
Secondary	17	13.4	59	23.4	p=0.012 4
High	5	4.0	20	8.0	
Occupation					
Housewife	38	30.2	80	31.7	
Agricultural worker	18	14.3	19	7.5	
Industrial worker	12	9.5	17	6.8	
Clerk	8	6.3	31	12.3	p>0.10
Retired	48	38.1	93	36.9	
Professional	2	1.6	12	4.8	
Marital status					
Single	4	3.2	2	0.8	
Married	99	78.5	228	90.4	p>0.10
Divorced	0	0	7	2.8	
Widowed	23	18.3	15	6.0	

*According to univariate logistic regression analysis

Univariate conditional logistic regression was first applied in the statistical analysis of data. In order to account simultaneously for the potential confounding effects of various risk factors, multivariate conditional logistic regression analysis was used.

RESULTS

Table 1 presents demographic characteristics of cases and controls. Women were more frequently than men anaplastic thyroid cancer cases (1.5:1). The age of cases varied from 37 to 88 years with a median age of 65 years. Two-thirds majority was from urban area.

There were no substantial differences between cases and controls in their marital status and occupation. A lot of them were married and houswife or retired.

Table 2 - Blood groups of anaplastic thyroid cancer patients and their controls

	Cases		Controls		p*
	No	%	No	%	
0+	49	38.9	112	44.4	
A+	52	41.3	118	46.8	
B+	**12**	**9.5**	**11**	**4.4**	
AB+	6	4.8	7	2.8	
O-	3	2.4	2	0.8	**P=0.0297**
A-	2	1.6	2	0.8	
B-	**1**	**0.8**	**0**	**0**	
AB-	1	0.8	0	0	

*According to univariate logistic regression analysis

Table 3 – Personal habits of anaplastic thyroid cancer patients and their controls

	Cases		CONTROLS		p*
	No	%	No	%	
Actual smoker					
Yes	43	34.1	98	38.9	p>0.10
No	83	65.9	154	61.1	
Former smoker					
Yes	6	7.1	15	9.7	p>0.10
No	77	92.9	139	90.3	
Alcohol consumption					
Yes	3	2.4	2	0.8	p>0.10
No	123	97.6	250	99.2	
Coffee consumption					
Yes	110	87.3	222	88.1	p>0.10
No	16	12.7	30	11.9	

*According to univariate logistic regression analysis

Data about blood groups of anaplastic thyroid cancer patients and their controls are shown at Table 2. A lot of participants had A or 0 blood groups (44.9% - A, 41.3% - 0 blood group among anaplastic thyroid cancer patients and 47.6% - A, 45.2% - 0 blood group among their controls). However, we found significantly more frequently blood group B among anaplastic thyroid cancer patients than their controls (10.3% : 4.4%).

Cases and control did not significantly differ either in smoking or in coffee and alcohol consumption. (Table 3) A lot of participants were not smokers and only a few were drunkard.

Table 4 shows some data from family history of cases and controls. There were no substantial differences between cases and controls in family history of thyroid disease, residence in endemic goiter area and malignant tumors.

Table 4 - Family history of anaplastic thyroid cancer patients and their controls

	Cases		Controls		p*
	No	%	No	%	
Thyroid diseases					
Yes	5	4.0	12	4.8	p>0.10
No	121	96.0	240	95.2	
Endemic goiter area					
Yes	27	21.4	52	20.6	p>0.10
No	99	78.6	200	79.4	
Malignant tumors					
Yes	16	12.7	25	9.9	p>0.10
No	110	87.3	227	90.1	

*According to univariate logistic regression analysis

Table 5 presents thyroid disorders in personal history of participants.

Thyroid nodule or goiter was reported only among cases, in 38 (30.2%) of them. They were present longer than a year (minimum 1, maximum 50, median 18 years) before rapid growth and before diagnosis of anaplastic thyroid cancer was made. Eight of anaplastic thyroid cancer patients had thyroid operation in personal history (4 for thyroid cancer and 4 for goiter).

Residence in endemic goiter area was reported by 29 (23.0%) cases and by 47 (18.7%) controls. All of them were in endemic goiter area for more than 10 years period of life, and majority were even born in region of goiter endemia. There were no substantial differences between participants in residence in endemic goiter area because of cases and controls were individually matched by actual place of residence.

Hyperthyroidism, thyroiditis, radioiodine therapy and thyroxin therapy in personal history were reported only by a few anaplastic thyroid cancer patients and non by controls, but the difference was not statistically significant. No one among cases and controls had hypothyroidism.

Table 5 - Thyroid disorders in personal history of anaplastic thyroid cancer patients and their controls

	Cases		Control		p*
	No	%	No	%	
Residence in endemic goiter area					
Yes	29	23.0	47	18.7	p>0.10
No	97	77.0	205	81.3	
Goiter					
Yes	38	30.2	0	0	p=0.0000
No	99	69.8	252	100.0	
Hyperthyroidism					
Yes	1	0.8	0	0	p>0.10
No	125	99.2	252	100.0	
Radioiodine therapy					
Yes	1	0.8	0	0	p>0.10
No	125	99.2	252	100.0	
Thyroxin therapy					
Yes	5	4.0	0	0	p>0.10
No	121	96.0	252	100.0	
Thyroiditis					
Yes	1	0.8	0	0	p>0.10
No	125	99.2	252	100.0	

*According to univariate logistic regression analysis

In the group of previous diseases, in personal history of participants, endocrine gland disease (diabetes mellitus) and the other malignant non-thyroid tumors were significantly related to anaplastic thyroid cancer. Out of 126 cases 15 (11.9%) had diabetes mellitus (3 had diabetes mellitus type 1). In the control group diabetes mellitus was reported in 15 (6.0%) participants.

Other malignant tumors were reported in 11 (8.7%) cases and 11 (4.4%) controls. Among malignant tumors preceding anaplastic thyroid cancer, the most frequent was cervix cancer - in 4 women, followed by skin cancer - in 3 cases (2 women and 1 man) and breast cancer - in 2 women. One case (man) had lung cancer and the other one had prostate cancer.

The frequency of mumps and immulogical disorders were similar in both groups.

Anaplastic thyroid cancer patients, statistically significant more frequently than controls (19.8% cases and 12.3% controls), had tonsillectomy in their personal histories.

Table 6 – Other disease in personal history of anaplastic thyroid cancer patients and their controls

	Cases		Controls		p*
	No	%	No	%	
Breast cancer					
Yes	2	1.6	0	0	p>0.10
No	124	99.2	252	100.0	
Other malignant tumors					
Yes	11	8.7	11	4.4	p=0.0936
No	115	91.3	241	95.6	
Endocrine gland disease					
Yes	15	11.9	15	6.0	p=0.0476
No	111	88.1	237	94.0	
Immunologic disorders					
Yes	1	0.8	1	0.4	p>0.10
No	125	99.2	251	99.6	
Mumps					
Yes	8	6.3	15	6.0	p>0.10
No	118	93.7	237	94.0	
Tonsillectomy					
Yes	25	19.8	31	12.3	p=0.0537
No	101	80.2	221	87.7	

*According to univariate logistic regression analysis

Table 7 – Exposure to various factors in personal history of anaplastic thyroid cancer patients and their controls

	Cases		Control		p*
	No	%	No	%	
Professional exposure to chemicals					
Yes	3	2.4	12	4.8	p>0.10
No	123	97.6	240	95.2	
Diagnostic radiation of head and neck					
Yes	15	11.9	21	8.3	p>0.10
No	111	88.1	231	91.7	
Radiotherapy					
Yes	2	1.6	1	0.4	p>0.10
No	124	98.4	251	99.6	
Immunotherapy					
Yes	1	0.8	0	0	p>0.10
No	124	98.4	251	99.6	

*According to univariate logistic regression analysis

There were no substantial differences between cases and controls in professional exposure to various chemicals (including agricultural chemicals) and diagnostic radiation of head and neck. Radiotherapy and immunotherapy were reported only by a few participants. (Table 7).

Table 8 – Menstrual, hormonal and reproductive characteristics of anaplastic thyroid cancer patients and their controls

	Cases		Controls		p*
	No	%	No	%	
Age at menarche					
<15	61	79.2	140	90.9	p=0.0151
15+	16	20.8	14	9.1	
Regular menstrual cycle					
Yes	73	94.8	149	96.8	p>0.10
No	4	5.2	5	3.2	
Pregnancies					
Yes	73	94.8	152	98.7	p>0.10
No	4	5.2	2	1.3	
Deliverance					
Yes	73	100.0	152	100.0	p>0.10
No	0	0	0	0	
Number of live born children					
1 and 2	61	83.5	137	91.3	p>0.10
3+	12	16.5	15	8.7	
Miscarriage					
Yes	4	5.5	4	2.7	p=0.0941
No	69	94.5	148	97.3	
Outcome of first pregnancy					
Lifebirth	68	93.2	148	97.4	p>0.10
Abortion	5	6.8	4	2.6	
Use of oral contracetives					
Yes	20	26.0	34	22.1	p>0.10
No	57	74.0	120	77.9	
Estrogen use in menopause					
Yes	5	7.0	8	5.6	p>0.10
No	66	93.0	136	94.4	

*According to univariate logistic regression analysis

Menstrual, hormonal and reproductive characteristics of anaplastic thyroid cancer patients and their controls are presented in Table 8. Out of them, according to univariate logistic regression analysis, two characteristics were significantly related to anaplastic thyroid cancer. Cases more frequently than their controls reported older age at menarche - after 15 year (20.8% : 9.1%). Anaplastic thyroid cancer patients two time more frequently reported miscarriage than their controls (5.5% : 2.7%).

Iregular menstrual cycles were almost the same in compared groups.

No significant differences in the number of pregnancy, number of deliverance, outcome of the first pregnancy, age at first full pregnancy, number of live-born children, age at menopause and thyroid enlagred during pregnancy, between anaplastic thyroid cancer patients and controls emerged.

Cases more frequently than their control were used oral contraceptives and hormonal replacement estrogen therapy during menopause (26.0% : 22.1% and 7.0% :5.6%). However, these differences were not statistically significant.

Out of 55 variables studied, according to univariate logistic regression analysis, 8 variables (education level, blood group B, history of goiter, history of other non-thyroid malignant tumors, history of endocrine gland disease, tonsillectomy, age at menarche and miscarriage) were related to anaplastic thyroid cancer at significance level of $p \leq 0.10$. All these variables were entared into models of multivariate logistic regression analysis, the results of which are presented in Table 9. According to multivariate logistis regression analysis the following factors were found to be independently related to anaplastic thyroid cancer: education level, history of goiter, history of other non-thyroid malignant tumors, blood group B and age at menarche.

Table 9 – Risk factors for anaplastic thyroid cancer – multivariate conditional logistic regression analysis

Factor	Coefficient	S.E.	P	Odds ratio	(95%CI)
Educational level	0.3514	0.1374	0.0105	1.42	1.09-1.86
History of goiter	3.6258	1.0431	0.000	37.55*	4.86- 290.11
History of malignant tumor	0.8828	0.4603	0.0551	2.42	0.99-5.95
Blood group "B"	0.8808	0.4354	0.0431	2.41	1.03-5.66
Age at menarche	1.4010	0.5846	0.0156	4.06	1.74-9.46

*Corrected by 1.

DISCUSSION

In the last few decades the distribution of malignant tumors of the thyroid gland has changed. Today, anaplastic carcinoma occupies a smaller portion than it did before. It contributes to 1-2% of thyroid cancer patients, while it used to contribute to over 10%. (63-

68) It is presumed that this is a result of several factors. The main factor that reduced the amount of patients with anaplastic carcinoma would be prophylactic iodinating of salt, particularly in endemic goiter regions, which has been conducted successfully in most of the well developed countries. (69-72) The earlier the prophylaxis was undertaken, the incidence of anaplastic carcinoma in that region was reduced sooner, which by itself demonstrates its successfulness. (73, 74) Today, the highest incidence of anaplastic cancer (nearly 20%) is in fact in countries with goiter endemic areas and with an inappropriate health system. (75-78) The total number of patients with anaplastic cancer has reduced due to the increased number of operations of goiter and a better recognition of well differentiated tumors, preventing its anaplastic transformation. Furthermore, the number of other malignant tumors of the thyroid gland is increased and so the anaplastic cancer fraction was relatively reduced at the same time. Many small cell lymphomas and medullar cancers were incorrectly placed in the group with anaplastic cancer of the thyroid gland (79, 80)

Anaplastic cancer of the thyroid gland usually appears in the seventh or eighth decade of life, as is the case with this study. (81) The average age of the patients is around 65 years. (82-84) More than 90% is older than 50 years (85) It scarcely appears before the age of 40 years. (86, 87) Cases of anaplastic cancer appearing in childhood have been described and then it has the same fatal result as with older patients with anaplastic cancer. (88-90)

All the histo-pathological types of cancer of the thyroid gland appear more often in women than in men. Anaplastic cancer affects men and women at a ratio 2:1, which statistically is in favor of women but is in fact worse. (91) In this study the ratio is 1.5:1 in favor of women. The ratio difference is smaller than with other histo-pathological types. The reason is that anaplastic cancer appears in elderly people, and in this period, as in childhood before puberty, the difference between the sexes is, as with the other histo-pathological types, the least. (92) Anaplastic cancer of the thyroid gland evolved, in 25% to 75% cases according to histo-pathological analysis, from an already existent well differentiated cancer of the thyroid gland, the commonest being papillary cancer (83, 93, 94) In this study the mentioned percentage is 33%. Dedifferentiation occurs usually after 10 to 15 years after the first operation of well differentiated cancer. (95, 96) To recognize this group of patients is important, since they have a slightly better prognosis than do de novo anaplastic cancers of the thyroid gland have. (97) The anaplastic transformation may be the result of p53 tumor suppressor gene point mutation. (98-100)

Nearly half of the patients with anaplastic cancer of the thyroid gland have had goiter for years before the anaplastic transformation. (84, 101, 102) This risk is even greater with elderly people who have had goiter longer than ten years. (103, 104) An early on operation on patients with an altered goiter is the only prophylactic measure available against anaplastic cancer of the thyroid gland. (105)

There is a fine difference between the occurrences of certain histo-pathological types in areas that are endemic and areas that are not. (106) In endemic goitreeareas there is a higher incidence of follicular and anaplastic cancer of the thyroid gland. Along with the implementation of iodine prophylaxis their incidence has gone down. (107-109) Anaplastic cancer appears three times more in endemic goiter regions. (110) Except the active iodine prophylaxis there is silent prophylaxis going on thanks to the consumption of industrially conserved food. (111)

According to the results of the shown study the most common risk factors for the development of anaplastic cancer of the thyroid gland are goitre, previous malignant non-thyroid tumors, lower degree of education, persons with blood goup B and late menarche. The results of our previous pilot study indicated to goiter, life on an endemic goiter area, previous malignant non-thyroid tumors, diabetes mellitus and a lower degree of education as hypothetical risk factors for the development of anaplastic cancer of the thyroid gland. We can see that three factors repeat and they are goiter, previous malignant non-thyroid tumors and a lower degree of education (a complete or incomplete primary education).

The link between anaplastic cancer of the thyroid gland and other malignant tumors is fortified by the fact that the former appears in women with breast cancer. (112) Late menarche has been described as one of the factors for development of cancer of the thyroid gland. (15, 113) A low social and economic status is responsible for a high incidence of anaplastic cancer of the thyroid gland since three quarters of people with goitre are from under developed countries. (114) According to the results of our study we did not retrieve a link connecting anaplastic cancer of the thyroid gland with radiotherapy. This link has been described in literature as such, but it is mainly a characteristic of papillary cancer of the thyroid gland, after effect of radiotherapy of Hodgkin's lymphoma or enlarged thymus or haemangioma. (115-117)

The development of anaplastic cancer of the thyroid gland after therapy with radioactive iodine because of hyperthyroidism has been described too. (118) Ten or more years after therapy can pass before the development of anaplastic cancer. (119) Excluding Graves disease, the development of anaplastic cancer of the thyroid gland after therapy with radioactive iodine because of a toxic adenoma or hyperthyroidism caused by Amiodaron, has been described in literature. (120, 121)

In addition to well-known disadvantages of case-control studies, the main drawback of this investigation is a relatively small number of participants and consequently insufficient study power to discover some risk factors. Having this in mind, this study should be repeated with a greater number of subjects and possibly using subjects from various other centers.

REFERENCES

[1] Gaitan, E; Nelson, NC; Poole, GW. Endemic gitre and endemic thyroid disorders. *World J Surg, 1991* 15, 205-215.

[2] Gharib, H; Goelner, JR; Johnson, DA. Fine-needle aspiration cytology of the thyroid. A 12-year expirience with 11000 biopsies. *Clin Lab Med, 1993* 13, 699-709.

[3] Brander, A; Viinkikoski, P; Nickels, J; Kivisaari, L. Thyroid gland: US screening in a random adult population. *Radiology, 1991* 181, 683-687.

[4] Hundahl, SA; Fleming, ID; Fremgen, AM; Menck, HR. A National Cancer Data Base report on 53,856 cases of thyroid carcinoma treated in the U.S., 1985-1995. *Cancer, 1998 83*, 2638-2648.

[5] Correa, P; Chen, VW. Endocrine gland cancer. *Cancer, 1995* 75, 338-352.

[6] Pettersson, B; Adami, HO; Wilander, E; Coleman, MP. Trends in thyroid cancer incidence in Sweden, 1958-1981, by histopathologic type. *Int J Cancer, 1991* 48, 28-33.

[7] Devesa, SS; Silverman, DT; Zoung, JL; Pollack, ES; Brown, CC; Horm, JW; Perey, CL; Myers, MH; McKay, FW; Fraumeni, JF. Cancer incidence and mortality trends among whites in the United States, 1974-1984. *JNCI, 1987* 79, 701-707.

[8] Boone, RT; Fan, CY; Hanna, EY. Well-differentiated carcinoma of the thyroid. *Otolaryngol Clin North Am, 2003* 36, 73-90.

[9] Quimby, EH; Werner, SC. Late radiation effects in rontgen therapy for hyperthyreoidism. *JAMA, 1949* 140, 1046-1047.

[10] Duffy, BJ; Fitzgerald, PJ. Thyroid cancer in childhood and adolescence. A report of twenty-eight cases. *Cancer, 1950* 3, 1018-1032.

[11] Sako, K. Haed and neck irradiation in childhood: increased risk of developing thhyroid disease. *Semin Surg Oncol, 1991* 7, 112-114.

[12] Tucker, MA; Jones, PH; Boice, JD; Robinson, LL; Stone, BJ; Stovall, M; Jenkin, RD; Lubin, JH; Baum, ES; Siegel, SE. Therapeutics radiation at a young age is linked to secondary thyroid cancer. The late effects study group. *Cancer Res, 1991* 51, 2885-2888.

[13] Hol, LE. Radiation induced thyroid neoplasia. *Soz Preventivmed, 1991* 36, 266-275.

[14] Schneider, AB; Ron, E; Lubin, J; Stovall, M; Gierlowski, TC. Dose-response relationships for radiation-induced thyroid nodules: evidence for the prolonged effects of radiation on the thyroid. *J Clin Endocrinol Metab, 1993* 77, 362-369.

[15] Shore, RE; Hildreth, N; Dvoretsky, P; Andersen, E; Moseson, M; Pasternack, B. Thyroid cancer among persons given x-ray treatment in infancy for an enlagred thymus gland. *Am J Epidemiol, 1993* 137, 1068-1080.

[16] Lundell, M; Hakulinen, T; Holm, LE. Thyroid cancer after radiotherapy for skin hemangiona in infancy. *Radiat Res, 1994* 140, 334-339.

[17] DeYong, SA; Demeter, JG; Jarosz, H; Lawrence, AM; Paloyan, E. Thyroid carcinoma and hyperthyroidismus after radiation therapy for adolescent acne vulgaris. *Surgery, 1991* 110, 691-695.

[18] Hanckok, SL; Cox, RS; McDougall, IR. Thyroid disease after treatment of Hodgkins disease. *N Engl J Med, 1991* 325, 599-605.

[19] Ron, E; Modan, B. Benign and malignant thyroid neoplasms after childhood irradiation for tinea capitis. *JNCI, 1980* 65, 7-11.

[20] Shimaoka, K; Shibata, Y; Akiba, S. Thyroid disease in cohort studies of A-bomb survivors. *Thyroid Clin Exp ,1994* 6, 37-41.

[21] Ezaki, H. Thyroid cancer: epidemiological study of thyroid cancer in A-bomb survivors from extended life span study cohort in Hiroshima. *J Radiat Res, 1993* 32, 193-200.

[22] Abelin, T; Averkin, JI; Egger, M; Egloff, B; Furmanchuk, AW; Gurtner, F; Korotkewich, JA; Marx, A; Matveyenko, II; Okeanov, AE. Thyroid cancer in Belarus post Chernobyl: improved detection or increased incidence. *Soz Preventivmed, 1994 39,* 189-197.

[23] Douglas, AJ. Cancer mortality and morbidity among workers at the Sellafield plant of British Nuclear Fuels. *Br J Cancer, 1994* 70, 1232-1243.

[24] Nmadu, PT; Mabougunje, OA. The risk of cancer in endemic multinodular goitre. *Centr Afr J Med, 1991* 37, 242-244.

[25] Wahner, HW; Cuello, C; Correa, P; Uribe, LF; Gaitan, E. Thyroid carcinoma in an endemic goitre area. Cali, Colombia. *Am J Epidemiol, 1996 40*, 58-66.

[26] Levi, F; Franceschi, S; La Vecchia, C; Negri, E; Gulie, C; Duruz, G; Scazziga, B. Previous thyroid disease and risk of thyroid cancer in Switzerland. *Eur J Cancer, 1991* 27, 85-88.

[27] D Avanzo, B; La Vecchia, C; Franceschi, S; Negri, E; Talamini, R. History of thyroid disease and subsequent thyroid cancer risk. *Cancer Epidemiol Biomarkers Prev, 1995* 4, 193-199.

[28] Galanti, MR; Sparen, P; Karlsson, A; Grimelius, L; Ekbom, A. Is residence in areas of endemic goiter a risk factor for thyroid cancer? *Int J Cancer, 1995*, 61, 615-621.

[29] Franceschi, S; Fassina, A; Talamini, R; Mazzolini, A; Vianello, S; Bidoli, E; Serriano, D; La Vecchia, C. Risk factors for thyroid cancer in northern Italy. *Int J Epidemiol, 1989* 18, 578-584.

[30] Clark, OH; Duh, QY. Thyroid cancer. *Med Clin North Am 1991* 75, 211-234.

[31] Salabe, GB. Aetiology of thyroid cancer: an epidemiological overview. *Thyroidal Clin Exp, 1994* 6, 11-19.

[32] Grimalt, JO; Sunyer, J; Moreno, V; Amaral, OC; Sala, M; Rosell, A; Anto, JM; Albaiges, J. Risk excess of soft-tissue sarcoma and thyroid cancer of community exposed to airboneorganochlorinatd compound mixtures with a high hexachlorbenzene content. *Int J Cancer, 1994* 56, 200-203.

[33] Sokic, S; Adanja, B; Vlajinac, H; Jankovic, R; Marinkovic, J; Zivaljevic, V. Risk factors for thyroid cancer. *Neoplasma, 1994* 41, 371-374.

[34] Stein, M; Lachter, J; Bartal, A; Rennert, G; Kuten, A. Thyroid cancer and multiple primary malignancies in Israel. *J Surg Oncol, 1991* 47, 221-224.

[35] Valdina, EA. Association of cancer of the thyroid with other malignant tumors. *Vopr Oncol, 1986* 32, 49-53.

[36] Ron, E; Cutris, R; Hoffman, AD; Flannery, TJ. Multiple primary breast and thyroid cancer. *Br J Cancer, 1984* 49, 87-92.

[37] Wingren, G; Harschek, T; Axelson, O. Determinants of papillary cancer of the thyroid. *Am J Epidemiol, 1993* 138, 482-491.

[38] Hallquist, A; Hardel, L; Degerman, A; Boquist, L. Thyroid cancer: reproductive factors, previous disease, drug intake, family history and diet. A case-control study. *Eur J Cancer Prev, 1994* 3, 481-488.

[39] Hoermann, R; Quadbeck, B. Medullary thyroid carcinoma. *Oncol Pract, 1999* 1, 8-10.

[40] Grossman, RF; Tu, SH; Duh, QY; Siperstein, AE; Novosolov, F; Clark, OH. Familial nonmedullary thyroid cancer. An emerging entity that warrants aggressive treatment. *Arch Surg, 1996* 130, 892-897.

[41] Alsanea, O. Familial nonmedullary thyroid cancer. *Curr Treat Options Oncol, 2000* 1, 345-351.

[42] Uchino, S; Noguchi, S; Kawamoto, H; Yamashita, H; Watanabe, S; Shuto, S. Familial nonmedullary thyroid carcinoma characterized by multifocality and a high recurrence rate in a large study population. *World J Surg, 2002* 26, 897-902.

[43] Zivaljevic, V; Vlajinac, H; Jankovic, R; Marinkovic, J; Dzodic, R; Grujicic, S; Paunovic, I; Diklic, A; Zivaljevic, B. Case-control study of female thyroid cancer – menstrual, reproductive and hormonal factors. *Eur J Cancer Prev, 2003* 12, 63-66.

[44] Kravdal, O. Positive corelation between parity and incidence of thyroid cancer: new evidence based on complete Norwegian cohorts births. *Int J Cancer, 1991* 49, 831-836.

[45] Gallanti, MR; Lambe, M; Ekbom, A; Sparen, P; Petterson, B. Parity and risk of thyroid cancer: a nested case-control study of a nation wide Swedish cohort. *Cancer Causees Control, 1994* 6, 37-44.

[46] Kolonel, LN; Hankin, JH; Wilkens, LR; Fukunaga, FH; Hinds, MW. An epidemiological study of thyroid cancer in Hawaii. *Cancer Causes Control, 1990* 1, 223-234.

[47] Levi, F; Franceschi, S; Gulie, C; Negri, E; LaVecchia, C. Female thyroid cancer: the role of reproductive and hormonal factors in Switzerland. *Oncology, 1993* 50, 309-315.

[48] Asklen, LA; Nilssen, S; Kvale, G. Reproductive factors and risk of thyroid cancer. A prospective study of 63090 women from Norwey. *Br J Cancer, 1992* 65, 772-774.

[49] Preston-Martin, S; Jin, F; Duda, MJ;, Mack, WJ. A case-control study of thyroid cancer in women under age 55 in Shanghai. *Cancer Causes Control, 1993* 4, 431-440.

[50] Franceschi, S; Fassina, A; Talamini, R; Mazzolini, A; Vianello, S; Bidoli, E; Cizza, G; La Vecchia, C. The influenze of reproductive and hormonal factors on thyroid cancer in women. *Rev Epidemiol Sante Publique, 1990* 38, 27-34.

[51] Glattre, E; Haldorsen, T; Berg, JP; Stensvold, I; Solvoli, K. Norwegian case-control study testing the hypothesis that seafood increases the risk of thyroid cancer. *Cancer Causes Control, 1993* 4, 11-16.

[52] Picchi, P; Faloci, C; Salabe, GB. Hormonal end reproductive factors and cigarete smoking as risk factors for thyroid cancer in women. A case-control study. *Minerva Endocrinol, 2001* 26, 53-57.

[53] Dal Maso, L; La Vecchia, C; Franceschi, S; Preston-Martin, S; Ron, E; Levi, F; Mack, W; Mark, SD; McTiernan, A; Kolonel, L; Mabuchi, K; Jin, F; Wingren; G; Galanti, MR; Hallquist, A; Glattre, E; Lund, E; Linos, D; Negri, E. A pooled analysis of thyroid cancer studies. V. Anthropometric factors. *Cancer Causes Control, 2000* 11, 137-144.

[54] Franceschi, S; Preston-Martin, S; Dal Maso, L; Negri, E; La Vecchia, C; Mack, WJ; McTiernan, A; Kolonel, L; Mark, SD; Mabuchi, K; Jin, F; Wingren, G; Galanti, R; Hallquist, A; Glattre, E; Lund, E; Levi, F; Linos, D; Ron, E. A pooled analysis of case-control studies of thyroid cancer. IV. Benign thyroid diseases. *Cancer Causes Control, 1999* 10, 583-595.

[55] La Vecchia, C; Ron, E; Franceschi, S; Dal Maso, L; Mark, SD; Chatenoud, L; Braga, C; Preston-Martin, S; McTiernan, A; Kolonel, L; Mabuchi, K; Jin, F; Wingren, G; Galanti, MR; Hallquist, A; Lund, E; Levi, F; Linos, D; Negri, E. A pooled analysis of case-control studies of thyroid cancer. III. Oral contraceptives, menopausal replacement therapy and other female hormones. *Cancer Causes Control, 1999* 10, 157-166.

[56] Negri, E; Dal Maso, L; Ron, E; La Vecchia, C; Mark, SD; Preston-Martin, S; McTiernan, A; Kolonel, L; Yoshimoto, Y; Jin, F; Wingren, G; Rosaria Galanti, M; Hardell, L; Glattre, E; Lund, E; Levi, F; Linos, D; Braga, C; Franceschi, S. A pooled analysis of case-control studies of thyroid cancer. II. Menstrual and reproductive factors. *Cancer Causes Control, 1999* 10, 143-155.

[57] Negri, E; Ron, E; Franceschi, S; La Vecchia, C; Preston-Martin, S; Kolonel, L; Kleinerman, RA; Mabuchi, K; Jin, F; Wingren, G; Hallquist, A; Levi, F; Linos, A; Fraumeni, JF Jr. Risk factors for medullary thyroid carcinoma: a pooled analysis. *Cancer Causes Control, 2002* 13, 365-372.

[58] Haigh, PI; Ituarte, PH; Wu, HS; Treseler, PA; Posner, MD; Quivey, JM; Duh, QY; Clark, OH. Completely resected anaplastic thyroid carcinoma combined with adjuvant chemoterapy and irradiation is associated prolonged survival. *Cancer, 2001* 91, 2335-2342.

[59] Haigh, PI. Anaplastic thyroid carcinoma. Curr Treat Options Oncol, 2000 1, 353-357.

[60] Clark, OH. Predictors of thyroid tumor aggressiveness. *West J Med, 1996* 165, 131-138.

[61] Ain, KB. Anaplastic thyroid carcinoma: a therapeutic chalenge. *Semin Surg Oncol, 1999* 16, 64-69.

[62] Zivaljevic, V; Vlajinac, H; Jankovic, R; Marinkovic, J; Diklic, A; Paunovic, I. Case-control study of anaplastic thyroid cancer. *Tumori, 2004* 90, 10-13.

[63] Busnardo, B; Girelli, ME; Nacamulli, D; Pelizzo, MR; Daniele, O; Rigon, A. Undifferentiated carcinoma of the thyroid gland. *Chir Ital, 1994* 46, 37-41.

[64] Pomorski, L; Bartos, M. Metastasis as the first sign of thyroid cancer. *Neoplasma, 1999* 46, 309-312.

[65] Pasieka, JL. Anaplastic thyroid cancer. *Curr Opin Oncol, 2003*, 15, 78-83.

[66] Burgess, JR. Temporal trends for thyroid carcinoma in Australia: an increasing incidence of papillary thyroid carcinoma (1982-1997*). Thyroid, 2002* 12, 141-149.

[67] Castillo, L; Haddad, A; Meyer, JM; Sadoul, JL; Santini, J. Predictive malignancy factors in thyroid nodular disease. *Ann Otolaryngol Chir Cervicofac, 2000* 117, 383-389.

[68] Hundahl, SA; Cady, B; Cunningham, MP; Mazzaferri, E; McKee, RF; Rosai, J; Shah, JP; Fremgen, AM; Stewart, AK; Holzer, S. Initial results from a prospective cohort study of 5583 cases of thyroid carcinoma treated in the United States during 1996. U.S. and German Thyroid Cancer Study Group. An American College of Surgeons Commission on Cancer Patient Care Evaluation study. *Cancer, 2000* 89, 202-217.

[69] Demeter, JG; De Jong, SA; Lawrence, AM; Paloyan, E. Anaplastic thyroid carcinoma: risk factors and outcome. *Surgery, 1991* 110, 956-963.

[70] Ain, KB. Anaplastic thyroid carcinoma: behavior, biology, and therapeutic approaches. *Thyroid, 1998* 8, 715-726.

[71] Tan, RK; Finley, RK3rd; Driscoll, D; Bakamjian, V; Hicks, WL Jr; Shedd; DP. Anaplastic carcinoma of the thyroid: a 24 year expirience. *Head Neck, 1995* 17, 41-46.

[72] Bubenhofer, R; Hedinger, C. Thyroid neoplasms before and after the prophylactic supplementation of table salt with iodine. *Schweiz Med Wochenschr, 1977* 107, 733-741.

[73] Ratnatunga, PC; Amarasinghe, SC; Ratnatunga, NV. Changing patterns of thyroid cancer in Sri Lanka. Has the iodination programme helped? *Ceylon Med J, 2003* 48, 125-128.

[74] Feldt-Rasmussen, U. Iodine and cancer. *Thyroid, 2001* 11, 483-486.

[75] Pacheco-Ojeda, LA; Martinez, AL; Alvarez, M. Anaplastic thyroid carcinoma in Ecuador: analysis of prognostic factors. *Int Surg, 2001* 86, 117-121.

[76] Mulaudzi, TV; Ramdial, PK; Madiba, TE; Callaghan, RA. Thyroid carcinoma at King Edward VIII Hospital, Durban, South Africa. *East Afr Med J, 2001* 78, 242-245.

[77] Muthuphei, MN. Carcinoma of the thyroid in Ga-Rankuwa Hospital, Pretoria. *East Afr Med J, 1999* 76, 700-702.

[78] Omran, M; Ahmed, ME. Carcinoma of the thyroid in Khartoum. *East Afr Med J, 1993* 70, 159-162.

[79] Holting, T; Moller, P; Tschahagrane, C; Maybier, H; Buhr, H; Herfarth; C. Immunohistochemical reclassification of anaplastic carcinoma reveals small and giant cell lymphoma. *World J Surg, 1990* 14, 291-295.

[80] Tobler, A; Maurer, R; Hedinger, CE. Undifferentiated thyroid tumors of diffuse small cell type. *Virchows Arch A Pathol Anat Histopathol, 1984* 404, 117-126.

[81] Miccoli, P; Iacconi, P; Cecchini, GM; Caldarelli, F; Ricci, E; Berti, P; Puccini, M. Thyroid surgery in patients aged over 80 years. *Acta Chir Belg, 1994* 94, 222-223.

[82] McIver, B; Hay, ID; Giuffrida, DF; Dvorak, CE; Grant, CS; Thompson, GB; Van Heerden, JA; Goellner, JR. Anaplastic thyroid carcinoma: a 50-year experience at a single institution. *Surgery, 2001* 130, 1028-1034.

[83] Spires, JR; Schwartz, MR; Miller, RH. Anaplastic thyroid carcinoma. Association with differentiated thyroid cancer. *Arch Otolaryngol Head Neck Surg, 1988* 114, 40-44.

[84] Sierra, M; Gamboa-Dominguez, A; Herrera, MF; Barredo-Prieto, B; Alvarado dela Barrera, C; Llorente, L; Perez-Enriquez, B; Rivera, R; Gonzalez, O; Rull, JA. Anaplastic carcinoma of the thyroid at the Instituto Nacional de la Nutricion Salvador Zubiran. *Rev Invest Clin, 1997* 49, 97-103.

[85] Hadar, T; Mor, C; Shvero, J; Levy, R; Segal, K. Anaplastic carcinoma of the thyroid. *Eur J Surg Oncol, 1993* 19, 511-516.

[86] Fadare, O; Sinard, JH. Glandular patterns in a thyroid carcinoma with insular and anaplastic features: a case with possible implications for the classification of thyroid carcinomas. *Ann Diagn Pathol, 2002* 6, 389-398.

[87] Bezos Capelastegui, J; Morales Angulo, C; Garcia Mantilla, J; Carrera Herrero, F; Ondiviela, R. Anaplastic carcinoma of the thyroid in a young man. A report of a case. *An Otorrinolaringol Ibero Am, 1999* 26, 413-419.

[88] Parlowsky, T; Bucsky, P; Hof, M; Kaatsch, P. Malignant endocrine tumours in childhood and adolescence-results of a retrospective analysis. *Klin Padiatr, 1996* 208, 205-209.

[89] Meller, J; Conrad, M; Behr, T; Gratz, S; Becker, W. Differentiated thyroid gland carcinoma in children and adolescents. *Klin Padiatr, 1998* 210, 373-378.

[90] Jocham, A; Joppich, I; Hecker, W; Knorr, D; Schwarz, HP. Thyroid carcinoma in childhood: management and follow up of 11 cases. *Eur J Pediatr, 1994* 153, 17-22.

[91] Junor, EJ; Paul, J; Reed, NS. Anaplastic thyroid carcinoma: 91 patients treated by surgery and radiotherapy. *Eur J Surg Oncol, 1992* 18, 83-88.
[92] Stio, F; Battisti, G; Felici, A; Franco, P; Iavarone, C; Marigliani, M; Maceroni, M; Brescia, A. Thyroid cancer and its incidence in nodular thyroid diseases: our experience. *G Chir, 1990* 11, 487-490.
[93] Venkatesh, YS; Ordonez, NG; Schultz, PN; Hickey, RC; Goepfert, H; Samaan, NA. Anaplastic carcinoma of the thyroid. A clinicopathologic study of 121 cases. *Cancer, 1990* 66, 321-330.
[94] Wallin, G; Backdahl, M; Tallroth-Ekman, E; Lundell, G; Auer, G; Lowhagen, T. Co-existent anaplastic and well differentiated thyroid carcinomas: a nuclear DNA study. *Eur J Surg Oncol, 1989* 15, 43-48.
[95] Mooradian, AD; Allam, CK; Khalil, MF; Salti, I; Salem, PA. Anaplastic transformation of thyroid cancer: report of two cases and review of the literature. J Surg Oncol, 1983 23, 95-98.
[96] Gal, I; Hathazi, L; Nemes, Z; Solymosi, T. Anaplastic transformation of papillary carcinoma of the thyroid. *Orv Hetil, 1994* 135, 581-584.
[97] Rodriguez, JM; Pinero, A; Ortiz, S; Moreno, A; Sola, J; Soria, T; Robles, R; Parrilla, P. Clinical and histological differences in anaplastic thyroid carcinoma. *Eur J Surg, 2000* 166, 34-38.
[98] Fogelfeld, L; Bauer, TK; Schneider, AB; Swartz, JE; Zitman, R. p53 gene mutations in radiation-induced thyroid cancer. *J Clin Endocrinol Metab, 1996* 81, 3039-3044.
[99] Shingu, K; Kobayashi, S; Yokoyama, S; Fujimori, M; Asanuma, K; Ito, KI; Hama, Y; Maruyama, M; Kusama, R; Amano, J. The likely transformation of papillary thyroid carcinoma into anaplastic carcinoma during postoperative radioactive iodine-131 therapy: report of a case. *Surg Today, 2000* 30, 910-913.
[100] Sera, N; Ashizawa, K; Ando, T; Ide, A; Abe, Y; Usa, T; Tominaga, T; Ejima, E; Hayashi, T; Shimokawa, I; Eguchi, K. Anaplastic changes associated with p53 gene mutation in differentiated thyroid carcinoma after insufficient radioactive iodine (131I) therapy. *Thyroid, 2000* 10, 975-979.
[101] Agrawal, S; Rao, RS; Parikh, DM; Parikh, HK; Borges, AM; Sampat, MB; Histologic trends in thyroid cancer 1969-1993: a clinico-pathologic analysis of the relative proportion of anaplastic carcinoma of the thyroid. *J Surg Oncol, 1996* 63, 251-255.
[102] Abeatici, S; Palestini, N; Durando, R; Fortunato, A. Precedents of benign thyroid pathology in carcinoma of the thyroid. *Chir Ital, 1994* 46, 75-77.
[103] Mathai, V; Idikula, J; Fenn, AS; Nair, A. Do long-standing nodular goitres result in malignancies? *Aust N Z J Surg, 1994* 64, 180-182.
[104] Lam, KY; Lo, CY; Chan, KW; Wan, KY. Insular and anaplastic carcinoma of the thyroid: a 45-year comparative study at a single institution and a review of the significance of p53 and p21. *Ann Surg, 2000* 231, 329-338.
[105] Wahl, RA. Preventive operation of the thyroid gland. *Langenbecks Arch Chir Suppl Kongressbd, 1991* 2, 203-210.
[106] Bacher-Stier, C; Riccabona, G Totsch, M; Kemmler, G; Oberaigner, W; Moncayo, R. Incidence and clinical characteristics of thyroid carcinoma after iodine prophylaxis in an endemic goiter country. *Thyroid, 1997* 7, 733-741.

[107] Hedinger, C. Geographic pathology of thyroid diseases. *Pathol Res Pract, 1981* 171, 285-292.

[108] Lind, P; Langsteger, W; Molnar, M; Gallowitsch, HJ; Mikosch, P; Gomez, I. Epidemiology of thyroid diseases in iodine sufficiency. *Thyroid, 1998* 8, 1179-1183.

[109] Franceschi, S. Iodine intake and thyroid carcinoma--a potential risk factor. *Exp Clin Endocrinol Diabetes, 1998* 106, 38-44.

[110] Belfiore, A; La Rosa, GL; Padova, G; Sava, L; Ippolito, O; Vigneri, R. The frequency of cold thyroid nodules and thyroid malignancies in patients from an iodine-deficient area. *Cancer, 1987* 60, 3096-3102.

[111] Regalbuto, C; Salamone, S; La Rosa, GL; Calaciura, F; Buscema, M; Vigneri, R. Iodine deficiency and iodine prophylaxis experience in Sicily. *Ann Ist Super Sanita, 1998* 34, 429-436.

[112] Ohsumi, S; Urakami, J; Matsumori, H; Sasaki, S; Murakami, M; Nose, S. A case of two primary carcinomas: thyroid papillary carcinoma with anaplastic transformation of metastatic cervical lymph node and breast cancer. *Gan No Rinsho, 1990* 36, 2439-2444.

[113] Franceschi, S; Fassina, A; Talamini, R; Mazzolini, A; Vianello, S; Bidoli, E; Cizza, G; La Vecchia, C. The influenze of reproductive and hormonal factors on thyroid cancer in women. *Rev Epidemiol Sante Publique, 1990* 38, 27-34.

[114] Bakiri, F; Djemli, FK; Mokrane, LA; Djidel, FK. The relative roles of endemic goiter and socioeconomic development status in the prognosis of thyroid carcinoma. *Cancer, 1998* 82, 1146-1153.

[115] Getaz, EP; Shimaoka, K; Rao, U. Anaplastic carcinoma of the thyroid following external irradiation. *Cancer, 1979* 43, 2248-2253.

[116] Komorowski, RA; Hanson, GA; Garancis, JC. Anaplastic thyroid carcinoma following low-dose irradiation. *Am J Clin Pathol, 1978* 70, 303-307.

[117] Lemaire, M; Lejeune, G; Lambermont, B. Radiation-induced thyroid cancer. *Acta Otorhinolaryngol Belg, 1988* 42, 606-611.

[118] Wiener, JD; Thijs, LG; Meijer, S. Thyroid carcinoma after 131I treatment for hyperthyroidism. Report of a case. *Acta Med Scand, 1975* 198, 329-330.

[119] Peters, J; O'Reilly, S; Barragry, JM. Anaplastic carcinoma of the thyroid following radio-iodine therapy. *Ir J Med Sci, 1993* 162, 3-4.

[120] Gorowski, T; Gabryelewicz, MB; Jastrzebska, H. Anaplastic thyroid carcinoma developed after treatment of "hot" thyroid nodule with radioiodine. *Endokrynol Pol, 1992* 43, 308-313.

[121] Bridges, AB; Davies, RR; Newton, RW; McNeill, GP. Anaplastic carcinoma of the thyroid in a patient receiving radio-iodine therapy for amiodarone-induced thyrotoxicosis. *Scott Med J, 1989* 34, 471-472.

In: Trends in Thyroid Cancer Research
Editor: Carl A. Milton, pp. 241-251

ISBN 1-59454-627-4

Chapter XII

Hurthle Cell Tumors of the Thyroid Personal Experience and Review of the Literature

***M. Appetecchia*[1,*]*, A. Barnabei*[1]*, E. Ferretti*[1] *and A. Procaccini*[2]**

[1]Endocrinology Unit, Regina Elena Cancer Institute, Rome, Italy,
[2]Otorinolaringology Unit, S. Camillo de Lellis Hospital, Rieti, Italy.

Abstract

Hurthle cell carcinoma represents about 5% of differentiated thyroid carcinomas [1]. When Hurthle cell population represents more than 75% of cell population, the lesion can be considered a Hurthle cell tumor. Hurthle cell tumor can be classified as malignant when capsular or vascular invasion is reported or if there is a perithyroid infiltration or distant metastases occur. Until now, there is a controversy about its classification; in fact, the World Health Organization (WHO) Committee considers this tumor the oxyphilic variant of follicular thyroid cancer, while for the Armed Forces Institute of Pathology (AFIP) Hurthle cell carcinoma should be separated into a category of thyroid neoplasm, different from true follicular cancer. The prognosis of the malignant variant of the tumor is still under debate as some authors have reported that Hurthle cell adenoma occasionally behaves like Hurthle cell carcinoma. The purpose of the current study was to evaluate previous reported data and our own experience on the clinical and pathological features of patients affected by Hurthle cell tumor that can predict disease progression and death. Factors potentially associated with decreased survival for all patients were identified as: age, disease stage, tumor size, extraglandular invasion, lymphnodes disease, distant metastases, extensive surgery, radioiodine therapy and external beam radiation therapy. From 1992 to 2003, the authors identified 28 patients affected by Hurthle cell tumor, 9 patients with Hurthle cell adenomas and 19 patients

* Correspondence concerning this article should be addressed to Prof. M Appetecchia MD, Endocrinology Unit – Regina Elena Cancer Institute – Rome – Italy. Via Elio Chianesi, 53 – 00128 Rome, Italy. Fax: +390652666024; e-mail: appetecchia@ifo.it.

with Hurthle cell carcinomas. Twenty-two were females and 6 males. Mean age of patients affected by adenoma was 49.7 years (30-72 yrs) versus 49.3 years (15 –72 yrs) of Hurthle cell carcinoma patients. In all patients a total thyroidectomy was performed. At hystology 9 adenomas, 5 “minimally invasive” and 14 invasive carcinomas were found. Average size of primary tumor was: 28.8 mm medium diameter in Hurthle cell adenoma versus 25.8 mm in Hurthle cell carcinoma. None patient had lymph nodes metastases. Postoperatively, in Hurthle cell carcinoma patients TNM staging showed 9 patients stage I, 5 stage II, 4 stage III and 1 stage IVa (UICC, 2002). All invasive carcinomas underwent ^{131}I therapy (91-150 mCi). One Hurthle cell carcinoma patient received external beam radiotherapy. The average follow-up period was 62 months (range 6-324). In none of our cases with adenoma a relapse was observed. Only one Hurthle cell carcinoma patient showed distant lung metastases at 60 months of follow up. She was submitted to repeated ^{131}I treatments and she is still in follow-up. In conclusion, several clinical and pathologic prognostic factors were rewieved from literature and from our own series of patients with Hurthle cell adenoma and Hurthle cell carcinoma in order to analyze factors that could be associated with worse prognosis. Hurthle cell carcinoma was not found to have an aggressive behaviour when risk factors, including extent of tumour invasion, were taken into account. None of Hurthle cell adenoma showed a relapse or death caused by the tumor.

Keywords: Hurthle cell tumors, thyroid carcinoma, prognostic factors.

INTRODUCTION

Hurthle cell tumor (HCT) is a rare thyroid neoplasm of follicular cell origin composed over 75% of cell with oncocytic features. Since the first description of this entity in 1907 by Langhans [2] the ability to categorize each tumor with oncocytic features as either benign or malignant has been extensively debated. As a consequence, even in recent years several studies have been focused on this topic. Hurthle cell carcinoma (HCC) accounts for approximately 3-7% of well–differentiated thyroid carcinomas [3]. In fact, small series of patients with Hurthle cell carcinoma have been reported in the literature during the past years. Because of its relative rarity, its pathologic and clinical significance has not been well documented [4,5,6,26,44] and little is known about the long-term survival of the patients with this tumor. Some authors affirmed that Hurthle cell carcinoma have a worse prognosis than papillary and follicular thyroid hystotype, only an estimated 10% of Hurthle cell carcinoma metastases take up radioiodine, more frequently involves regional lymph nodes than does follicular carcinoma, shows a higher mortality rate and a greater tendency to metastatize to distant sites [7,8,9,49] while others reported a relative benign course and showed that when the tumor is treated aggressively the patients have survival rates close to those for follicular carcinoma [26,44]. Moreover, many controversies exist in distinguishing benign from malignant Hurthle cell variants. The two entities are distinguished based on identification of capsular or vascular invasion or the presence of metastatic disease [28,31,32]. However, the prognosis of the malignant variant of the tumor remains controversial as some authors reported that patients with benign lesions subsequently developed malignant behaviour with metastatic disease [13].

Stemming from these differences in experiences, controversies have emerged as to the best therapeutic strategy for Hurthle cell carcinoma. Some researchers recommend a conservative management whereas others claimed an aggressive treatment [10,13, 26, 44].

The purpose of the current study was to evaluate the clinical and pathological features of our patients with Hurthle cell neoplasms, in order to analyze the clinical and pathologic prognostic factors rewieved from literature that could be associated with a worse prognosis.

PATIENTS AND METHODS

Twenty-eight patients with Hurthle cell tumors were followed from 1992 to 2003 at the Endocrinology Unit of Regina Elena Cancer Institute, in Rome, were retrospectively reviewed. Thyroid hormonal profile (TSH: normal value 0.3 – 3.5 mcUI/ml; FT_3: normal value 2.2 – 5.00 pg/ml; FT_4: normal value 8.00 -18.50 pg/ml), Thyreoglobulin (normal value 0.2-50 ng/ml) and serum thyroid autoantibodies (Tg-Ab: normal value. 0-115 U7ml; TPO-Ab: normal value 0-32 U/ml), ultrasonography and scintiscan information were obtained for all patients. In all patients a thyroid nodule or neck node fine needle ago-biopsy (FNAB) was performed. A diagnosis of "follicular lesion" was considered suspicious for malignancy. In all patients with a suspicious or certain cytological diagnosis of malignancy surgery was performed. Cervical lymph nodes dissection was added if lymph nodes involvement was proved at preliminary imaging staging or at surgical examination. The tumors were classified as "carcinoma" on the basis of the presence of vascular or capsular invasion and in "adenoma", in the absence of these features. Information of tumor size was obtained mainly from pathologic specimens and, occasionally, from operative notes, imaging reports or clinical examination notes. The extent of the tumor at presentation was stated according to TNM staging classification system for thyroid cancer (International Union Against Cancer - UICC, 6th Ed, 2002). Surgery was followed by radioactive iodine administration in all invasive carcinomas. External radiotherapy was given in only one patient with Hurthle cell carcinoma. Metastatic tumor was treated with repeated radioactive iodine therapy.

After primary treatment, levothyroxine TSH-suppressive therapy was started in all patients.

RESULTS

Nineteen patients with Hurthle cell carcinoma and 9 patients with Hurthle cell adenoma were included in this study. None of them had a familial history of thyroid cancer or a personal history of external beam radiation therapy. Average age of patients affected by adenoma was 49.7 years (30-72 yrs) versus 49.3 years (15-72 yrs) of Hurthle cell carcinoma patients. Twenty-two patients were females and 6 males. Pre-operatively, thyroid hormonal profile (TSH, free-T_3 and free-T_4) were in the normal range in all patients. Thyreoglobulin serum levels were elevated in 5 out of 19 patients with Hurthle cell carcinoma (range 110-34.000 ng/ml). Two out of 28 patients had detectable serum Tg and TPO autoantibodies. At ultrasonography a multinodular goitre was found in 21 patients, a single nodule was found in

7 patients. All nodules resulted "cold" at scintiscan examination. Sixteen patients had a cytological finding positive or suspicious for malignancy. Twelve patients were submitted to surgery for obstructive symptoms. All patients but one underwent total thyroidectomy; who was treated with lobo-isthmectomy. Only one patient was submitted to neck lymph nodes dissection for neck node metastases at presentation. The neoplasms ranged in size from 5 mm to 58 mm, (greatest diameter). Medium diameter was 28.8 mm in Hurthle cell adenoma patients and 25.8 mm in Hurthle cell carcinoma patients. At histology 9 adenomas, 5 "minimally invasive" and 14 invasive carcinomas were found. In 2 Hurthle cell carcinoma patients with an ultractustructural growth pattern a foci of papillary microcarcinoma was associated. Two Hurthle cell carcinoma patients also showed histological findings of chronic inflammation with detectable serum thyroid antibodies. One patient had neck nodes metastases. In 2 Hurthle cell carcinoma patients the tumor was multifocal. After surgery, six patients had persistent hypo-parathyroidism and 2 patients had a permanent vocal cord injury. At post-operative TNM staging 9 patients were stage I, 5 stage II, 4 stage III and 1 patient was stage IVa (UICC, 2002). A ^{131}I whole body scan (WBS) was performed in all invasive carcinomas. No Hurthle cell invasive carcinoma showed distant metastases at whole body scan examination. In 1 Hurthle cell carcinoma patient a computed tomography detected distant lung metastases 60 months after total thyroidectomy. Due to the evidence of high levels of serum thyroglobulin, repeated radioiodine treatments (range of radiation dose 91-585 mCi) were performed and the patient is still in follow-up. The median follow-up period was 62 months (range 6–324). In none of our adenoma a relapse was observed.

Discussion

Hurthle cell neoplasms are heterogeneus tumors that may play many clinical behaviours. They arise from follicular cells and are predominantly or exclusively composed of cells exhibiting oncocytic features, also called oncocytes. Oncocytes are microscopically characterized by an abundant granular cytoplasm. Ultrastructural studies showed that this granularity is due to a lot of intracytoplasmatic mitochondrias [11].

Oncocytic cells have been variously called such as Hurthle cells, Askanazy cells and oxyphilic cells. They are usually considered a variant of follicular epithelial cells as sustained by the thyreoglobulin immunoreactivity found at cytological or histological specimens and as confirmed by the presence of a functional activity of thyreotropin receptor-adenylate cyclase [12]. The World Health Organization (WHO) Committee prefers to define them as oxyphilic cells [13]. However, the most widely used definition among endocrinologist is "Hurthle cells", although the cells that Hurthle firstly described in 1894 in a dog's thyroid, were more likely C cells [14].

Since Hurthle cells can be found in both neoplastic and non-neoplastic thyroid lesions, it is difficult to differentiate benign Hurthle cell hyperplasia from true Hurthle cell neoplasm. There is general agreement that the cut-off parameter useful to distinguish between true Hurthle cell tumor and Hurthle cells hyperplasia, is 75% of Hurthle cells of cell population. Usually, as for the follicular type, a Hurthle cell tumor can be classified as malignant (HCC) when capsular or vascular invasion is reported or if there is a perithyroid infiltration or distant metastases are found [15,16]. At histology Hurthle cell carcinoma is distinguished in "minimally invasive Hurthle cell carcinoma", if only capsular invasion is reported or "invasive Hurthle cell carcinoma", when both vascular and capsular infiltration are present.

Consequently, the cytological diagnosis obtained by fine needle aspiration biopsy (FNAB) is not able to differentiate between true follicular and Hurthle cell neoplasms and between the benign and malignant variants of Hurthle cell tumor [17]. As in the case of the follicular thyroid neoplasms, even intraoperative frozen sections have low sensitivities in Hurthle cell cancer detection [17,18].

Only histological analysis can differentiate between adenoma and carcinoma. For that reason some authors claimed to treat all thyroid nodular lesions with a cytological finding of more 50% Hurthle cells [19]. Neverthless, a recent work reported that, despite a high risk of malignancy, clinical features such as nodule size, patient age and sex should be part of the decision making process[17].

Hurthle cell neoplasm was first decribed in 1907 by Langhans who reported 5 cases of patients with thyroid neoplasms composed of oncocytes [2]. Although 2 out of 5 patients died for distant metastases, he did not describe any microscopic evidence of malignancy. Twenty years later, Wegelin et al. stated that most of the Hurthle cell tumors were benign [20], while in 1941, Harry et al. described these tumors as moderate malignancy carcinomas [21] and Warren et al. classified them as benign tumors potentially malignant [22]. In 1951, the American Cancer Society claimed that surgical treatment of Hurthle cell neoplasms should be aggressive because of their malignant potential [23]. More recently, some authors reported that as Hurthle cell thyroid lesions are usually aggressive malignant neoplasms and even adenomas could metastasize [24,25], all Hurthle cell lesions should be submitted to total thyroidectomy. In 1988, McLeod et al. again allowed that treatment of Hurthle cell neoplasms was controversial because of the absence of a clear correlation between the microscopical features and the clinical behavior of the tumor [26]. From literature data less than 1% of thyroid Hurthle cell adenoma act as cancer [27]. Thompson et al. said that Hurthle cell neoplasms should be considered malignant irrespective of size and pathological features and advocated total thyroidectomy for all such lesions [17]. Grant et al. reported that only one of 272 patients affected by benign Hurthle cell adenoma had evidence of malignancy and no patients died of thyroid carcinoma [28].

In the last twenty years many studies have been performed in order to find histopathological and clinical factors reliable in predicting malignancy in patients with Hurthle cell neoplasm [29,30,31]. Since Hurthle cell tumors may exhibit a follicular or papillary growth pattern, they have been often classified only on the basis of their architectural features independently of the presence of Hurthle cells. At present, there is general agreement in considering Hurthle cell neoplasms as a subset of all differentiated thyroid cancer, irrespectively of papillary or follicular growth pattern. The World Health Organization Committee considers this tumor the oxyfilic variant of follicular thyroid cancer, while for the Armed Force Institute of Pathology (AFIP) Hurthle cell carcinomas should be separeted into a subset of thyroid neoplasms different from true follicular cancers [32,33].

Recently, in a large series of patients affected by Hurthle cell carcinoma with papillary growth pattern, the authors found worse characteristics than in classic papillary thyroid carcinoma, similar to tall cell variant, in terms of vascular invasion, distant metastases and prognosis [34].

If Hurthle cell carcinoma prognosis is worse than follicular histotype is still a matter of debate. Some authors consider this neoplasm aggressive and unpredictable, with a mortality rate as high as 25% in 30 years while others find it no more aggressive than similary staged follicular carcinoma without Hurthle cells [35,36,37].

The pathogenesis of these lesions seems joined to alterations of mithocondrial DNA (mtDNA)[38]. Systematic analysis of the primary structure of mtDNA in 79 benign and malignant tumors (43 Hurthle and 36 non-Hurthle cell neoplasms) and respective normal parenchyma displayed a relatively high percentage (up to 16%) of mtDNA common delection (CD) in Hurthle cell tumors, independently of the lesion's histotype. The percentage of deleted mtDNA molecules was significantly higher in tumors with D-loop mutations than in mtDNA stable tumors. Sequence variants of the ATPase 6 gene, one of the complex V genes thought to play a role in mtDNA maintenance and integrity in yeast, were significantly more prevalent in patients with Hurthle cell tumors than in patients with non-Hurthle cell neoplasms. The authors concluded that germline polymorphisms of the ATPase 6 gene are associated with the occurrence of mtDNA CD, the hallmark of Hurthle cell tumors [39].

In 2001, Erickson et al. [40] analysed Hurthle cell neoplasms by interphase fluorescence in situ hybridization to evaluate the diagnostic and prognostic utility of numerical anomalies by DNA fluorescent probes for cyclin D1 and p53 gene loci and chromosomes 5, 7, 11, 12, 17, and 22. They showed that chromosomal imbalances as gains are common in both benign and malignant Hurthle cell neoplasms, but Hurthle cell carcinomas tend to have more chromosome losses than adenomas and that the loss of chromosome 22 may have prognostic value in Hurthle cell carcinoma of the thyroid.

Musholt PB et al. in 2003 suggested that "the expression of rearranged RET hybrid oncogenes is present in a similar percentage of Hurthle cell carcinomas when compared with the literature on nonoxyphilic papillary thyroid carcinomas, defines papillary thyroid carcinoma-like Hurthle cell carcinomas better than histomorphologic characterization, excludes Hurthle cell carcinomas as a subgroup of follicular thyroid carcinomas, and may play a role in the early tumorigenesis of oncocytic tumors [41].

Recent reports suggested the use of some proliferative cellular markers such as PCNA and Ki-67 in cytological differential diagnosis of Hurthle cell tumors. Augustynowicz et al. reported a significant difference in all proliferative activity markers between malignant and benign tumors (HCC:HCA $p<0.01$; HCC:HCM $p<0.001$) [42].

As rare as Hurthle cell carcinoma is, prognostic scoring systems have been criticised for not taking into account the possible differences among Hurthle cell carcinoma and follicular cancer with their variable behaviour.

Many studies have shown that there are several differences between Hurthle cell carcinoma and follicular thyroid carcinoma [43]. Hurthle cell carcinoma is an aggressive disease; patients frequently present with Hurthle cell carcinoma with intrathyroid multifocality (33%), extrathyroid invasion (39%), lymph node (25%) or distant metastasis (18%). It has been reported that some of these features are increased in Hurthle cell carcinoma patients compared to follicular thyroid carcinoma patients. Hurthle cell carcinoma patients are significantly older, have larger nodules, a higher mortality associated with recurrence, and a higher treatment failure rate compared with follicular thyroid carcinoma patients. Cervical lymph node metastases are common in Hurthle cell carcinoma patients, but uncommon in follicular thyroid carcinoma patients. Hurthle cell carcinoma usually does not take up radioactive iodine, whereas most follicular thyroid carcinomas do. In some reports on Hurthle cell carcinoma and follicular thyroid carcinoma it has been stated that an older patient's age, large tumor size, extra-thryoid invasion are of negative prognostic significance [44,45,46]. The purpose of our study was to identify the clinical and pathologic features of Hurthle cell carcinoma that can predict disease progression or death.

We compared 19 Hurthle cell carcinoma patients with 9 Hurthle cell adenoma patients. None had previous exposure to external beam radiation.

Age is the most important risk factor in all risk factor systems for well-differentiated thyroid carcinoma. In our study, the age of the Hurthle cell carcinoma group was younger than the reported series [47]. No gender differences were seen in either group, nor were there seen significant differences in the age or size of primary tumors. Multifocality rate, which was observed in 2 Hurthle cell carcinoma patients and extrathyroid invasion rate, which was found in 3 Hurthle cell carcinoma patients, were lower than that reported in other series. Vascular invasion was not associated with a worse survival rate.

In reported cases, the incidence of males is 20-30%, but there has been a female predominance among Hurthle cell carcinoma patients in most reports [1]. In our study, the male-female ratio among Hurthle cell carcinoma patients was about 1:3 versus about 1:2 among those with Hurthle cell adenoma.

Without prospective trials, due to the small number of Hurthle cell carcinomas, conclusions about the effects of different treatments are not available. The large part of our patients was submitted to total thyroidectomy, so we did not evaluate the impact of surgery treatments on survival.

The use of radioactive iodine is still controversial since most metastases of these tumors do not take up radioactive iodine [48]. But if these tumors do take up radioactive iodine as in our invasive patients, this treatment is advisable as even low risk patients who have Hurthle cell carcinoma or follicular thyroid carcinoma and major blood vessels invasion are at some risk of recurrence and death. This does not apply to patients with minimal capsular invasion alonc. In our series, all invasive cancers received radioactive iodine, independently by ^{131}-Iodine whole body scan uptake.

They were treated at least with one course of radioiodine, for which the main indication was adjuvant thyroid remnant ablation. The range dose of radioiodine was 91-585 mCi. In 1 Hurthle cell carcinoma patient, who was treated with radioactive iodine for adjuvant ablation of remnant thyroid tissue (150mCi), 60 months after primary radioiodine treatment a computed tomography (CT) scan showed lung metastasis negative at ^{131}I-whole body scan in spite of high Tg serum levels.

A series of reports from Cleveland Clinic, Lahey Clinic, and Memorial Sloan-Kettering Cancer Center comparing Hurthle cell carcinoma and follicular thyroid carcinoma often showed that Hurthle cell carcinoma is more aggressive in behaviour with poorer patient survival. Carcangiu et al. were also of this opinion, although they did not have a comparison group of follicular thyroid carcinoma [49,50].

However, in other reports, patients with Hurthle cell carcinomas were said to have better survival than those with follicular thyroid cancer.

In the Memorial Sloan-Kettering Cancer Center series, patients with follicular thyroid cancer had a higher rate of regional lymph node metasases than found in patients with Hurthle cell carcinoma, but these reported data (30%) are also considerably higher than what neoplasm has been generally found to have. Data from the Mayo Clinic demonstrated a higher rate of regional lymph node metastasis in Hurthle cell carcinoma than follicular thyroid cancer [35]. In our study, lymph node dissection was undergone only by one Hurthle cell carcinoma patients with extra thyroid invasion, which is lesser than the number reported in other series.

In the series of Memorial Sloan-Kettering Cancer Center and the earlier series from the Mayo Clinic, Hurthle cell carcinoma had a higher rate of distant metastasis than follicular thyroid cancer [35]. Recent publications from the Mayo Clinic stated that the survival of Hurthle cell carcinoma patients and follicular thyroid cancer patients were similar, while earlier series from the same institution revealed poorer Hurthle cell carcinoma patient survival [51,52]. We did not find this to be true, in fact we observed distant metastases only in 4.5% of our Hurthle cell carcinoma cases.

In agreement with the results of other authors, the recurrence was observed within the first 5 years after surgery. In our series of patients neither adenoma nor minimally invasive Hurthle cell carcinomas exhibited malignant behaviour. We compared patients with only minimal capsular invasion versus those with blood vessel invasion or major capsular invasion. Recurrence was present only among invasive Hurthle cell carcinomas.

Although, in our population, the follow-up was relatively short, we did not find age, sex, primary tumor size, extraglandular invasion, or neck node at presentation to have a significant prognostic value in Hurthle cell carcinoma patients overall.

In all patients, blood vessel invasion and/or major capsular invasion did not represent a significant risk of death. All risk factors we examined were not associated with all-cause mortality nor disease specific mortality.

In conclusion, in our study, Hurthle cell carcinoma was not found to have an aggressive behaviour, as otherwise reported by other authors when risk factors, including the extent of tumour invasion were were taken into account. None of our Hurthle cell adenoma patients showed a relapse or death caused by the disease.

REFERENCES

[1] Bhattacharyya N. Survival and Prognosis in Hurthle cell carcinoma of the thyroid gland. *Arch Otolaryngol*, 2003. 129, 207-210.

[2] Langhans T. Uber die epithelialen Formen der malignen Struma. *Virchows Arch (Pathol Anat),* 1907, 189, 69-152.

[3] Har-El G, Hadar T, Segal K et al Hurthle cell carcinoma of the thyroid gland. A tumor of moderate malignancy. *Cancer* 1986, 57, 1613-1609.

[4] Hundahl Sa, Fleming ID, Fremgen AM, Menck HR. A National Cancer Database report on 53856 cases of thyroid carcinoma treated in the U.S., 1985-1995. *Cancer* 1998, 83, 2638-2648.

[5] Chen H, Nicol TL, Geiger MA et al Hurthle cell neoplasm of the thyroid: are there factors predictive of malignancy? *Ann Surg* 1998; 227, 542-546.

[6] Sugino K, Itto K, Mimura T, Kameyama K, Iwasaki H, Ito K. Hurthle cell tumor of the thyroid: analysis of 188 cases. *World J Surg* 2001; 25, 1160-1163.

[7] Sanders LE, Silverman M. Follicular and Hurthle cell carcinoma: predicting outcome and directing therapy. *Surgery* 1998; 124: 967-974.

[8] Shaha AR, Loree TR, Shah JP. Prognostic factors and risk group analysis in follicular carcinoma of the thyroid. *Surgery* 1995; 118, 1131-1136.

[9] McDonald MP, Sanders LE, Silverman ML, Chan HS, Buyske J, Hurthle cell carcinoma of the thyroid gland: prognostic factors and results of surgical treatment. *Surgery* 1996; 120, 1000-1005.

[10] McHenry CR, Sandoval BA. Management of follicular and Hurthle cell neoplasms of the thyroid gland. *Surg Oncol Clin N Am* 1998; 7, 893-910.

[11] Maximo V, Sobrinho-Simoes M: Hurthle cell tunors of the thyroid. A review with emphasis on mitochondrial abnormalities with clinical relevance. *Vierchow Arch*, 2000, 437: 107-115.

[12] Clark OH, Gerend PL. Thyreotropin receptor-adenylate cyclase system in Hurthle cell neoplasms. *J Clin Endocrinol Metab* 1985, 61, 773-778.

[13] Hedinger CE, Williams ED, Sobin LH. Histological typing of thyroid tumors, in Hedinger CE (Ed), *International histological classification of tumors*, 11, Berlin, Springler-Verlag, 1988.

[14] Hurthle K. Beitrage zur Kenntnis des Sekretionsvorgangs in der Schilddruse. *Arch Gesamte Physiol,* 1984, 56, 1-44,.

[15] LiVolsi VA. *Surgical pathology of the thyroid*. Ed. Philadelphia, Saunders 1990.

[16] Hedinger C, Williams ED, Sobin LH. The World Health Organization histhological classification of thyroid tumors: a commentary on the second edition. *Cancer* 1989, 63, 908-911.

[17] Giorgadzc T, Rossi ED, Fadda G, Gupta PK, LiVolsi VA, Baloch Z. Does the fine-needle aspiration diagnosis of "Hurthle-cell neoplasm/follicular neoplasm with oncocytic features" denote increased risk of malignancy? *Diagn Cytopathol* 2004, 31 (5), 307-312.

Dahl LD, Myssiorek D, Heller KS. Huthle cell neoplasms of the thyroid. *Laryngoscope* 2002, 112 (12), 2178-2180.

[18] Kauffmann PR, Dejax C, de Latour M, Dauplat J. The meaning and predicitivity of Hurthle cells in fine needle aspiration cytology for thyroid nodular disease. *Eur J Surg Oncol* 2004, 30(7), 786-789.

[19] Wegelin C. Die Schilddruse. In Henke F, Lubarsch O (Eds), *Handbuch der spieziellen Pathologischen Anatomie und Histologie.* Bd VIII. Berlin: Springer-Verlag, 1926.

[20] Harry NM. Hurthle cell tumors of the thyroid gland. *Roy Melbourne Hosp Clin Rep* 1941, 12, 18-22.

[21] Warren S. The classification of tumors of the thyroid. *Am J Roentgenol* 1941, 46, 447-450.

[22] Manual of Tumor Nomenclautre and Coding: Prepared by the Subcommittee of the Statistics Committee, American Cancer Society, New York 1951.

[23] Ruchiti C, Komor J, Konig MP. Grosszellige Tumoren (so genannte Hurthlezellen-tumoren) der Schilddrusse. *Helv Chir Acta* 1976, 43, 129-132.

[24] Thompson NW, Dunn EL, Batasakis JG, Nishiyanna RH. Hurthle cell lesions of the thyroid gland. *Surg Gynecol Obstet*. 1974, 139, 155-160

[25] McLeod MK, Thompson NW, Hudson JL, Gaglio JA, Lloyd RV, Harness JK, Nishiyama R, Cheung PS. Flow cytometric measurements of nulcear DNA and ploidy analysis in Hurthle cell neoplasms of the thyroid. *Arch Surg* 1988, 123, 849-854.

[26] Yutan E, Clarck OH. Hurthle cell carcinoma.*Curr Treat Opt Oncol* 2001, 2, 331-335.

[27] Grant CS, Barr D, Goellner JR et al. Benign Hurthle cell tumors of the thyroid: a diagnosis to be trusted? *World J Surgery* 1988,12, 488-495.

[28] Bronner MP, LiVolsi VA. Oxyphilic (Askanazy/Hurthle cell) tumors of the thyroid: microscopic features predict biologic behaviour. *Surg Pathol* 1988, 1, 137-150.

[29] Carangiu ML, Bianchi S, Savino D, Voynick IM, Rosai J. Follicular Hurthle cell Tumors of the thyroid gland. *Cancer*. 1998, 68, 1944-1953.

[30] Stojadinovic A, Ghossein RA, Hoos A, Urist MJ, Spiro RH, Shah JP, Brennan MP, Shaha AR, Singh B. Hurthle cell carcinoma: a critical histopathologic appraisal. *J Clin Oncol*. 2001, 19, 2616-2625.

[31] Rosai J, Carcangiu ML DeLellis RA. *Tumors of the thyroid gland. Atlas of tumor pathology*. Washinghton DC, AFIP, Third series fascicles 5, 1992.

[32] Frassila KO, Ackerman LV, Brown CL et al. Follicular carcinoma. *Semin Diagn Pathol* 1985, 2, 101-105.

[33] Mai KT, Thomas J, Yazdi J, Commons AS, Lamba M, Stinson AW. Pathologic study and clinical significance of Hurthle cell papillary thyroid carcinoma. *Appl Immunoistochem Mol Morphol.* 2004, Dec; 12 (4): 329-37.

[34] Watson RG, Brennan MD, Goellner JR, van Heerden JA, McConahey WM, Taylor WF. Invasive Hurthle cell carcinoma of the thyroid : natural hystory and managment. *Mayo Clinic Proceedings* 1984, 59, 851-855.

[35] Shaha Ar, Shah JP. Loree TR. Patterns of nodal and distant metastases based on histologic varieties in differentiated carcinoma of the thyroid. *Am J Surg* 1996, 172, 692-694.

[36] Brennan MD, Bergstralhb EJ, van Heerden JA, McConahey WM. Follicular thyorid cancer treated at Mayo clinic 1946 trough 1970: initial manifestations, pathological findings, therapy and outcome. *Mayo Clinci Proceedings*, 1991, 66, 1-22.

[37] Rogounovitch T, Saenko V and Yamashita S. Mitochondrial DNA and Human Thyroid Disease. *Endocrine J* 2004, 51, 265-277.

[38] Maximo V, Soares P, Lima J, Cameselle-Teijeiro J, Sobrinho-Simoes M. *Am J Pathol.* 2002 May;160(5), 1857-1865.

[39] Erickson LA, Jalal SM, Goellner JR, Law ME, Harwood A, Jin L, Roche PC, Lloyd RV. *Am J Surg Pathol.* 2001 Jul;25(7):911-917.

[40] Musholt PB, Imkamp F, von Wasielewki R, Scmidt KW, Musholt TJ. RET rearrangements in archival oxyphilic thyroid tumors: new insights in tumorigenensis and classification of Hurthle cell carcinomas? *Surgery* 2003, 134(6), 881-889.

[41] Augustynowicz A, Dzieciol J, Barwijuk-Machala M, Dadan J, Puchalski Z, Sulkowski S. Assessment of proliferative activity of thyroid Hurthle cell tumors using PCNA, Ki-67 and AgNOR methods. *Folia Histochem Cytobiol*, 2004, 42 (3), 165-168.

[42] Khafif A, Khafif RA, Attie JN. Hurthle cell carcinoma: a malignancy of low grade potential. *Head and Neck* 1999 21, 506-511.

[43] Shaha AR, Ferlito A, Rinaldo A. Distant metastases from thyroid and parathyroid cancer. *ORL J Otorhinolaryngol Relat Spec*, 2001, 63, 243-249.

[44] Tallini Gcarcangiu ML, Rosai J. Oncocytic neoplasms of the thyroid gland. *Acta Pathol Jpn*, 1992,42,305-315.

[45] DeGroot LJ, Kaplan EL, Shukla MS et al Morbidity and mortality in follicular thyroid cancer. *J Clin Endocrinol Metab*, 1995, 80, 2946-2953.

[46] Lopez-Penabad L, Chiu AC, Hoff AO, Schultz P, Gaztambide S, Ordonez NG, Sherman SI. Prognostic factors in patients with Hurthle cell neoplasms of the thyroid. *Cancer* 2003, 597 (5), 1186-1194

[47] Soh EY, Clark OH Surgical consideration and approach to thyroid cancer. *Endocrinol Metab Clin North Am* 1996, 25, 115-139.

[48] Nishiyama RH. Overview of surgical pathology of the thyroid gland. *World Journal of Surgery* 2000, 24,: 898-906.

[49] Crile G, Pontius Kl, Howk WA. Factors influencing the survival of patients with follicular carcinoma of the thyroid gland. *Surgery, Gynecology & Obstetrics* 1985 160, 409-413.

[50] Grebe SKG, Hay ID. Follicular thyroid cancer. *Endocrinological Metababolism Clinics of North America* 1995 24, 761-801.

[51] Grant CS. Operative and postoperative management of the patient with follicular and Hurthle cell carcinoma. Do they differ? *Surgical Clinics of North America*, 1995, 75, 395-403.

In: Trends in Thyroid Cancer Research
Editor: Carl A. Milton, pp. 253-341

ISBN 1-59454-627-4

Chapter XIII

SEARCHING SUSCEPTIBILITY GENES FOR GRAVES' DISEASE: AN UPDATE

Dimitry A. Chistiakov*

Department of Pathology and Laboratory Medicine, University of Cincinnati Medical Center, Cincinnati OH 45267-0529.

ABSTRACT

Graves' disease (GD) is a complex organ-specific autoimmune pathology that affects thyroid gland. A specific clinical outcome of GD is the presence of autoantibodies, which activate thyroid-stimulating hormone receptor and cause thyroid hyperfunction, or hypertyroidism. Clinical and subclinical hyperthyroidism is widely distributed in humans affecting up to 2% of Caucasians and occurs mostly in women. GD has a strong genetic background, which accounts up to 80% of the predisposition to disease. During last five years, with the availability of the complete human genome sequence, a significant progress was made in the identification and functional characterization of genes conferring susceptibility to GD. In this review, we summarized recent findings in searching the susceptibility loci. To date, strong and consistent evidence for the involvement in GD pathogenesis was shown for HLA class II (chromosome 6p21), CTLA-4 (2q33), thyroglobulin (8q24) and CD40 (20q11) genes. The list of GD susceptibility genes can be extended by including of the VDR (12q12) and PTPN22 (1p13) genes, a role of which in thyroid autoimmunity is rather general, since they are shown to be involve in several autoimmune diseases. These loci are likely to interact, and their interactions could determine disease severity and clinical outcome. The review is also focused on recent advances in the identification of common susceptibility genes responsible for shared genetic background between several autoimmune disorders. In the near future, additional GD-specific and general susceptibility loci will be found that will

* Correspondence concerning this article should be addressed to Dimitry A. Chistiakov Department of Pathology and Laboratory Medicine, University of Cincinnati Medical Center, PO Box 670529 231 Albert Sabin Way, Cincinnati OH 45267-0529. Phone: (513) 558 4402; Fax: (513) 558 2141; E-mail: dmitry.chistyakov@uc.edu.

help to clarify tight pathogenic mechanisms of the induction and progression of this disease as well as to dissect common pathways in the etiology of autoimmune diseases.

Keywords: Graves' disease, susceptibility, genetic markers, thyroid autoimmunity

INTRODUCTION

Graves' disease (GD) is one of clinical outcomes of autoimmune thyroid disease (AITD). Other clinical manifestations of thyroid autoimmunity include Hashimoto's thyroiditis (HT), thyroid-associated orbitopathy (TAO), postpartum thyroiditis and atrophic autoimmune thyroiditis. These forms of thyroid autoimmunity can occur independently or simultaneously. The most frequent combination is between GD and TAO. This is a reason why TAO is often called Graves' ophtalmopathy and considered as an extrathyroidal complication of GD [1].

Hyperthyroidism is a major clinical feature of GD. In overt GD, the hyperfunction of the thyroid gland is associated with the increased volume and goiter of the thyroid, lower levels of serum thyroid-stimulating hormone (TSH < 0.3 mU/l) and higher levels of thyroid hormones (serum thyroxine, T_4 > 170 nmol/l; serum tri-iodothyronine, T_3 > 50 nmol/l). This results from the activating influence of self-antibodies against TSH receptor (TSHR). The antibodies called TSAbs are detectable in 80-100% of GD patients and able to stimulate the thyrotropin receptor that leads to Graves' hyperthyroidism. Another clinical characteristics of overt GD are higher serum levels of other thyroid antibodies (Tabs) directed against thyroglobulin (Tg, > 1.0 IU/l) and thyroid peroxidase (TPO, > 100 IU/l) [2]. TPO-Abs are presented in 45-80% of GD subjects, while Tg-Abs are less common and can be found in up to 30% of individuals affected with GD [3]. Patients with subclinical hyperthyroidism demonstrate low levels of TSH, but normal range of serum concentrations of thyroid hormone [4]. For subclinical hyperthyroidism, diagnostic criteria for determining the cut-off TSH level can vary. A recent panel of experts classified patients with subclinical hyperthyroidism into two categories: those with mildly low but still detectable serum TSH (0.1-0.4 mU/l) and those with an undetectable serum TSH (< 0.1 mU/l) [5]. Depending of these criteria, the prevalence of subclinical hyperthyroidism can vary. For the TSH cut-off point of 0.1 mU/l, the prevalence was 0.7% [2], whereas the cut-off value was 0.3 mU/l, the disease prevalence was estimated to be 2.1% [6].

GENETIC EPIDEMIOLOGY OF GRAVES' DISEASE

Population Studies

Hyperthyroidism, or thyrotoxicosis, is a common form of thyroid disfunction, which is widely distributed in a world population. For example, in USA, according to the National Health and Nutrition Examination Survey (NHAHES III), reported in 2002, the prevalence of thyrotoxicosis in a general population was 1.3%, including 0.7% subclinical and 0.5% clinical disease [2]. The occurence of thyrotoxicosis is significantly higher (2.6-19.5-fold) in women than in men (Li et al. 2000; Vanderpump et al. 1995; Table 1) [7,8]. GD is the commonest form of thyrotoxicosis in iodine-sufficient countries, accounting for 60-90% of cases in both Caucasians and Asians [8-10] (Table 1). Dietary iodine is a major environmental factor influencing the incidence of thyrotoxicosis (and GD). For instance, epidemiological survey of populations living in three regions of China with low (region of Panshan), mild (Zhangwu) and higher iodine intake (Huanghua) showed significant prevalence of subclinical hyperthyrodism in Panshan (3.7%) and Zhangwu (3.9%) compared to Huanhua (1.1%), while there were no significant differences in clinical hyperthyroidism and GD [11]. However, in high iodine intake areas, the increased incidence of hyperthyroidism and GD is often occurred, suggesting on a predisposing role of excess dietary iodine for thyroid hyperfunction [12,13]. From data presented in Table 1, the annual incidence of GD in different Caucasian and Asian populations, living in mostly iodine-sufficient regions, is relatively similar and usually ranges between 15-25 per 100,000.

Table 1. Epidemiological data of the incidence and prevalence of clinical thyrotoxicosis and GD in different countries and regions

Country/region	Clinical outcome	Survey, years	Incidence per 100,000/year (F/M)	Prevalence (F/M, %)	Reference
US/Rochester, MN	GD	1935-1967	(36.8/8.3)	N/A[1]	[504]
USA/Oakland, CA	Thyrotoxicosis	1977	N/A	0.31[2]	[505
USA/Colorado	Thyrotoxicosis	1995	N/A	0.1[2]	[6]
USA (metaanalysis)	Thyrotoxicosis	1965-1995	13.9	1.2	[506]
USA/NHANES III	Thyrotoxicosis	1988-1994	N/A	0.5[1]	[2]
UK/Whickham 1	Thyrotoxicosis	1972-1974	N/A	2.7/0.16	[507]
UK/Whickham 2	Thyrotoxicosis	1972-1992	(80/0)	3.9/0.2	[8]
New Zealand/ North Canterbury	Thyrotoxicosis	1983-1985	25.8 (40.7/10.5)	N/A	[9]
Sweden/Malmo	GD	1970-1974	17.7 (27.2/7.4)	N/A	[508]
Sweden/Malmo	GD	1988-1990	22.2 (34.4/8.8)	N/A	[14]
Iceland	Thyrotoxicosis	1980-1982	23.6 (38.4/8.9)	N/A	[509]
Spain/Vigo	GD	1990-1992	24.24	N/A	[510]
Austria	GD	1987-1989	10.4	N/A	[17]
Japan	Thyrotoxicosis	1999	12.2	0.07-0.11 (GD)[3]	[10]
Korea	Thyrotoxicosis	2002	N/A	0.5	[511]
China/Daqing	GD	1984-1999	20.0 (27.8/10.8)	0.41/0.16	[7]
China/ Hong Kong[4]	GD	1989-1998	5.0 (9.5/0.9)	N/A	[15]

[1] N/A, data nonavailable

[2] Clinical hypo/hyperthyroidism

[3] Estimated prevalence for GD, assuming that the disease occurs in 60-90% cases of thyrotoxicosis in different regions of Japan

[4] The survey includes children at age before 15 years

Since GD represents a complex disorder, resulted from harmful interactions between genetic and environmental factors, the incidence of this disease should vary with time. For example, a number of follow-up observations reported a significant growth in the incidence of GD with time [8,14,15]. In Malmo (Sweden), the incidence of GD increased from 17.7/100,000/yr in 1970-1974 to 22.2/100,000/year in 1988-1990 [14]. In Hong Kong, overall annual incidence of GD was 3.2/100,000 in 1989-93 and 6.5/100,000 [15]. The incidence rates for girls from Hong Kong have particularly increased from 3.8/100,000/year in 1989 to 14.1/100,000/year in 1998 [15]. The average incidence of hyperthyroidism in an iodine-deficient region of China, Panshan, was reported to jump up from 27.6/100,000/year in 1991-1995 to 80.6/100,000/year in 1996-1999 after implementation of the universal salt iodization (USI) program in 1995 [11]. Similar observations on the growth of the incidence of hyperthyroidism in local inhabitants were obtained from previously iodine-deficient areas after the increment of iodine intake in frames of USI in other countries [16,17]. This can reflect a role of environmental influence (e.g., dietary iodine) on the etiology of Graves' hyperthyroidism.

Family and Twin Studies

GD segregation in members of affected families could indicate the presence of genetic component in the development of Graves' disease. A high frequency of thyroid abnormalities was observed in relatives of patients with GD, most commonly the presence of thyroid antibodies [18-20]. The calculation of sibling risk ratio (λs) helps to determine, whether familial clustering of disease is resulted from genetic or non-genetic factors. The λs represents a ratio of the prevalence of the disease in siblings of affected subjects to the frequency of the disease in the general population and therefore reflects the increased risk of developing the disease in an individual, who has a sibling with the disease [21]. A λs higher than 5 usually suggests a significant genetic contribution in the etiology of the disease [21]. In the Japanese Nationwide Epidemiologic Survey (2001), the prevalence of familial GD was estimated as 2.1%-3.1% of hyperthyroidism, providing an approximate sibling risk to be 19-42 [10]. In Caucasians, λs values of familial GD of the proband's first-degree relatives were reported to be 16-26, suggesting for a strong genetic influence in the pathogenesis of GD [22-24].

Twin studies estimate cooccurence (concordance) of the disease among monozygotic (MZ) twins with the concordance among dizygotic (DZ) twins, assuming that MZ twins are almost genetically identical, whereas DZ twins share 50% of their genes like siblings. If the concordance is higher in the MZ twins than in DZ twins, it suggests that the disease has an inherited component. Twin study in Denmark showed that MZ twins with GD were concordant in 22% of cases, while no concordant DZ twins were observed [25]. A study in the second Danish twin cohort replicated previous results showing 22% of the concordance in MZ twins against 1.7% in DZ twins [26]. Twin study in California confirmed a significant prevalence of the concordance in MZ (17%) compared to DZ twins (1.9%), supporting an evidence for strong genetic contribution in GD [27]. According to the estimates by Brix et al. [26], 79% of the susceptibility to develop GD can be attributable to genes, while environmental factors contrubute the remaining 79%. Potential environmental factors and ways, by which these factors influence pathogenic mechanisms of thyroid autoimmunity, are considered in several recent reviews [28-31].

APPROACHES TO MAP, IDENTIFY AND CHARACTERIZE A SUSCEPTIBILITY GENE

Genetic Linkage and Association Analyses

GD is a typical complex disease and hence genetic strategies and techniques, using for the identification of a predisposing locus, can be applied for the search of GD susceptibility genes. The dominant methodologies used to locate GD susceptibility genes are association and linkage studies. The linkage analysis by genome scanning with polymorphic genetic markers is the preferred strategy. Genome-wide scanning may be coupled with parametric linkage analysis based on recombinant/nonrecombinant information in family pedigrees. Alternatively, genome scans may use nonparametric analysis based on identity-by-descent (alleles are shared by descent from a common ancestor) or identity-by-state (alleles are the same but are not known to be derived from a common ancestor) allele sharing. Both methods of analysis look at association between disease phenotype and polymorphic genetic markers within families, with the goal of locating chromosomal regions, which harbor susceptibility genes for GD. Linkage mapping by this method requires no theory of disease etiology, nor does it require that known genes be tested. Detection will depend on the number of loci involved in disease susceptibility and their interaction, frequency of risk-causing alleles, the density of the marker map, the size of the sample analyzed, and the degree of polymorphism of the chosen markers [32]. If genome scanning provides sufficient evidence for linkage between disease phenotype and a particular locus, high-resolution genetic mapping can serve to localize a gene to <1 centiMorgan (cM), so that molecular techniques may be applied to identify it [33]; however, this may require much larger sample sizes than presently achieved (e.g., thousands of sib pairs).

Association studies look for disease risk with exposure to a specific genotype in individuals from different families. Test genotypes may be polymorphic genetic markers, candidate genes or a combination of these. Of current interest are linkage disequilibrium studies, which look for nonrandom association of alleles at different loci. Specific alleles in an individual haplotype (alleles derived from the same gamete) can be assumed to occur independently, and deviation from this independence is termed linkage disequilibrium. This method of analysis requires no assumptions about mode of inheritance and has sufficient power to detect linkage of loci with moderate phenotypic effect, as defined by the genotypic risk ratio (λs). Statistics formulated to analyze linkage disequilibrium (LD) studies, such as haplotype relative risk [34], haplotype-based haplotype relative risk [35] and the transmission disequilibrium test (TDT) [36] examine disease risk as a function of genotype or allele frequency differences between affected individuals and appropriate control groups.

Because genome scans by linkage disequilibrium analysis require genotyping of large numbers of marker or candidate gene loci, DNA pooling has been suggested as a means to reduce the size of this task [37]. In linkage disequilibrium studies, allele frequency estimates may be made from pooled multiple individual DNAs, provided that appropriate measures are taken to avoid artifactual differences between pools [37]. Such pooling is not possible in standard linkage analysis, which requires that identity by descent be established through construction of individual genotypes, using family data. Particularly suitable for linkage disequilibrium studies are candidate genes, because test marker loci may be chosen that are either within the candidate gene or very close to the chromosomal location of the candidate gene under study.

Results are reported with an ever-increasing number of statistical terms, stemming from parametric and nonparametric methods of analysis, considerations of sample heterogeneity and from the different computer packages designed to extract information from study samples. Parametric linkage analysis requires assumptions of certain values for unknown genetic parameters, such as mode of inheritance, allele frequencies and penetrance. The LOD score (log of the odds ratio) method of parametric linkage analysis is the most widely used [38] and under correct genetic parameters is considered the gold standard in linkage analysis [39]. This method looks at the relative likelihood that a particular set of family genotype data would be obtained if two loci are linked, rather than if they are segregating independently (null hypothesis). For two-point (disease vs. marker) LOD score calculations, constant values are first assigned to certain parameters, then LOD scores are calculated for different possible recombination fractions (θ), probabilistic representations of distance between the hypothetical disease locus and a genetic marker locus. Multiplex nuclear or extended pedigrees (including additional informative relatives other than sibs) offer information on pattern of inheritance within a family and may provide additional insight into the number of contributing loci [32]. Because observations in different pedigrees are statistically independent, LOD scores may be summed for each value of θ yielding a maximum LOD score for each genetic marker tested, at a specific recombination fraction. Testing for genetic heterogeneity is often reported with a heterogeneity LOD score (HLOD) [40], accompanied by an estimated percentage of families, segregating the locus in question.

Pairs of affected relatives of different degrees of relationship may also be used as the basis for nonparametric, allele-sharing-based analyses. Nonparametric linkage analysis requires no assumptions about mode of inheritance. Affected sib-pair studies in particular require no prior assumptions about penetrance, allele frequency or phenocopy rate, and sib pairs tend to be more closely matched for nongenetic covariates, such as environment, age and cohort effects [41]. The relative merits (power afforded by different relative pairs, ease of ascertainment, etc.) of sib-pair or other affected relative pair nonparametric analyses are widely discussed in the literature [21,32,41-43]. LOD scores generated in nonparametric analyses represent the log-likelihood ratio of the data under the hypothesis that the allele-sharing proportion has the observed value, as compared to the hypothesis of no excess (e.g, random) sharing [44].

Plots of the maximum multipoint LOD score (MLS) versus the chromosomal distance in cM are common in linkage data reports. The Z score (nonparametric LOD; NPL_{pairs} or Z_{pairs}), in sib-pair studies, is the number of standard deviations by which the average proportion of alleles shared identical-by-descent exceeds its null expectation of 0.50 (no linkage), and the P value reflects the pointwise (nominal) chance of observing a deviation as high as that observed under independent assortment [44]. The Z score and P value can be reported for each marker location tested in a map of markers. To increase statistical power over the sib-pair statistics, allele sharing among several affected relatives may be considered, resulting in a statistic called NPL_{all} or Z_{all}. Although arguments have been made that nonparametric analysis lacks power when compared with traditional parametric linkage analysis, performance of NPL, when evaluated by Lander & Kruglyak [44], was roughly comparable to parametric LOD score analysis under the correct model (approximately correct models are determined empirically). NPL requires neither consideration of multiple inheritance models, which necessitate corrections for multiple testing, nor prior knowledge of the correct model of inheritance [45].

To keep the chance of encountering false positives at no more than 5%, Lander & Kruglyak [44] have proposed "significant linkage" thresholds for sib-pair studies defined to be a $Z \geq 4.1$, $LOD \geq 3.6$, and $P = 2 \times 10^{-5}$ with the term "suggestive linkage" applied to LOD = 2.2 and $P = 7.4 \times 10^{-4}$, and include thresholds for other study designs. They recommend that the term "replication study" be reserved for situations, in which significant linkage has been obtained in a previous study or combination of studies [44].

Candidate Gene Approach

The approach includes selection and evaluation of candidate genes with known sequence and location, which may be involved in the development of disease due to their physiological functions. Typically, this strategy is used to test positional candidate genes located within the chromosomal region that showed significant evidence for linkage to a given disease. Otherwise, if the candidate gene is not situated at the susceptibility locus but demonstrates a strong functional relationship to the disease, it could be also chosen for subsequent analysis. For example, genes, encoding target autoantigens in AITD (Tg, TPO, TSHR) or regulating immune response (Human Leucocyte Antigens (HLA), immunoglobulines and others), can be included into consideration as functional candidates. If a candidate gene is indeed the cause of a disease, then marker in that locus should show association and linkage with the disease [46].

If microsatellites are markers of choice for genome-wide scans and linkage mapping of susceptibility loci, single nucleotide polymorphisms (SNPs) are ideal for fine-mapping genes in linked regions, using association studies. The significance of SNPs stems from the fact that many of them located within the coding regions and have the potential to change the amino acid sequence of a gene product and hence influence gene function [47].

If the allele tested is associated with the disease, it will appear significantly more frequently in patients than in controls. The probability of having the disease in an individual positive for the allele compared with an individual negative for the allele is estimated by the relative risk (RR) or odds ratio (OR). The existence of an association between an allele and disease can be explained that the allele itself contributes to the increased risk of the disease or this allele is in LD with other genetic variant, which causes the disease [48].

Actually, SNPs are not independent of one another and exist within extended LD blocks. In human genome, the length of a LD block usually varies between 20 and 100 kilobases (kb), and therefore several genes can lie within the same LD block [49]. The International HapMap project is now underway to characterize patterns of LD in the human genome [50]. Within the block, alleles of every SNP will be a part of several extended haplotypes. It is possible to select a subset of SNPs, presenting in the most of haplotypes. This subset is generally called "tag SNPs" and can be effectively used for genotyping in association studies [51,52]. Genotyping only several haplotype tagging (ht SNPs) per block is sufficient to determine the state of all other variants and hence ensures that all of the common variation within a region of LD is surveyed in a disease association study [53]. This cannot be guaranteed, when an association map is based on SNP spacing alone (such as one SNP per 10 kb) or when adjacent SNPs are combined in a two-locus LD analysis without determining the underlying haplotype structure of a region at the outset [54].

Functional Studies

Functional evaluation of the disease-associated allele is necessary to show that this allele is able to affect gene function in a way that increases the risk of developing disease. For example, a dinucleotide repeat polymorphism at the 3' untranslated region (UTR) of the CD154 gene, encoding an important immune regulator, showed association with systemic lupus erythematosus (SLE) and functional effect to the protein expression [55]. SLE patients, carrying two alleles of the microsatellite with >24 CA repeats, had more prolonged CD154 expression in activated lymphocytes compared to control subjects, containing the allele with 24 repeats; this allele is associated with lower risk of SLE [55]. The SNP in the NOD2 gene that is associated with Grohn's disease was found to affect the activation of nuclear factor-kB, thereby influencing the activation of intestinal T cells [56]. Thus, the evidence for functional effect of the disease-associated allele to the disease indirectly suggests that it may be the true predisposing allele for the disease.

Another important application of functional studies is the identification and characterization of susceptible genetic variants that could represent a potential therapeutic target for drugs. This promotes a research in new fields of pharmacogenetics and pharmacogenomics, such as analysis of the response and behavior of this genetic variant depending on the treatment with different drugs, dissecting a molecular mechanism, with which a drug influences and interacts with its target, and selection of drugs with best clinical effects [57]. Disease pathway genes and drug-metabolizing enzymes can be used as primary predictors of drug efficacy or toxicity. For GD, several attempts to find a correlation between polymorphic variants of different immunomodulatory genes and efficiency of antithyroid drug therapy have been reported [58-62]. P-glycoprotein, a product of the multidrug resistance (MDR1) gene, can serve as an example of the protein, involved in drug metabolism. P-glycoprotein is a membrane protein that functions as an ATP-dependent efflux pump, transporting exogenous and endogenous substrates from the inside of cells to the outside [63]. P-glycoprotein has significant impact on therapeutic efficacy and toxicity as it plays a key role in absorption of oral medications from the intestinal tract, excretion into bile and urine, and distribution into protected tissues such as the brain and testes. Numerous

Table 2. Genetic mapping of susceptibility loci for AITD and GD.

Chromosome (locus)	Phenotype	Marker/susceptibility gene	Position, cM[1]	Evidence for linkage[2]	Reference
2q33	GD	D2S117/CTLA-4	194.45	NPL = 3.46 P = 0.0003	64
2p21	AITD	D2S171	45.3	MLS = 3.03	512
3q27	AITD	D3S1580	207.73	LOD = 2.1[3]	138
5q31-q33	GD	D5S436	147.49	MLS = 3.14	137
5q33	GD	D5S2090	150.34	LOD = 4.31 MLS = 4.12 NPL = 2.66 P = 0.001	334
6p21	GD	D6S273/HLA	47.0	NPL = 1.95 P = 0.026	64
6p11 (AITD-1)	AITD	D6S257	79.92	MLS = 2.9	130
6p11 (AITD-1)	AITD	D6S422	35.66	HLOD = 2.0	131
7q11	GD	D7S502	78.65	HLOD = 2.3	131
8q24	AITD	D8S272/Tg	154.02	MLS = 2.0	137
8q24	AITD	D8S284/Tg	143.82	MLS = 3.5	178
8q24	AITD	D8S284/Tg	143.82	HLOD = 3.5	131
9q21	AITD	D9S175	70.33	LOD = 2.05 MLS = 2.01 NPL = 7.5 $P < 10^{-6}$	364
11q12	AITD	D11S4191	60.09	LOD = 2.31 MLS = 2.13 NPL = 6.1 $P < 10^{-6}$	364
14q24.3-q31 (GD-1)	GD	D14S81	108.22	LOD = 2.1	209
14q24.3-q31 (GD-1)	GD	D14S81	108.22	MLS = 2.5	210
18q21 (IDDM6)	GD	D18S487	76.15	NPL = 3.09 P = 0.001	353
18q21 (IDDM6)	AITD	D18S487	76.15	NPL = 3.46 P = 0.0003	353
20q11.2 (GD-2)	GD	D20S195/CD40	50.81	MLS = 3.2 NPL = 2.4 P = 0.00043	284
20q11	GD	D20S106/CD40	50.81	NPL = 2.02 P = 0.023	285
Xq21.33-q22 (GD-3)	GD	DXS8020	65.5	MLS = 2.5	306
Xp11 (IDDMX)	GD	DX8083	46.54	NPL =2.21 P = 0.014	211

Abbreviations: LOD, two-point LOD score; HLOD, heterogeneity LOD; MLS, multipoint LOD score; NPL, non-parametric LOD. [1] Marker position is shown as a distance from the p-terminus of the chromosome according to the Marshfield sex-averaged genetic map. [2] LOD or MLS >2.2, HLOD > 2.5 and NPL > 3.2 correspond to P < 0.0007 ("suggestive linkage"); LOD or MLS > 5.4, HLOD > 6.0 and NPL > 7.1 are equivalent to $P < 3 \times 10^{-7}$ ("highly significant linkage") [45, 513, 514]; [3] The linkage was shown in the subset of DR3-positive families affected with AITD.

genetic polymorphisms in MDR1 have been described, some of which have been shown to determine P-glycoprotein expression levels and substrate transport. Furthermore, some of these polymorphisms have an impact on pharmacokinetic and pharmacodynamic profiles of drug substrates and directly influence outcome and prognosis of certain diseases that explains increasing interest in the possible role of genetic variation in MDR1 in drug therapy [63].

Genetic Determinants of Graves' Disease

An Overview

To date, several genome-wide screens for loci linked to susceptibility to AITD and specifically to GD were performed in different populations. Also, there are a number of studies including linkage analysis of genetic markers around a selected candidate gene. Results of the above analyses summarized in Table 2 revealed a total of 15 loci for AITD and GD located on 12 different chromosomes. Among them, only a few true susceptibility genes (HLA, CTLA-4, thyroglobulin and CD40) have been found within the regions of linkage (Fig. 1). A role of these genes in the etiology of GD and AITD was additionally supported by association and functional analyses and in experiments using animal models. The detailed information on the mapping and identification of GD-specific and general AITD susceptibility loci/genes is described below.

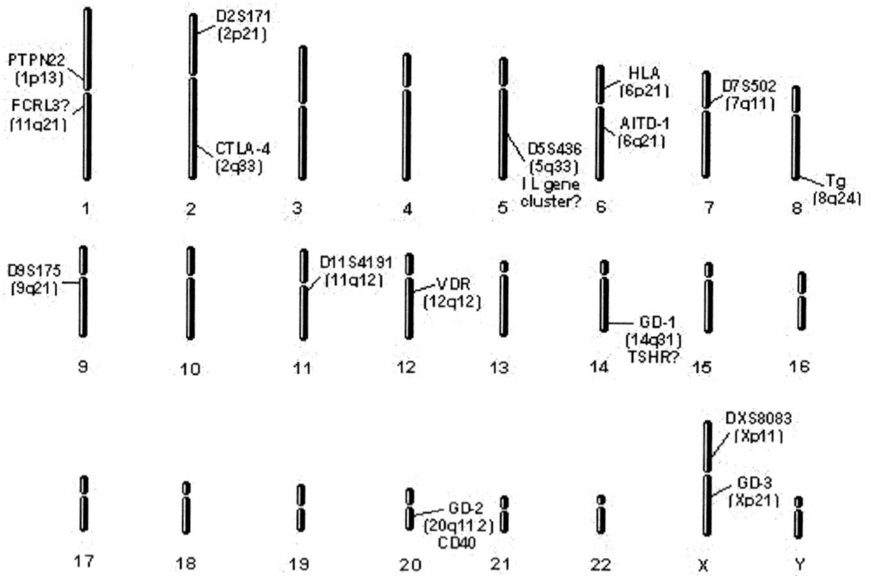

Fig. 1. Susceptibility loci for Graves' disease (GD) and autoimmune thyroid disease (AITD) mapped in the human genome. Putative susceptibility genes are marked with a sign question. The chromosomal location of the loci is shown in brackets. Abbreviations: CTLA-4, cytotoxic T lymphocyte associated antigen-4; FCRL3, Fc receptor-like 3; HLA, Human Leucocyte Antigens; IL, interleukin, PTPN22, lymphoid protein tyrosine phosphatase; Tg, thyroglobulin; TSHR, thyroid-stimulating hormone receptor; VDR, vitamin D receptor.

The 2q33 Locus and the Cytotoxic T-Lymphocyte-Associated Antigen-4 (CTLA-4) Gene

Genetic Linkage and Association Studies

Vaidya et al. [64] found in 77 Caucasian affected sib-pairs with AITD from the UK an evidence for linkage to GD for markers surrounding the cytotoxic T-lymphocyte-associated antigen-4 (CTLA-4) locus, an important immunomodulatory gene on chromosome 2q33, with a peak NPL score of 3.43 at the marker D2S117. Later, a whole-genome search for susceptibility genes linked to thyroid antibody (TAb) production was conducted in 56 multiplex Caucasian AITD families [65]. The search found marker D2S325 on chromosome 2q33, which showed a highest two-point LOD score of 3.6. The 2q33 locus showed no evidence for linkage to GD or HT, demonstrating that the gene in this region conferred susceptibility to TAbs, but that clinical disease development required additional genetic and/or environmental factors. Fine mapping showed a maximum LOD score of 4.2 obtained for marker D2S155, which is situated in the vicinity to the CTLA-4 locus harbouring a cluster of three immune modulatory genes encoding CTLA-4, CD28 antigen and inducible costimulator (ICOS) [65,66]. Association analyses of these positional candidate genes revealed that CTLA-4 only represents a true gene, which confers susceptibility to AITD [65,67,68].

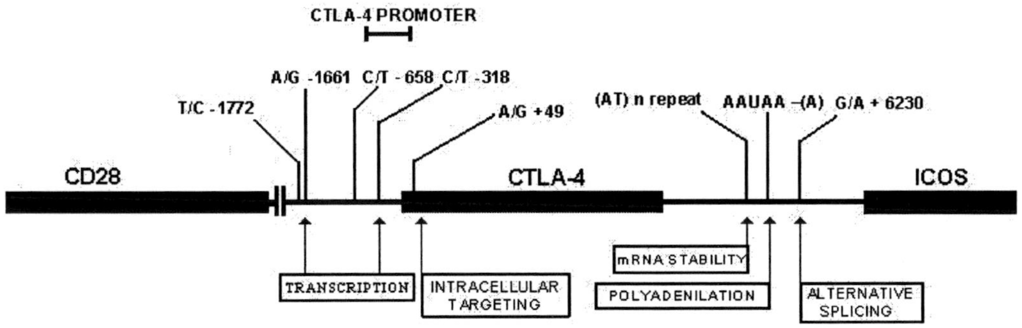

Fig. 2. Three genes encoding costimulatory molecules, CD28, CTLA-4 (cytotoxic T lymphocyte associated antigen-4) and inducible costimulator (ICOS) located on cromosome 2q33, with positions of functional and potentially functional single nucleotide polymorphisms (SNPs) within the CTLA-4 gene. The –319 and +49 SNPs lie within a highly conserved region (approximately 400 bp), which includes a promoter of the CTLA-4 gene (marked). Potential functional roles of the SNPs are shown in boxes.

Case-control studies in different populations consistently suggested in favour of a strong association between the CTLA-4 gene and GD, demonstrating RR range between 1.5 and 3.0 (reviewed in [69-72]). The data have been mostly obtained for three polymorphic sites within the CTLA-4. There are the A/G+49 nucleotide substitution causing threonine-to-alanine change at codon 17, the C/T(-318) polymorphism of the promoter region and the $(AT)_n$ dinucleotide microsatellite at the 3' untranslated region (Fig.2). However, a large population and family-based study (882 GD individuals and 210 GD families) in the UK showed that the etiological variant for GD does not include any of the above polymorphisms but lies within the noncoding 6.1-kb 3'region of CTLA-4 [68]. The susceptibility to both GD and HT was determined by the disease-predisposing haplotype, comprising four single nucleotide polymorphisms (SNPs), CT60, JO31, JO30 and JO27-1, at the 6.1-kb region, with functionally relevant CT60 (A/G+6230) SNP that showed a relationship with the efficiency of splicing and production of a soluble CTLA-4 isoform. Similar findings have also been obtained for murine CTLA-4 [68].

No significant difference was found between frequencies of susceptibility alleles of CTLA-4 A/G(49) and CT60 SNPs in the subsets of patients with familial and sporadic GD [73]. Therefore, this suggests that the CTLA-4 confers a general increased risk for both familial and sporadic GD. In addition, the relationship between this gene and susceptibility to other clinical forms of AITD, such as HT and Tab production [65,67,68], provides the evidence that CTLA-4 could be considered as a common susceptibility gene for thyroid autoimmunity. Multiple genetic studies demonstrated strong association between CTLA-4 and a variety of autoimmune diseases, including type 1 diabetes (T1D) [68,74], celiac disease [75], multiple sclerosis (MS) [76], SLE [77], rheumatoid arthritis (RA) [78,79] and biliary cirrhosis [80]. Case-control studies showed association of genetic variants of CTLA-4 with susceptibility to autoimmune Addison's disease [81-83] and autoimmune polyglandular endocrinopathy type 2, which comprises Addison's disease coexisting with T1D and/or AITD [83,84]. Taken together, these data strongly suggest that CTLA-4 represents a general autoimmune locus, and genetic variations within this gene are associated with general defects in the immune regulation and response [84,85-87]. Finding common susceptibility loci for different autoimmune disorders, such as CTLA-4, may explain the majority of the coexistence of different autoimmune disorders in the same patients or their families as well as a shared genetic background for these diseases [68,88]. Gene-gene interactions are shown to occur between predisposing alleles of common susceptibility loci that result in significant strengthening genetic risk of the development of autoimmune disorder. For example, the interaction between predisposing variants of the CTLA-4 and HLA genes increasing RR up to of 5.1 was described in US Caucasian patients affected with GD [73] or within a large North Swedish pedigree with multiple cases of T1D, GD and HT [84].

Functional Analyses and Mechanism of the Involvement of CTLA-4 Molecular Variants in GD Etiology

Ueda et al. [68] observed less levels of soluble CTLA-4 in patients with the CT60G susceptibility haplotype than in individuals carrying the CT60A haplotype, therefore suggesting that lower levels of soluble CTLA-4 mRNA are associated with the susceptible haplotype (G49/G6230). However, this observation is in controversy with biochemical data showing significantly increased serum levels of soluble CTLA-4 in patients affected with T-cell mediated autoimmune and allergic disorders, such as AITD [89], SLE [90,91], cutaneous systemic sclerosis [92] and allergic asthma [93]. It is unlikely that genetic susceptibility to GD at the CTLA-4 locus can be attributed and explained exclusively by nucleotide variations at the 3' CTLA-4 region. Some effects from causal variations 5' of CTLA-4 could not be excluded, since all polymorphic markers in the CTLA-4 gene were found to lie within the same linkage disequilibrium (LD) block, which is 100-kb long [51,94]. Thus, several CTLA-4 polymorphisms constituting an extended haplotype or several haplotypes are likely to contribute to genetic predisposition to AITD at the CTLA-4 locus, including +49 exon 1

SNP, (-318) promoter SNP and the 3' UTR microsatellite, e.g. polymorphic sites, which are reported to be functionally significant.

The G49 allele of the exon 1 polymorphism encoding alanine-17 in the signal peptide of CTLA-4 molecule showed consistent association with higher risk of the development of GD providing RR of 1.5-2.0 in multiple populations [71]. Functional evidence in support of this association was initially obtained by Kouki et al. [95], who found increased proliferation of T lymphocytes in patients homozygous for the predisposing G49 allele. This finding was confirmed by observations of Maurer at al. [96], who showed a reduced up-regulation of CTLA4 from G/G donors upon T-cell activation in response to IL-2, if compared with wild-type T lymphocytes.

The exon 1 polymorphism of CTLA-4 was found to influence production of thyroid antibodies. Zaletel et al. [97] measured significantly higher levels of TAb in GD patients carrying the G49 allele. Therefore, this observation confirmed data of Tomer at al. [65], who observed linkage between the A/G +49 CTLA-4 polymorphism and TAb production in AITD families. In addition, Kinjo et al. [59] showed association of the codon 17 SNP with remission of GD after anti-thyroid drug treatment demonstrating significantly higher frequencies of the GG genotype and the G allele in patients with persistently positive TAb over 5 years of anti-thyroid drug treatment than in individuals, who had TAb disappeared within 5 years of chemotherapy.

Finally, Anjos et al.[98] reported a defect in targeting of CTLA-4 to the cell surface in CTLA-4 Ala17 individuals. The authors found an inefficient glycosylation of the CTLA-4 molecule with alanine-17 in its signal peptide. This might affect the intracellular processing of the peptide chain and explain poor expression of CTLA-4 on the surface of T cells of patients homozygous for the Ala17 allele, which was 3-fold less than the surface expression of CTLA-4 in Thr17 homozygotes [99,100]. The defect in targeting of CTLA-4 to the cell surface can also explain quantitative differences in intracellular CTLA4 distribution between the two genotypes observed by Maurer et al. [96] using confocal fluorescence microscopy. The less efficient function of CTLA-4 in Ala17 homozygous patients could therefore promote T-cell proliferation leading to autoimmune disease.

For the C/T(-318) promoter polymorphism of CTLA-4, the first evidence for functional activity was obtained by Ligers et al. [101], who observed significantly increased expression both of cell-surface CTLA-4 after cellular stimulation and of CTLA-4 mRNA in non-stimulated T cells from individuals with multiple sclerosis, carrying T(-318) and homozygous for adenine at position 49. In a luciferase gene reporter assay, Wang et al. [102] then showed the ability of the promoter SNP at position –318 to affect CTLA-4 transcription. The T(-318) allele was associated with a higher promoter activity [102]. Anjos et al. [103] further confirmed the ability of the C/T(-318) polymorphism to influence the transcriptional activity of the CTLA-4 promoter. The T promoter variant was found to direct higher luciferase transcription in Jurkat T cells and be associated with greater expression levels of CTLA-4 mRNA in human lymphocytes [103]. This can explain association of the T(-318) allele with lower genetic risk of GD.

The –318 polymorphism is located within the 400-bp highly conserved region, which includes the 335-bp promoter sequence essential for the expression of CTLA-4 [104,105]. A thymidine-to-cytosine substitution at position –318 affects the binding sequence for transcription factor LEF-1 and hence could mediate regulatory effects of the factor on the transcription of CTLA-4 but this needs further investigations [103,106].

The $(AT)_n$ repeat at the 3'UTR of the CTLA-4 gene could be involved in mRNA stability playing a role of AU-rich elements, which participate in mRNA degradation [107]. Two alleles of the $(AT)_n$ microsatellite, referred as 88- and 106-bp allele, are the most common in Caucasians. The 88-bp allele is in strong LD with the A49 allele, while the 106-bp allele is tight LD with the G49 allele of the exon 1 SNP [94]. The 106-bp allele showed significant association with higher risk of GD (RR=1.8-2.8) [86].

The increased mRNA stability is one of the major mechanisms, by which synergistic induction of the expression of cell surface CTLA-4 occurs in T cells after stimulation by T-cell receptor (TcR) and CD28 signals [108]. Wang et al. [109] found negative correlation between the number of repeats in the 3'UTR mucrosatellite and stability of CTLA-4 mRNA. The authors observed a 1.5-fold increase in steady-state level of CTLA-4 mRNA for the 86-bp allele, compared to the longer alleles [109]. The 86-bp allele was shown to be associated with a lower risk of myasthenia gravis. Lymphocytes from patients homozygous for this allele demonstrated the lowest level of T-cell proliferative responses upon the addition of anti-CD28 antibodies, which block stimulation of T cells, compared to cells from patients with longer microsatellite alleles [110]. The association of the long AT-repeat allele with reduced control of T-cell proliferation compared to the 86-bp allele was also showed in Japanese patients with Graves' disease [111]. These observations could be explained by longer stability of CTLA-4 mRNA in case of the 86-bp allele, which supports elongated suppressive effect of CTLA-4 to the proliferation of T cells.

Recently, Anjos et al. [112] functionally reanalyzed the CT60 (A/G+6230) SNP located 3' to the known polyadenylation site of CTLA-4. The authors found no effect of this SNP on the expression of either CTLA-4 or ICOS but confirmed an influence of the C/T(-318) promoter polymorphism on the transcription of both full-length and soluble CTLA-4 isoforms. In addition, no CTLA-4 transcript containing the CT60 SNP or alternatively polyadenylated CTLA-4 mRNA was found [112]. Thus, the functional background for the association of CTLA-4 with autoimmune disease on the basis of implication of the +6230 polymorphism only remains questionable and hence needs further clarification.

Transcripts for both full-length and soluble CTLA-4 maintain the exon 1 SNP and the $(AT)_n$ microsatellite at the 3'UTR but do not contain +6230 SNP, since this polymorphism lies 3' the polyadenylation site of the CTLA-4 mRNA. Therefore, the +49 and the $(AT)_n$ repeat could modulate CTLA-4 properties including cell surface targeting and mRNA stability. Studies of Anjos et al. [112] showed no relationship between the CT60 SNP and steady-state mRNA of any known CTLA-4 isoform.

The soluble CTLA-4, expression of which is markedly increased in a variety of autoimmune and allergic disease, may reflect the dysregulation of T cell activation and should play a role in the pathogenesis of autoimmunity [90,93]. However, the function of soluble CTLA-4 is at present poorly characterized. The soluble isoform is produced by alternative splicing of the transmembrane domain and is expressed mainly in non-simulated T cells, while the full-length CTLA-4 has the transmembrane domain and presented on the surface of activated CD4+ and CD8+ T lymphocytes [113,114]. Since soluble CTLA-4 maintains the ability to bind CD80/CD86 molecules, this molecule could compete with membrane-bound CTLA-4 for CD80/CD86 binding sites and cause a reduction of inhibitory signaling. Further work on the dynamics of full-length versus soluble isoform expression and needed to resolve this issue.

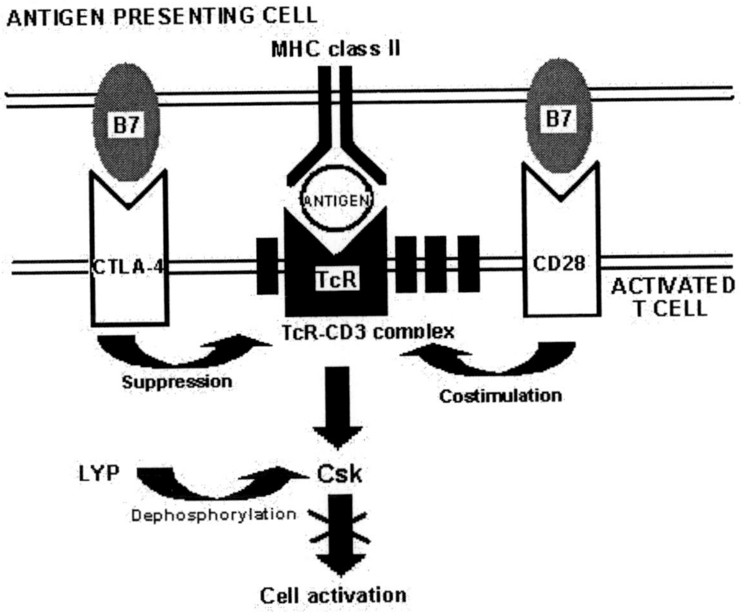

Fig. 3. Schematic representation of T helper cell activation. The activation includes two steps: the initial activation signal from the T cell receptor-CD3 complex (TcR), which interacts with the presented antigen binded to the Human Leucocyte Antigen (HLA) class II molecule on the surface of the antigen-presenting cell, and costimulatory signal from the complex between the CD28 molecule and B7 (CD80 or CD86) molecule. On the other hand, binding the cytotoxic T lymphocyte associated antigen-4 (CTLA-4) molecule to B7 suppress activation of the T cell. Due to the negative control function of CTLA-4, functional alterations of the sequence of the CTLA-4 gene could increase susceptibility to Graves' disease. Stimulating signal from TcR leads to T cell activation through the recruitment of a number of intracellular signaling molecules and regulatory proteins, including carboxy-terminal SPC kinase (Sck). Lymphoid protein tyrosine phospatase (LYP), a product of the PTPN22 gene, is able to phosphorylate the Sck molecule, so that arresting the stimulation of the T cell. A disease-associated tryptophane-to-arginine amino acid substitution in codon 620 (R620W) of LYP prevents binding of LYP to Sck that results in the hyperreactivity of pathogenic T cells.

The CTLA-4 molecule together with another co-stimulator (CD28) plays a crucial role in T-cell response to antigen presentation. T lymphocytes can be activated through the two-way mechanism, including first signal from the presentation of the complex between the antigen and a Major Histocompatibility Complex (MHC) class II molecule on the surface of the antigen-presenting cell (APC) to the TcR and second signal from costimulatory molecules (Fig. 3). The absence of costimulatory signal causes the T cell to be refractory (anergy) or induces apoptosis of the cell [115].

Both CTLA-4 and CD28 bind to similar ligands, CD80 (B7.1) and CD86 (B7.2), on APC. The interaction between CD28 and its ligands stimulates T cells. In contrast, binding CTLA-4 to CD80/CD86 molecules results in inhibitory signals to T-cell activation. In addition, CTLA-4 has a much greater affinity for B7 molecules than CD28 [115]. In non-activated cells, CTLA-4 is mostly stored in intracellular vesicles. In stimulated T cell, the vesicles move to the cell surface and resolve CTLA-4 molecules, allowing expression of CTLA-4 on the outer membrane and competition with CD28 for engaging B7-binding sites [116]. A dramatic evidence for the inhibitory function of CTLA-4 came from the CTLA-4-knockout mice, which rapidly developed fatal lymphoproliferative disorder and died, due to the massive lymphocytic infiltration into non-lymphoid tissues [117].

The role of CTLA-4 in autoimmunity is consisted in maintaining peripheral T-cell tolerance and homeostasis but not central tolerance, once thymocyte development appears normal in CTLA-4-deficient mice [118]. The mechanism, by which CTLA-4 maintains peripheral tolerance of T cells, is not clear in details. Where B7 levels are low and TcR signal are weak, the amount of CTLA-4 induced is low but may be sufficient to minimize costimulation and prevent activation. Under these conditions CTLA-4 may set a treshold for activation. Two scenarios, in which CTLA-4 may play a role in establishing a threshold for CD28 and/or TcR signals needed for activation of naïve T cells, are proposed. The first scenario suggests the role for CTLA-4 for maintaining tolerance for T cells with specificity to tissue-specific antigens that are not expressed in the thymus and have not be deleted as a consequence of negative selection. This scenario may explain the observation that CTLA-4 blockage or deficiency accelerates an onset and severity of insulitis and diabetes in non-obese diabetic (NOD) mice expressing a transgenic αβTcR cloned from the islet-β-cell-specific CD4+ T cell clone isolated from a NOD mouse [119]. T cells, bearing this TcR, are efficiently selected, rather than deleted in the thymus, demonstrating that central tolerance is not effective for T cells with this specificity. A bispecific antibody capable of simultaneously binding to CTLA-4 and a tissue-specific antigen (murine TSHR) inhibited the T cell alloresponse in CBA/J (H2(k)) mice injected with murine TSHR cDNA, suggesting a protective role of CTLA-4 against proliferation and immune attack by tissue-antigen specific T cells [120].

The second scenario deals with the regulation of the response of T cells to tonic signaling by self-peptide/MHC interactions [121]. These continuous TcR interactions with self-peptide/MHC provide important signal for the peripheral T lymphocytes. Some of these interactions, under conditions of low levels of CD28/B7 interaction, might be sufficient to activate CD4+ T cells and induce and/or mobilize CTLA-4. CTLA-4 might prevent the signals generated by these tonic interactions from leading to full activation of CD4+ T cells but would unable the T cells to receive partial signals [122]. In this scenario, due to limiting B7 levels, competition for ligand may be the primary mechanism of action, and CTLA-4 will predominantly affect the CD28-mediated signals.

The attenuation model assumes high levels of B7 and a possibility of the CD28-mediated costimulation to overwhelm the inhibitory effects of low levels of CTLA-4, allowing T-cell activation to proceed. This often happens in Th1-type immune response-mediated inflammatory and organ-specific autoimmune diseases, such as MS, T1D, posterior uveitis and others [123]. CTLA-4 has a role in inducing a T helper type 1 (Th1) response and suppressing Th2 cytokines, an effect, which is antagonized by CD28 [124]. The balance between CD28 and CTLA-4 expression by T lymphocytes could be a factor in the pathogenesis of autoimmune diseases. For thyroid autoimmunity, two clinical outcomes are possible depending on the predominance of Th1 or Th2 type cytokine profiles in the affected thyroid. The predominance of Th1 cytokines may result in the development of HT, whereas GD is considered to be Th2-mediated [125]. Using bispecific antibody (BiAb) enable to bind to both CTLA-4 and TSHR, experimental autoimmune thyroiditis (EAT), an animal model of human HT, in mice immunized with mouse Tg was prevented, suggesting that the engagement of CTLA-4 expressed on activated autoreactive T cells in close proximity to the thyroid can increase the number of regulatory T cells and their ability to produce tumor growth factor β1 (TGF-β1), with a concomitant reduction in interferon γ (IFN- γ) and TNF-α, e.g. Th1 type cytokines, resulting in suppression of EAT [126]. Thus, CTLA-4 also is able to suppress T cell activation through enhancing production of the inhibitory cytokine TGF-β1. This evidence was supported by results of experiments with cross-linking CTLA-4 [127,128].

Soluble CTLA4-Ig is known to block CD28 engagement with CD80 and CD86. This ability provides effective results in using of CTLA-4-Ig therapy at the induction of tolerance to pancreatic islets, skin and renal allografs [129]. The therapy induces global immunosuppression, since CTLA-4-Ig blocks both wanted and unwanted immune responses. This is a reason, why CTLA-4-Ig cannot be widely applied in the immunotherapy of an organ-specific pathology, such as AITD. The ultimate goal of any tissue-specific immune therapy is to suppress immune response against specific antigens in vivo, while preserving the global immune response. A bispecific antibody approach, such as BiAb coupling simultaneously TSHR and CTLA-4, could represent a potential immune therapeutic tool in the treatment of thyroid autoimmunity [120]. Targeting of the BiAb to a given antigen on a specific tissue (e.g., TSHR) and engagement of CTLA-4 on activated T cells that are in close proximity to the target tissue could inactivate these T cells specifically and limit unwanted global immunosuppression. Lack of significant CTLA-4 expression in non-activated T cells suggests that the BiAb approach would be ideal for targeting subsets of tissue-specific activated T cells. It was shown that the presence of CTLA-4 molecules on the surface of target cells is able to protect those cells from immune attack by antigen-specific T lymphocytes [120]. So, it is possible to induce tolerance to BiAb-coated cell and use this in the treatment of organ- and tissue-specific autoimmune pathology, such as thyroiditis, T1D and RA. For example, without knowing the precise autoantigenic peptide-MHC complex expressed on thyroid cells in HT, the BiAb-treated thyrocytes could induce tolerance to all major and minor antigens involved in stimulating the autoimmune response. Initial results with the murine experimental model suggest that a single administration of the antibody specific to TSHR and CTLA-4 can induce significant tolerance to thyroidspecific autoantigens and decrease the autoimmune response [126].

The AITD-1 Locus (Chromosome 6p11) and the Major Histocompatibility (MHC) Region

Genetic Linkage and Association Studies

A first whole-genome scan for susceptibility to thyroid autoimmunity performed in 56 multiplex multigenerational Caucasian AITD families resolved an evidence for linkage to disease on chromosome 6p [130]. The MLS was 2.9 obtained between markers D6S1610 and D6S257. The locus was linked to both GD and HT. The susceptibility locus spanning around 20 cM on chromosome 6p11 was designated AITD-1[131]. Later, the AITD-1 locus was confirmed by a second genome-wide scan in the expanded dataset of 102 multiplex families, with maximum MLS of 2.0 for marker D6S422 located approximately 30 cM telomeric to D6S257 [131].

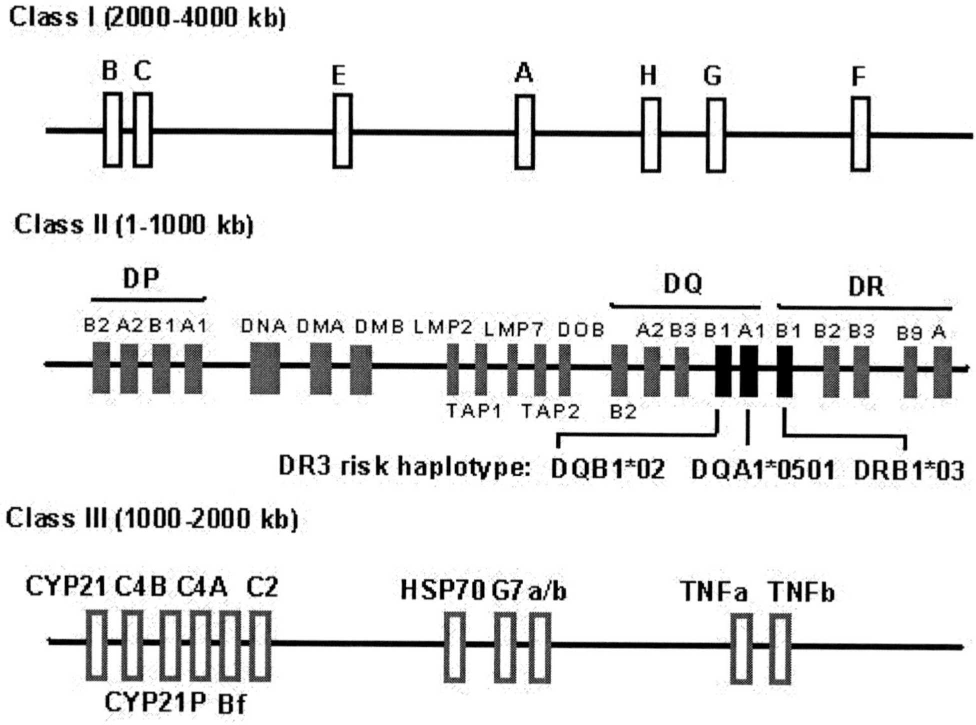

Fig. 4. Simplified scheme of the genomic organization of the human HLA gene cluster. HLA class II genes contributing to HLA-DR3, a risk haplotype for Graves' disease, are shown in solid black boxes. Abbreviations: TAP, transport associated with antigen processing; LMP, large multifunctional proteasome; HSP70, heat shock protein 70; TNF, tumour necrosis factor.

The AITD-1 locus is situated close but distinct from the MHC gene cluster, which located on chromosome 6p21. In humans, the cluster harbors a major complex of immune regulatory genes called Human Leucocyte Antigens (HLA). The HLA region includes three different gene subclusters, namely class I, class II and class II (Fig. 4). The class I region comprises the HLA-A, -B and –C genes encoding surface cell molecules, which participate in the presentation of endogeneous antigens to CD8+ T lymphocytes. The HLA class II genes encode a variety of proteins expressed on the cell surface of macrophages, B lymphocytes, dendritic cells and activated T cells and involved in the processing and presentation of exogeneous antigens to CD4+ T lymphocytes. The class II cluster contains the DQ and DR genes encoding the α and β peptide chains of the HLA class II molecules. Genes, products of which participate in the processing antigens (LMP2 and LMP7) and their transportation to the cell surface membrane (TAP1 and TAP2), lie in the center of the class II cluster, between the DP-DM and DQ-DR gene families. The DM genes are responsible for transfer of antigenic peptides onto class II molecules. The DP genes encode additional peptide chains that constitute the class II molecule and hence also envolve in the presentation of antigens to

CD4+ Th cells. The class III region lies between the class I and class II regions and contain eleven genes encoding tumour necrosis factor (TNF), heat shock protein (HSP70), complement components (C2, C4 and Bf) and other proteins [132].

Because the HLA cluster contains multiple immune modulatory genes, it was the first candidate genetic region to be evaluated for association and linkage with AITD. However, linkage analyses provided mostly negative results for linkage between the HLA region and GD or AITD [133-138]. Only a study in UK affected families revealed linkage between HLA and GD after stratification for carriage of HLA-DR3 [139]. Another study from the UK also reported a linkage of the HLA gene cluster to GD, with a peak NPL of 1.95 between D6S273 and TNFα [64].

In contrast to results of the linkage analyses, multiple case-control studies showed prominent association of the HLA genes with GD, with RR ranging from 1.1 to 5.7 (reviewed in [70,71,140]). In Caucasians, the HLA-DR3 (HLA-DRB1*03) allele is established to be a common risk marker for GD. The frequency of this allele generally ranges from 40 to 60% in GD patients that is 2-4-fold greater than the frequency of DR3 in healthy individuals, providing a RR for DR3 carriers of up to 5.7 [141,142]. In a mixed Brazilian population, the HLA-DRB1*0301 and HLA-DQA1*0501 alleles showed the most strong association with GD [143]. In non-Caucasian GD patients, other HLA alleles were shown to represent major risk markers. In Asians (Chinese and Japanese), there was HLA-Bw46, giving a RR of up to 4.8 [144]. In Indians, there was HLA-DQw2 (RR = 5.4) [145]. The frequency of the susceptible haplotype DRB3*0202- DQA1*0501 was found to be increased in African Americans affected with GD [146].

Because of the tight LD within the HLA region, several HLA alleles can show association with GD. For example, in Caucasian populations, the HLA-DQA1*0501 allele is significantly associated with higher risk of GD [147-149]. The susceptibility supported by DQA1*0501 is most likely, due to it being in LD the predisposing HLA-DR3 allele. The combination of both these alleles resulted in a shared susceptibility haplotype, which provides striking increase in the RR for development of Graves' disease (RR of up to 27.0 for females and RR of up to 8.4 for males) [150]. Haplotype analysis suggested that the DRB1*0301 allele conferred the primary susceptibility to GD and therefore represents the major genetic risk marker among HLA class II genes in Caucasians [151]

Lack of the linkage between HLA and GD assumes that HLA-DR3 does not significantly contributes to familial clustering of GD. Analysis of subsets of US Caucasians with sporadic and familial GD did not found significant difference in the frequency of HLA-DR3 between the subsets [73]. This observation suggests that the HLA-DR3 allele provides a generalized increase in risk for both sporadic and familial GD.

The HLA-DR3 allele has multiple sequence variations. In 2004, a total of 28 subtypes of the HLA-DRB1*03 allele was known [152]. To identify, which of the DRB1 sequences actually represents a primary etiological variant, the HLA-DRB1 gene was sequenced in Caucasian GD patients. Sequence analysis revealed that the frequency of DRB1variant encoding arginine at position 74 was significantly increased in GD patients compared to controls (OR = 4.6) [153]. In DR3-negative individuals, DRβ1-Arg74 was still significantly associated with GD, suggesting that the primary association of GD is with DRβ1-Arg74, whereas the association with HLA-DR3 is secondary [153]. Logistic regression analysis of each of 102 amino acid positions of the exon 2-encoded peptide-binding domain of DRB1 in the independent case-control study (871 affected and 621 control subjects from the UK) showed the strongest association with GD for codon 74 [154]. These findings suggest that an amino acid variation at position 74 of the DRβ1 chain could represent a primary etiological variant, which confers susceptibility to GD.

Except for arginine, other amino acids situating at position 74 include alanine and glutamine. The DRβ1-Gln74 variant is always observed on the DR7 allele, which was reported to be protective for GD in several populations [153,155,156]. This suggests, that position 74 plays a critical role in the pathogenesis of GD, presenting DRβ1-Gln74 as a protective variant and DRβ1-Arg74 as a causative variant for GD development.

Functional Analyses and Possible Mechanism of the Involvement of HLA Class II Molecules in the Pathogenesis of GD

A complex between a HLA class II molecule and processed thyroid autoantigen can be recognized by autoreactive T lymphocytes on the surface of APC through interaction with a T cell receptor. Different HLA alleles have different affinities for thyroid antigenic peptides. Some of these alleles can permit binding the antigenic peptide with peptide-binding pocket of the HLA molecule and further recognition by the T cell receptor, while others cannot [58]. Three-dimensional structure simulations showed that the amino acid position 74 lies within the antigen-binding pocket of the class II molecule [153]. The replacement of neutral alanine or glutamine amino acid residues by positively charged arginine-74 could influence charge and electrostatic potential in the binding cavity and therefore cause conformational changes in the DR3 molecule. This could affect antigen-binding properties of the HLA class II molecule. Similar role was already shown for an aspartic residue at position 57 of the DQβ chain, which is protective for T1D development [157]. Lack of aspartic acid at position 57 provides opportunity for immunogenic insulin peptides to fit the antigen-binding pocket of the HLA-DQαβ heterodimer and to be recognized by TcR [158]. The presence of the aspartate residue at position 57 prevents binding and further presentation of the insulin peptide to TcR.

Studies on a cleaved peptide from the invariant chain (CLIP), partipating in class II peptide-binding functions, demonstrated the ability of Arg74Gln mutation to enchance the interaction between CLIP and the DR3 molecule and increase the resistance of CLIP-DR3 complexes to dissociation by sodium dodecylsulfate [159]. In addition, position 74 participates in several structural compartments needed for antigen binding by DR3 and interaction between the peptide-DR3 complex and TcR [160]. These observations also support in favour of the significant role of this position in antigen-binding properties of the DRβ1 molecule.

Studies on animal models of experimental autoimmune thyroiditis showed a clear role of the HLA-DR3 allele in predisposing thyroid autoimmunity. Immunization of DR3 transgenic mice with human Tg resulted in severe thyroiditis [161,162]. Vaccination of DR3+ mice with a plasmid expressing human TSHR induced production of anti-TSHR antibodies [163]. The interaction between the DR3 allele and thyroid-specific antigenic peptides in DR3+ mice was demonstrated in several studies using specific peptides derived from thyroglobulin [164] and TSHR [165].

Thyroid autoantigens could be presented by HLA molecules in the thyroid through the expression of HLA class II molecules by professional APC, such macrophages and dendritic cells [166], and/or through the aberrant expression of HLA antigens by non-professional APC, such as thyrocytes [167,168]. The aberrant expression of HLA molecules by thyroid cells occurs in the thyroid of GD patients, but not in the normal thyroid gland [166]. This could happen as a consequence of viral infection [169,170], cytokine action [171-173], toxin influence [174], altered dietary iodine intake [175] and other reasons. The necessity of the aberrant HLA class II expression as a possible primary mechanism of the induction of thyroid autoimmunity was supported by studies on a murine model, which was enable to develop Graves-like disease after injection with fibroblasts co-transfected with TSHR and HLA class II DNA [176,177].

The 8q23-q24 Locus and the Thyroglobulin Gene

Genetic Linkage and Association Studies

A susceptibility locus for AITD on chromosome 8q was first found in Japanese [137]. Using 123 affected sib-pairs, Sakai et al. [137] showed evidence for the linkage of marker D8S272 on 8q24 to AITD (MLS = 2.31). The region of linkage to AITD on chromosome 8q24 was also identified in the independent data set of 102 Caucasian families (MLS = 3.5) [131,178]. A peak of linkage was obtained between markers D8S514 and D8S284 within the thyroglobulin gene [178]. A newly identified marker Tgms2 in intron 27 of the Tg gene showed linkage (MLS = 2.9) and association (RR = 1.4) with AITD in US Caucasians [178]. This marker also showed association with thyroid autoimmunity in UK Caucasians [179].

These results suggest that the Tg locus is likely to harbor the AITD susceptibility gene. Ban et al. [180] sequenced the coding region of the human Tg gene and found 14 new SNPs. Of these, four SNPs located in exon 10, 12 and 33 showed significant association with both AITD and GD, comprising a common susceptibility haplotype related to higher risk of AITD (OR = 2.5) and to each of thyroid autoimmunity phenotypes (GD and HT; OR = 2.54 and 2.38, respectively). In addition, the exon 33 SNP, representing an arginine-to-tryptophane amino acid substition in codon 1008, showed gene-gene interaction with a well established GD susceptibility allele HLA-DR3, providing a combined RR of 6.1 [180]. Analysis of the exon 10, 12 and 33 SNPs in a large cohort of 1214 AITD patients from the UK did not found significant association of these markers with disease [181]. In Japanese, no association between the exon 33 SNP and AITD was also found [182]. Howewer, in Japanese patients, the Tgms2 microsatellite showed relation to HT, but not to GD (OR = 2.60) [182]. Although results of the association analysis of the thyroglobulin gene are inconsistent, this gene is likely to represent a thyroid-specific AITD susceptibility gene, which seems to be specific for neither GD phenotype nor HT clinical outcome [183]. Moreover, the Tg locus was shown to implicate susceptibility to thyroid autoimunity not only in humans, but also in mouse. In the murine gene, a unique SNP haplotype at exon 10 and 12 associated with a high risk of the development of experimental autoimmune thyroiditis (EAT) was observed in 45% EAT-prone strains, but in none of the mouse strains that were resistant to thyroiditis [180].

A recent study in Japanese AITD patients found a putative alternative candidate gene for susceptibility to AITD on chromosome 8q23 [184]. The gene was designated ZFAT (zinc-finger gene in AITD susceptibility region; official name ZNF406). It encodes a zinc-finger protein TR-ZFAT, which functions as a transcription factor, and small antisense transcript (SAS-ZFAT) that probably regulates transcription of TR-ZFAT. SAS-ZFAT is exclusively expressed in CD19+ B lymphocytes. A SNP marker, Ex9-SNP10, located at 3' untranslated region (UTR) of TR-ZFAT and the promoter region of SAS-ZFAT, showed strong association with AITD in a Japanese population [184]. The T allele of Ex9-SNP10 was related to higher risk of AITD, increased expression of SAS-ZFAT and, subsequently, decreased expression of TR-ZFAT. This suggests that Shirasawa et al. [184] described a functional polymorphism of the ZFAT gene that alters the expression of this gene. Hence, these authors presented intriguing data on the self-regulation of the gene that can confer AITD susceptibility and reflect pathogenic mechanism, by which genetic alterations within the ZFAT gene contribute to the pathogenesis of the disease. The ZFAT gene is only situated 1.34 megabases (Mb) telomeric to the thyroglobulin gene and therefore could represent an AITD predisposing gene in the 8q23-q24 susceptibility locus. However, the association of ZFAT with thyroid autoimmunity was shown only by a single study in a single population from Japan and needs to be replicated by other investigations in different ethnic groups. To date, genetic data reporting a role of the Tg gene are consistently proven in several studies and are likely to suggest that this gene represents a true susceptibility gene within the AITD locus on chromosome 8q.

Animal Models of Thyroglobulin-Induced Autoimmune Thyroiditis and Possible Mechanisms, by which Thyroglobulin can Induce Susceptibility to AITD

Thyroglobulin is a thyroid-specific protein, which is iodinated and further digested in the thyroid gland to produce a prohormone thyroxine [185]. Iodination of specific tyrosine residues in the Tg molecule and coupling of these iodinated residues to form thyroxine depend on the thyroid peroxidase [186]. Iodination status and iodine content are crucial for antigenicity of Tg. Non-iodinated thyroglobulin is not able to initiate proliferation of autoreactive T lymphocytes. A highly iodinated thyroglobulin molecule is a better immunogen than Tg of low iodine content [187]. Autoantibodies against Tg represent a bulk of thyroid antibodies in patients with AITD, both GD and HT, although can be detected in healthy individuals [188,189]. Tg-antibodies in AITD patients are restricted in their epitope specificity compared to the polyclonal nature of the autoantibodies in non-affected individuals [190].

The NOD. $H2^{h4}$ mouse strain, an animal model for human autoimmune thyroiditis, is able to develop EAT, when immunized with murine or human Tg [191]. Immunization with mouse thyroglobulin can induce EAT in other genetically predisposing strains of mice, expressing susceptible class II molecules, such as the H-2A(k), H-2A(s), or H-2A(q) alleles [192]. The induction of EAT implies interaction between class II molecules and Tg as resulted from the immunization of HLA and H2 class II transgenic mice with a variety Tg peptides [193,194]. HLA-DR3+ mouse developes thyroiditis after injection of potential pathogenic peptides from either human or murine Tg, suggesting for the interaction between the susceptible DR3 allele and the immunogenic Tg peptide [162,164]. In addition, evidence for gene-gene interaction between the predisposing HLA-DR3 allele and molecular variants of Tg, resulting in significant increase of the relative risk of GD, is supported by results of genetic studies [180]. H2A-based mouse strains can develop EAT after immunization with certain peptides from murine Tg, demonstrating the importance of class II alleles in the molecular recognition of autogenic Tg epitopes [193,194]. The restricted TcR repertoire of intrathyroidal T lymphocytes detected in mice with human Tg-induced EAT provides evidence for specific character of molecular interaction between Tg epitopes and TcR molecules, which results in oligoclonal proliferation and expansion of the intrathyroidal T cell populations [195-197].

Studies on animal models of autoimmune thyroiditis revealed a unique and important role of thyroglobulin in the induction of thyroid autoimmunity [198]. MHC class II and T cell receptor molecules are shown to be directly responsible for the presentation and immune recognition of Tg epitopes [197,199,200]. Aberrant presentation of Tg peptides by thyroid cells can be induced by several ways including viral or bacterial infection [201], cytokine treatment [29] and iodine uptake [202]. Dietary iodine represents an important environmental trigger in the pathogenesis of AITD. Iodine might facilitate the uptake, processing and presentation of Tg by professional APC, such as dendritic cells, macrophages and B lymphocytes, through enchanded iodination of the Tg molecule [175,203]. This promotes unmasking cryptic Tg epitopes and generation of pathogenic T cell determinants, which are recognized by T lymphocytes through the interaction with TcR [187,204]. Finally, high concentrations of iodine can destruct thyrocytes, probably, via generation of oxigen radicals and hence resolve target antigens from the thyrocytes [205,206].

Sequence variations within the Tg gene can predispose to AITD influencing antigenic properties of Tg by increasing the affinity of critical peptides to MHC class II molecules and TcR. To date, unfortunately, no data, evaluating how thyroglobulin polymorphisms can affect its antigenicity have been reported. However, availability of monoclonal anti-Tg antibodies provide good opportunity for these studies [207]. In addition, sequence variations in Tg could presumably explain interactions between genetic and environmental (dietary iodine) factors in the pathogenesis of AITD, since iodination of Tg plays a vital role in the biosynthesis of the thyroid hormone and influences immunogenic properties of thyroglobulin in autoimmune thyroiditis [187,208]. Functional relevance of known Tg SNPs, particularly those, causing amino acid changes and showing association with AITD, remains unclear and hence needs to be functionally evaluated. This should greatly assist our further understanding of the role of Tg in thyroid autoimmunity.

The human Tg gene spans around 300 kb on chromosome 8 [185]. Since LD blocks in the human genome are 20-100-kb long, the Tg gene is likely to contain several LD blocks and therefore several extended haplotypes associated with AITD [49]. Future investigations should be focused on dissection of the fine haplotype structure of Tg to reveal all disease-associated variants and estimate their significance in conferring genetic susceptibility to AITD.

The GD-1 Locus (chromosome 14q31) and the Thyrotropin Receptor Gene

Genetic Linkage and Association Studies

The susceptibility locus (designated GD-1) on chromosome 14q was identified by Tomer et al. [209] in linkage analysis of 56 multiplex AITD families from the US using a set of polymorphic markers around a positional candidate gene, TSHR (chromosome 14q31). Several markers showed positive linkage to GD, but not to HT, with a peak of linkage (MLS = 2.5) for marker D14S81 located on chromosome 14q31[210]. The TSHR gene itself did not show significant linkage to GD [210]. The GD-1 locus was replicated in the extended dataset of 102 affected US families, with a MLS of 2.1 for marker D14S258 located 20 cM telomeric to D14S81 [131]. However, analysis of eight microsatellite markers spanning a 36-cM region on chromosome 14q31-q33 in 75 affected sibling pairs from the UK failed to show linkage to GD [211].

As mentioned above, TSHR represented an attractive positional candidate gene for susceptibility to GD, due to its function in the thyroid and exciting role in the pathogenesis of this disease [212]. However, several independent studies failed to find a linkage between this gene and GD [209,211,213]. Three SNPs within the coding region of TSHR have been evaluated for association to GD in multiple case-control studies. There are an aspartate-to-histidine substitution at codon 36 (D36H) and a proline-to-threonine amino acid change at position 52 (P52T) both located in the extracellular domain of the receptor and a glutamate-to-aspartate substitution at position 727 (D727E) within the intracellular TSHR domain [214].

In Caucasians, most studies found no association between the above TSHR polymorphisms and GD, except for the initial report of Cuddihy at al. [215], showing association of the P52T SNP with GD in US white females, and a study of Chistiakov et al. [216] reported on the association between the D727E dimorphism and GD in Russian patients. Ban et al. [217] found no major role of the D727E SNP in the development of GD in the US Caucasian dataset. However, when the authors made a meta-analysis combining their data with results of early investigations in other Caucasians, they showed a weak association of the D727E TSHR molecular variant with GD (RR = 1.6) [217].

In Japanese, a strong association with GD was shown for multiple polymorphic markers within the TSH receptor gene including two dinucleotide microsatellites [218,219] and an extended haplotype block [AATG$(CT)_6$(TT)AG] comprising alleles of seven SNPs in intron 7 [220]. The extended haplotype block was related to increased risk of GD (RR = 1.2). The study of Hiratani and co-authors [220] suggests that nucleotide changes in the coding region of TSHR do not seem to be driving the evidence of association. Non-coding SNPs are the source of evidence of association between TSHR and GD, at least in the Japanese population. What biological role that these non-coding SNPs may play remains unclear and needs further clarification. In summary, the above data suggest that the TSHR gene remains to be a GD-specific susceptibility gene for GD within the GD-1 locus, but likely with a minor genetic effect.

Among other potential candidate genes located within the GD-1 locus, the SEL1L gene encoding human ortholog of the Caenorhabditis elegans gene sel-1, a negative regulator of LIN-12/NOTCH receptor proteins, and the DIO2 gene encoding type II iodothyronine deiodinase have been analyzed. For SEL1L, no association between a $(CA)_n$ dinucleotide microsatellite located in intron 20 and AITD was shown in Japanese women [221]. In contrast, a threonine-to-alanine amino acid change in codon 92 (T92A) of the deiodinase 2 gene showed association with GD in Russian simplex families [222]. The codon 92 DIO2 SNP rather is non-functional [223,224] but could be in LD with another polymorphism within the DIO2 gene, which may affect an expression level or enzymatic activity of type II deiodinase. Recently, Peeters et al. [225] identified a new functionally relevant SNP, a glycine-to-aspartate substitution at position 3 (G3D) of DIO2 associated with serum iodothyronine levels. Due to the important role of type II deiodinase in the intrathyroidal iodine metabolism, alterations to the DIO2 gene could partially explain interactions between genetic and environmental factors such as dietary iodine in the etiology of Graves' disease and AITD [223]. However, more studies are required to estimate a role of DIO2 in the pathogenesis of thyroid autoimmunity.

Antigenic Properties of the TSHR Molecule, anti-TSHR Antibodies, Animal Models of TSHR-Induced Autoimmune Hyperthyroidism and Possible Mechanisms, by which TSH Receptor can Induce Susceptibility to GD

TSHR is a G-coupled transmembrane receptor expressed on the surface of thyroid epithelial cells. Binding TSH to TSHR results in stimulation of the thyroid growth and increasing thyroid hormone production [226]. The receptor molecule is heavily glycosylated and expressed on the cell surface as a single holoreceptor [227]. The mature TSHR undergoes intramolecular cleavage by a matrix metalloproteinase-like enzyme, resulted in loss of a 50-amino acid peptide on the C-terminus of the ectodomain and formation of a two-subunit (α and β) structure connected via disulfide bonds between cysteine clusters at the C-terminus of the ectodomain [228] (Fig. 5). The hormone-binding epitope involves a horseshoe conformational structure made up of the leucine-rich repeats in the α subunit and the N-terminus portion of the β subunit [229]. In thyrocytes, most of the TSHRs are fully glycosylated and cleaved, but β subunits on the plasma membrane are predominant, being 2.5-3 times more than α subunits [230]. This β predominance is likely resulted from the α subunit shedding catalyzed by protein disulfide-isomerase [231].

Since thyrotropin receptor represents a major GD autoantigen, the hallmark of GD is the production of the TSHR antibodies [212]. In GD, stimulating TSHR antibodies (TSHR-Abs) are able to mimic the activating action of binding TSH that leads to excessive and constitutional thyroid hormone production by the thyroid gland that therefore loses the regulation normally applied by TSH. The TSHR-antibody-induced hyperfunction of the thyroid gland causes autoimmune hyperthyroidism [232]. Properties of TSHR-Abs and immunogenic epitopes on the receptor molecule are extensively characterized and updated in several recent reviews [232-235].

Development of a mouse model of GD greatly helped in the discovery of antigenic functions and characterization of the role of TSHR in thyroid autoimmunity [236]. Contribution of HLA class II molecules needed to recognize antigenic TSHR epitopes and initiate production of stimulating but not blocking anti-TSHR-Abs was determined using the Shimojo murine model of GD induced with fibroblasts coexpressing HLA class II and TSHR [176,237]. The importance of the intact conformational structure of TSHR to induce stimulating self-antibodies was revealed in other mouse models of GD, which developed autoimmune hyperthyroidism after immunization with plasmid or adenoviral vectors expressing TSHR [238,239].

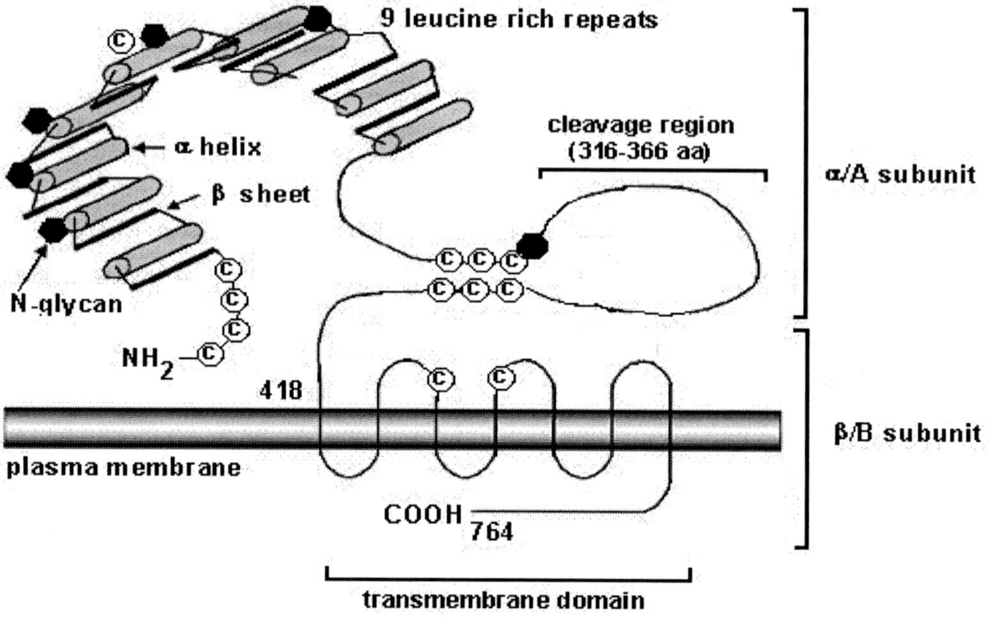

Fig. 5. Schematic representation of the thyroid-stimulating hormone receptor (TSHR) structure. The β/B subunit of the receptor molecule includes seven transmembrane domains crossing the plasma membrane and a short cytoplasmic tail. A posttranslational proteolysis results in splitting the TSHR molecule into the A and B subunits through the intramolecular cleavage of the 50 amino acid-long region (residues 316-366). Nine leucine-rich repeats, each containing of 20-24 amino acids, form a horschoe structure, which consists of α helices and β sheets and is responsible for binding TSH. This structure represents the receptor ectodomain, a major portion of the α/A subunit. N-glycosylation sites are indicated by solid pentagons. ©, cysteine residues.

Due to their conformational nature, the precise binding epitope(s) for stimulating TSHR-Abs are not recognized yet. However, the major binding region is located on the TSHR α subunit, where thyrotropin also binds, as resulted from studies on animal models [240,241], absence of binding TSHR-Abs to denaturated TSHR peptides [242-244], evidence on the ability of serum stimulating TSHR-autoantibodies from GD patients to recognize preferentially an intact α subunit of TSHR [245,246], and experiments with chimeric TSHR, a β subunit of which was replaced by a corresponding region from the lutropin/chorionic gonadotropin receptor [247]. The competition between TSH and TSHR-antibodies for binding to the TSHR was found in most patients with untreated GD. A linear correlation between the competing TSH activity and mouse TSHR-Ab binding inhibition was demonstrated [243]. Stimulating antibodies either from patients with GD or animal models of GD are able to recognize similar or closely related conformational binding site(s) as for thyrotropin on the TSHR α subunit [243,244,248]. These findings suggest the concept on a single epitope for stimulating TSHR-Abs. It is difficult to find a precise antibody-binding epitope(s) on the TSHR using TSHR-Abs from serum of GD patients, due to the heterogeneity (e.g., coexistence of stimulating and blocking TSHR-Abs) of these antibodies. To detect the individual epitopes, it is necessary to obtain monoclonal antibodies (and especially monoclonal stimulating TSHR-Abs) from GD patients. The isolation of these antibodies from GD sera was extremely complicated, since concentration of the TSHR-Abs is very low (less than 10 μg/ml) [245]. However, using an animal model of GD is the way to obtain monoclonal non-human TSHR antibodies. Early attempts to produce stimulating TSHR-Abs in mice resulted in generating TSHR-specific antibodies, which were neutral or blocked but never stimulated the TSHR-mediated signaling [249]. This happened, because most monoclonal Abs to the TSHR have been derived from rodents immunized with TSHR antigen from bacteria or insect cells. These antigens lacked the native conformation of the TSHR and the resulting monoclonal Abs were exclusively blocking or neutral TSHR-Abs [250].

Recent improvements in the antibody detection technique allowed to obtain mouse and hamster monoclonal TSHR-Abs with stimulating activity to human TSHR [242,243,248,251] and then isolate a monoclonal thyroid-stimulating antibody designated M22 from human lymphocytes [244]. These antibodies could effectively compete with TSH for coupling to TSHR and recognize the TSHR α subunit with high affinity. The epitopes of two mouse monoclonal antibodies (IRI-SAb2 and IRI-SAb3) were precisely mapped, at the amino acid level, to the N-terminal portion of the concave portion of the horseshoe structure of the TSHR ectodomain. They overlapped closely with each other and represented a three-dimensional conformational structure formed by discontinuous linear peptides and separate amino acids [252]. On the αsubunit of TSHR, Ando et al. [248] identified a conformational epitope A, which bound both stimulating and blocking monoclonal TSHR-Abs and a second epitope B specific to binding blocking Abs only. How the two conformational epitopes A and B are related to the TSH binding pocket defined by Jeffreys et al. [253] remains uncertain. In summary, these studies indicated that epitopes on the native TSHR by stimulating monoclonal TSHR-Abs are highly conserved and restricted rather than broadly distributed, and their stimulating potency is dependent on their binding affinity.

The structure of the Fab fragment of the human monoclonal antibody M22 was recently resolved [254]. The M22 Fab structure is standard although the hypervariable region of the heavy chain protrudes further from the framework than the hypervariable region of the light chain. The M22 antigen binding site is rich in aromatic residues and its surface is dominated by acidic patches on one side and basic patches on the other in agreement with an important role for charge-charge interactions in the TSHR-autoantibody interaction [254]. The availability of monoclonal TSHR-Abs greatly benefits further fine mapping and characterization of the antigenic epitope(s) of TSHR, resolving molecular mechanisms of the interaction between the TSHR and the antibody and precise structure of the TSHR-antibody complex to develop more sensitive and specific assays for antibody detection in early diagnosis of GD or for prediction of GD remission after treatment with anti-thyroid drugs [255-258].

TSHR-Abs are commonly oligoclonal and restricted to the IgG_1 subclass [259,260]. To isolate human IgG class monoclonal TSAbs Epstein–Barr-virus-transformed lymphocytes of GD patients have been developed [261,262]. However, antibodies isolated from these cells exhibited their thyroid-stimulating activity in concentrations, which were significantly higher than TSAbs levels in serum of affected patients [262]. Immunoglobulin (Ig) genes of two of these Epstein–Barr-virus-transformed B cells clones were reconstituted and characterized [263]. A significant number of somatic mutations were found in VH and VK regions of both clones, indicating the involvement of somatic mutations for the TSAb specificity. Analysis of the Ig heavy chain genes from four other monoclonal TSHR-antibodies derived from the Epstein–Barr-virus-transformed B cells clones showed using different VH gene families (VH-II, -III, -IV, and V) by each of those clones [264]. However, myeloma cells transfected with the reconstituted Ig genes could express IgG1 Abs that exhibited significant TSAb activities, but did not able to inhibit TSH binding to the receptor [263,265]. However, since true stimulating monoclonal TSHR-Abs are currently available, there will be no problem to analyze their Ig genes and hence find a true repertoire of VH and VL genes constituting these antibodies.

The detection of polyclonal TSHR-antibodies in sera of healthy individuals suggests on the possibility for TSHR or its structural components to initiate thyroid autoimmunity [266]. The shed α subunit may be at the origin of circulating antigenically active TSH receptor ectodomain detected in human blood [241,267]. In addition, expression of TSHR mRNA was found in fibroblasts from orbital tissues supporting an evidence for shared character of the TSHR-mediated immunoreactivity between the thyroid gland and the involved extrathyroidal sites in Graves' disease [268]. Analysis of the physico-chemical characteristics, e.g., hydrophobicity of the amino acids in the CDR3 (N) region of the TCR α chain, revealed a strong negative linear correlation between strength of stimulation and the average hydrophobicity of N-region amino acids [269]. This led to hypothesize that lower affinity T-cell clones were commonly more hydrophobic in their CDR3 α region amino acids in keeping with potential crossreactivity of such T cells as a consequence of promiscuous, hydrophobic CDR3 regions. This phenomenon would be analogous to polyreactive, natural autoantibodies, which tend to be crossreactive and 'sticky'. Thus, the physico-chemical characteristics of the TCR α CDR3 region supported the interaction with antigen/MHC by potentially cross-reactive T cells of low affinity [269]. It would seem likely that such low-affinity autoreactive T-cell populations serve as a pool of potentially pathogenetic cells. These cells would be able to respond to an insult, which, via a number of possible mechanisms such as molecular mimicry, would initiate a thyroid lymphocytic infiltration in an antigen-driven fashion with intrathyroidal T-cell expansion and a marked bias in the utilization of T-cell-receptor V genes [270].

As mentioned above, coexpression of HLA class II molecules and TSHR is crucial to induce GD-like autoimmune hyperthyroidism in mice [176,177]. In addition, GD thyrocytes are able to express aberrantly MHC class II molecules on their plasma membrane [166,167]. These findings suggest that the aberrant expression of MHC class II molecules by thyroid follicular cells followed by presentation of the complex between certain TSHR peptides and class II molecules could also contribute to the induction of immune response. The ability of the predisposing HLA-DR3 allele to bind TSHR autoantigenic peptides was shown in several studies [165,271]. Geluk et al. [272] proposed sequence for a DR3-specific peptide-binding motif. In the TSHR, two immunodominant epitopes corresponding to amino acids 207–222 and 357–376 have DR-3 specific binding motifs [273]. The GD-susceptible DR3 allele was shown to bind TSHR immunodominant peptide epitopes with intermediate affinity [165].

This is consistent with other studies indicating that most autoantigenic peptides show intermediate or low binding affinity to the disease-predisposing MHC class II molecules [273,274]. The relatively low affinity of autoantigenic peptides for MHC molecules may allow autoreactive T cells to escape from thymic deletion and initiate Tab production by B cells [275]. Thus, the pathogenic mechanism for thyroid autoimmunity discussed by Martin et al. [270] actually reflects a general way of inducing autoimmunity, which could be applicable to other organ- and tissue-specific autoimmune diseases.

The development of mouse models with TSHR-induced autoimmune hyperthyroidism transgenic for different HLA alleles but lacking murine MHC genes greatly helps in studying the potential value of these alleles for dissection of immune responses to the TSHR [163,276]. For example, Pichurin et al. [276] observed that approximately 30% of DR3-, but none of DQ6b-transgenic mice, developed detectable TSHR antibodies, therefore, suggesting for the permissive role of the DR3 allele in the pathogenesis of GD and production of thyroid-specific Abs. For the TSHR itself, genetic variations within the coding region of the TSH receptor gene, causing amino acid substitutions and altering sequence of immunogenic epitopes, could influence antigenic properties of the TSHR molecule. However, to date, no results, reporting how sequence alterations within the TSHR can affect immunoreactivity of the receptor, are available.

Both the D36H and P52T SNPs are situated in the extracellular TSHR domain, which harbor binding epitope(s) for TSHR-Abs. Functional analysis showed no relation of the D36H variant of the thyrotropin receptor to the TSH binding and cAMP formation, when expressed in NIH 3T3 cells [277]. For the other TSHR extracellular domain SNP, an enhanced cAMP accumulation was observed compared to the wild-type receptor, when the T52 variant was expressed in CHO cells [278]. However, this finding was not confirmed, when the P52T variant was expressed in other cells [279]. In addition, Cuddihy et al. [280] found two individuals with normal thyroid function who were homozygous for the T52 allele, suggesting that the altered receptor is able to respond normally to TSH with respect to the maintenance of the euthyroid state. Unfortunately, no immunologic studies were provided to verify whether the D36T and P52T molecular variants of the TSH receptor affect the binding between TSabs and the receptor molecule. Taking into account the fact that these polymorphisms are commonly detected in the general population, it would seem they represent simple polymorphisms and probably are not implicated in the pathogenesis of GD [214].

The D727E SNP, in the cytoplasmic tail of the TSHR molecule, might affect intracellular signal transduction. Gabriel at al. [281] showed that this molecular variant of the receptor is functionally relevant, and the E727 allele is associated with an increased cAMP responsiveness compared to that of the wild-type molecule, when expressed in COS-7 cells. However, this observation was not confirmed by further studies that did not reveal differences between the altered and wild type variants in relation to cAMP levels in TSH-stimulated thyroid cells [282, 283]. Meanwhile, since genetic analysis of a combined dataset from 3 different Caucasian populations showed a weak association between this polymorphism and GD [217], the codon 727 dimorphism maintained a chance to represent the etiological TSHR polymorphism for GD or be in LD with another disease-associated polymorphic marker.

To provide more details for understanding a role of TSHR on early stages of the pathogenesis of GD, further investigations of the physiological significance of TSHR cleavage and subunit shedding are required. The clarification of the role of extra-thyroidal TSHRs is needed, in particular their role in the maintenance of tolerance to the TSHR antigen in normal individuals.

The GD-2 Locus (chromosome 20q13) and the CD40 Gene

Genetic Linkage and Association Studies

The GD-2 susceptibility locus was first mapped on chromosome 20q11-q13 in a dataset of 56 multiplex US Caucasian families by Tomer et al. [284]. Interestingly, the locus showed strong linkage (MLS = 3.5) to GD only, but not to HT. Further fine mapping was enable to localize the susceptibility region within a 1-cM interval between markers D20S107 and D20S108 situated 55 and 56 cM apart from the p-terminus of chromosome 20, respectively [130]. Linkage analysis of the independent family dataset from the UK supported evidence for linkage with GD on chromosome 20q in the subset of families [285]. The GD-2 locus was confirmed in the expanded dataset of 102 multiplex families, with the most significant evidence for linkage in the subset of US Caucasian families of non-Italian origin (MLS = 3.3) [131,286].

The susceptibility locus harbors 17 known genes. Among those, the CD40 gene encoding an important immunomodulatory member of tumour necrosis factor receptor family is a likely candidate to be a GD susceptibility gene [287]. Sequencing of the human CD40 gene resulted in the identification of a C/T polymorphic substitution at position (-1) of the Kozak sequence of the gene. The C allele of the C/T SNP showed significant association (RR = 1.6) with GD in US Caucasians using 154 affected individuals and 118 controls [286]. The relationship of the CD40 Kozak dimorhism to GD, but not to HT, also was found in Koreans (132 affected patients and 164 normal controls), with significant association of the CC genotype with increased risk of the disease (OR = 1.93) [288].

However, studies in a large case-control sample (800 affected and 785 control subjects) from UK Caucasians failed to provide signifiacant evidence for association between the C/T CD40 SNP and GD [289,290]. Lack of association between the CD40 Kozak SNP and GD in the UK dataset is likely to suggest that the UK patients could represent a different phenotype of GD, and another unknown polymorphic marker within the CD40 gene can contribute to the pathogenic phenotype. A meta-analysis of all published data maintained a role of the CC genotype of CD40 in the pathogenesis of GD as a significant, but low-risk genetic factor (RR = 1.26) [291]. However, in the subgroup of GD patients, who was positive for thyroglobulin or thyroid peroxidase antibodies after treatment for GD, a carriage of the CC genotype was associated with significantly higher RR of 2.5 [291]. Taken together, these results strongly support that the CD40 gene can represent a susceptibility gene within the GD-2 locus.

Functional Analyses and Possible Mechanism of the Involvement of CD40 in the Pathogenesis of GD

Recently, Jacobson et al. [292] reported results of the functional evaluation of the CD40 Kozak SNP. An in vitro assay showed that the SNP affects CD40 expression on the translation level, but not on the transcription level. The C allele makes significantly more CD40 protein compared to the T allele [292]. Hence, this suggests that the C variant of the CD40 Kozak SNP could confer susceptibility to GD through increasing the translation efficiency of CD40 mRNA. In addition, GD patients carrying the C allele were reported to have higher TSHR antibody levels compared with those, carrying the T allele [288]. Therefore, this polymorphism also might contribute to the autoantibody production in GD patients.

The above results represent a strong evidence in favor of the involvement of the CD40 gene in the development of GD. CD40 is a tranmembraneous protein, which is expressed mainly in B cells, but also in monocytes, dendritic cells, epithelial cells and other cell types [293]. Thyroid follicular cells are known to be able coexpress both HLA-DRB1 molecules and CD40 in GD and hence aberrantly represent CD40 as an autoantigen [294]. CD40 binds to a CD40 ligand (CD40L or CD154) that is produced mainly on activated T cells. CD40-CD40L interaction plays a primary role in the induction of B cells to proliferate and produce immunoglobulins and rescue of B cells from apoptotic death and generation of B cell memory [293]. Therefore, CD40-CD40L-mediated signaling pathway is important in T cell-mediated immune responses and in the development of effector functions for many CD40-expressing cells.

Since the C/T polymorphism at the CD40 Kozak sequence may influence the ability of the ribosome to initiate translation and therefore increase CD40 expression levels, an excessive CD40 could overstimulate B lymphocytes and initiate GD. In vitro studies showed that extopic expression of a CD40L transgene in murine B cells causes overstimulation of murine B cells and induction of experimental SLE [295]. The overexpression of CD40 ligand is found in several immune-mediated disease, such as SLE, rheumatoid arthritis, multiple sclerosis, inflammatory bowel disease, allograf rejection and others [296]. Indeed, the CD40-CD40L interactions could represent a molecular trigger that switches towards either maintaining normal B cell function or inducing autoimmunity.

The role of CD40-CD154 in the development of Th2 type response, which plays a crucial role in inducing GD and several other autoimmune diseases, was shown in many studies. For example, anti-CD154 antibodies were shown to prevent Th1 type-mediated autoimmune disease, such as inflammatory bowel disease, by blocking IL-12 secretion and a mild up-regulation of IL-4 [297]. During co-stimulation of human T cells by anti-CD3, the administration of anti-CD154 antibodies was found to induce the production of Th2 type cytokines, such as IL-4 and IL-10 [296]. In monocytes from GD patients, T cell-dependent B-cell activation via a CD40 pathway resulted in the overproduction of IL-10 by mononuclear cells and a shift of the Th1/Th2 balance to Th2 dominance, a way that leads to the production of TSHR-stimulating antibodies and hyperthyroidism [298,299]. In the thyroid of GD patients, infiltrating lymphocytes coexist with thyroid epithelial cells expressing HLA-DR class II molecules and CD40 without visible apoptotic effects [300]. Reporting a lack of CD40 expression by thyrocytes from normal controls, Kie et al. [301] found a clear correlation between the expression of CD40 and the presense of lymphocyte infiltrates within the thyroid gland of GD pateints. Abberrant expression of CD40 and MHC class II antigen by thyroid cells can attract peripheral lymphocytes to infiltrate into the thyroid gland and initiate immune reponse [302]. As mentioned above, genetic analyses showed association between the CD40 gene and GD, a Th2 type-mediated autoimmune disease, but not with HT that is mediated by Th1 cells [130,288]. Therefore, this gene could represent the first defined susceptibility locus, which is specifically responsible for GD phenotype in thyroid autoimmunity.

CD40 antigen and its ligand (CD40L) were shown to play a major role in regulating both humoral and cellular immune responses [302]. The expression of CD40 was detected in the thymus that led to the hypothesis on a possible role of CD40 and its ligand in selection of the T cell respertoire [303]. This suggests for a therapeutic potential of CD40L-specific antibodies in prevention and early treatment of certain autoimmune disorders including GD. The antibodies are thought to act through the blockage of co-stimulation, confirming the important concept in immunology that antigen exposure in the absence of costimulation alters T-cell response leading to the development of tolerance [304].

Non-Defined Susceptibility Loci for GD

The GD-3 Locus (Chromosome Xq21) and a Phenomenon of Sex-Linked Predominance of GD

AITD is known to be up to 10 times more frequent in females compared to males [305]. To find a possible explanation of this phenomenon, chromosome X was screened for susceptibility to GD in the Caucasian AITD family dataset from the US. A susceptibility locus designated GD-3 was identified on chromosome Xq21 [130]. The maximum MLS value of 2.5 was obtained for marker DXS8020 located at position of 114 cM from the p-terminus of chromosome X [130,306]. However, this finding has not been later confirmed in the enlarged US family dataset [131]. A genetic study in the UK population revealed evidence for linkage on chromosome X but in another arm of this chromosome (Xp11), with a maximum NPL of 2.2 for marker DXS8083 [211], and in the region, where a T1D susceptibility locus was previously mapped [307]. So, the results of genetic linkage analyses for chromosome X are highly inconsistent and need further investigation.

There were no studies reported on the evaluation of the positional candidate genes on chromosome X for association to GD. One of the attractive positional candidate genes is the CD154 gene encoding CD40 ligand, which plays an important role in T cell costimulation [296]. The gene is located on chromosome Xq26.3 that is 36 Mb telomeric to DXS8020, a peak marker for GD-3 locus [308]. An increased serum level of soluble CD154 was reported several autoimmune diseases, such as SLE, RA, and Sjogren's disease, in correlation with the relevant autoantibodies and with the clinical disease severity [296]. Genetic variants of the CD154 gene have been reported to show association with SLE [55] and inflammatory Kawasaki disease [309]. Finally, CD40 ligand mediates costimulatory effects of CD40, which plays a crucial role in the pathogenesis of GD, as mentioned above.

If the increased AITD predominance in females could not be only explained by genetic background, it might results from the effects of sex steroid hormones in autoimmunity [310]. Meanwhile, genetic studies showed no association with GD for polymorphic markers of genes controlling metabolism and function of estrogens, such as CYP19 [306], ESR1 [216,311] and ESR2 [216,306,312]. In addition, functional studies on the influence of steroid hormones to thyroid autoimmunity provided conflicting results [310,313,314].

Fetal microchimerism was suggested to be another putative pathogenic mechanism, explaining sex-related predominance of AITD. The pregnancy is known to influence the course and severity of AITD, as evidenced by disease suppression during pregnancy and initiation, or exacerbation, of disease postpartum [315,316]. Fetal microchimerism represents transplacental passage of fetal cells followed by engraftment into maternal tissues, including thyroid gland, which could induce autoimmune response and therefore play a role in the pathogenesis of AITD (for more details, see recent reviews of Ando & Davies [317] and Sarkar & Miller [318]). This phenomenon was recently shown to be more frequent in mother-child pairs, carrying the susceptibility alleles HLA DQA1*0501-DQB1*0201 or DQB1*0301, and in the thyroid of mothers with sons [319]. An observation of maternal circulating cells in the fetus during pregnancy suggested an association of maternal HLA DQB1*0301 with microchimerism [320]. Therefore, immune reaction against microchimeric cells could be targeted on the immunogenetic basis of an HLA-restricted peptide/antigen recognition leading in some cases to cross-immunity against thyroid cells. The immunogenetic susceptibility markers, DQA1*0501-DQB1*0201 or DQB1*0301, would thereby enhance the likelihood of an immune reaction targeted in the thyroid, thus explaining the high risk in women with the predisposing HLA specificities of experiencing thyroid autoimmunity after childbirth. The exciting findings reported by Renne et al. [319] are based on the analysis a limited number of cases (n=49) and hence need to be extended to larger numbers to confirm these conclusions and elucidate the mechanism, by which microchimerism is linked to thyroid autoimmunity and immunogenetic risk. On the other hand, several population-based studies failed to show a significant relationship between the parity and AITD, that does not support a key pathogenic role for fetal microchimerism in chronic autoimmune thyroid disease [321-323]. However, fetal microchimerism can represent a pathogenic factor in specific AITD, such as postpartum thyroiditis and postpartum GD.

Genetic defects of the X chromosome (X cromosome monosomy or X-inactivation) may also constitute the pathological mechanism leading to female predominance in thyroid autoimmunity. The theory of X-inactivation was proposed by Stewart [324] to explain the phenomenon of X-inactivation antigenic mosaicism observed in SLE. X-inactivation in females results in the production of two classes of cells that differ in a subset of transcribed genes. One cell class transcribes those X-encoded genes inherited from the father while the other class transcribes those X-encoded genes inherited from the mother. Thus, the self-proteins expressed and presented by these cell types will also differ. If these two cell classes extend to the tolerizing cells of the thymus, some lymphocytes will, in theory, be tolerized by only one of the two self-antigen classes [325]. Such lymphocytes will be ignorant of the second antigenic class and thus may be autoreactive to self-antigens expressed solely by that second antigenic class. Recent studies showed that the frequency of X chromosome monosomy was significantly increased in peripheral white blood cells from women affected with systemic sclerosis, scleroderma and AITD, e.g., autoimmune diseases demonstrating strong predominance in females [326,327]. In addition, higher titres of autoantibodies, including those against thyroid-specific autoantigens, have been detected in patients with pathologies altering chromosome X, such as X-linked chronic granulomatous disease [328], Turner's syndrome [329], premature ovarian failure [330] and others. Finally, X-linked pathologies often cooccured with autoimmune diseases. For example, 83% women with an X-isochromosome, a phenotypic outcome of Turner's syndrome, are reported to be positive for Tabs, and 57% females with Turner's syndrome developed AITD [331]. Thus, abnormalities in chromosome X could represent a common mechanism for autoimmune diseases. Molecular mechanisms of the X-chromosome inactivation are not clear but can be initially associated with different patterns of DNA methylation that regulates gene expression [332].

The 5q31-q33 Locus

A genome-wide scan in 123 Japanese affected sib pairs found a suggestive linkage for AITD on chromosome 5q31-q33 [137]. The highest MLS was 3.14 for marker D5S436. The latest association study in 440 Japanese AITD patients and 218 controls using 6 microsatellites on chromosome 5q confirmed the susceptibility locus on 5q23-q33 [333]. The susceptibility locus on chromosome 5q was also replicated in a whole-genome screen of 54 Chinese Han multiplex GD pedigrees, with MLS of 4.12 for marker D52090 [334]. This region showed genetic linkage to several autoimmune and inflammatory diseases, such as MS [335], asthma [336], seasonal allergic rhinitis [337], Grohn's disease [338], atopic dermatitis [339] and celiac disease [340], therefore suggesting for the location of a common susceptibility gene for autoimmunity on chromosome 5q31-33. A number of genes located within this chromosomal region can be considered as positional candidates to represent the general succeptibility gene. These include the CARD15 and SLC22A4/SLC22A5 genes, encoding caspase-recruitment domain containing protein 15 and organic cation transporters, respectively, certain variants of which showed association with Grohn's disease [341-343], atopy [344] and psoriatic arthritis [345,346].

The 5q31-q33 locus contains a cytokine cluster gene, including IL-3, IL-4, IL-5, IL-9, IL-13, granulocyte-macrophage colony-stimulating factor (GM-CSF) and colony-stimulating factor-1 (CSF-1) [347]. Cytokine secretion profiles are considered to play a key role in triggering AITD as either Th1 responses, promoting the development of HT, or Th2 responses, leading to the pathogenesis of GD [348]. IL-4, IL-5 and IL-13 mediate the humoral immune response in Th2 pathway [349] and hence represent strong positional candidate genes for GD susceptibility on chromosome 5q31-q33. Case-control studies showed an association between GD and several nucleotide variations within these genes, such as C/T(-590) IL-4 in British Caucasians [350] and IL-13 polymorphisms (C/T(-1112) and Arg/Gln 130) in Japanese [351]. However, reevaluation of the C/T(-590) SNP of the IL-4 gene in the extended population sample (384 GD patients and 288 control subjects) from the UK did not replicate the association [352]. In addition, both IL-13 SNPs showed a lack of association with GD in UK patients [60]. These results could suggest for the strong genetic effects of the cytokine gene cluster 5q31 polymorphisms to the development of GD in Asian populations but not in Caucasians since the region of linkage to GD on chromosome 5q was mapped in

Asians only. However, disease-associated polymorphic markers within the IL-13 gene showed no relation to serum levels of thyroid hormone and Tabs, severity of disease and serum IgE levels [60,351]. To date, a GD susceptibility gene on chromosome 5q31 remains unclear. Additional studies are required to find this gene and the etiological and functionally active polymorphism within the gene, which actually predisposes to Graves' disease.

Other Loci

The AITD susceptibility locus on chromosome 18q21 was mapped in affected sib pairs from the UK, providing a maximum NPL score of 3.46 in the dataset of 81 AITD sib pairs and NPL score of 3.19 in the subset of 74 GD sib pairs for marker D18S487 [353]. Previously, this region showed a strong evidence for linkage to several autoimmune diseases, including T1D (IDDM6 locus) [354], RA [355] and SLE [356]. These findings provide evidence that this region is likely to harbor an important autoimmunity locus. A number of positional candidate genes are situated within the 18q21 susceptibility locus. Among them, the BCL2 gene, encoding an anti-apoptotic protein expressed in B lymphocytes [357], represents a strong candidate. Histological and biochemical data demonstrated the involvement of a Bcl2-dependent apoptotic process in determining the evolution of AITD towards either HT or GD, suggesting that increased levels of Bcl-2 should favor the thyrocyte survival and hyperfunction [358,359]. The Thr allele of the Ala/Thr43 polymorphism of bcl-2 was associated with lower risk of autoimmune pathology in Japanese [360]. In vitro studies showed that the inhibition of the programmed cell death function of 43Thr bcl-2 protein is suppressed compared with that of normal 43Ala bcl-2 protein, suggesting on a functional role of this SNP [360]. Genetic variations within the BCL2 gene need to be evaluated for association with GD. Another likely positional candidate gene is the deleted in colorectal carcinoma (DCC) gene, which also plays a role in apoptosis [361]. However, evaluation of the R201G amino acid substitution located in the extracellular immunoglobulin-like domain of DCC in a large cohort of individuals from New Zealand and UK affected with T1D, GD and RA showed lack of association with autoimmunity [362]. The 18q21 region also harbors the immunoglobulin-transcription factor-2 (ITF-2) gene, which encodes a regulatory protein, controlling expression of both heavy and light immunoglobulin chains, and hence can be another putative candidate gene [363].

A genome scan of a large multiplex Chinese-American family (27 members from three generations, six of whom were affected with GD and two had HT, resulted in the mapping of two new susceptibility loci on chromosome 9 and 11 [364]. For chromosome 9, a MLS of 2.01 and NPL of 7.5 were obtained for D9S175 located on 9q21. For chromosome 11, a peak marker D11S4191 was situated on 11q11, in the vicinity to centromere (MLS = 2.13; NPL = 6.1) [364]. Because these loci have not been previously found in Caucasians, these observations suggest that different susceptibility loci exist between different ethnic groups. Additionally, this also reflects genetic heterogeneity of AITD, when different genes contribute to similar phenotypes. To date, no positional candidate genes have been estimated in AITD susceptibility loci on chromosome 9 and 11. Among them, the 9q21 locus harbors two potential candidates, CD5 and CD6, encoding lymphocyte surface receptors of the scavenger receptor cysteine-rich superfamily, which show highly homologous extracellular regions [365]. Both molecules are expressed on the same lymphocyte populations (thymocytes, mature T cells, and B1a cells) and share similar co-stimulatory properties on mature T cells [366]. Increased levels of (CD5+)B lymphocytes producing Tabs were found in blood of patients with GD [367], supporting an evidence on the possible involvement of CD5 in the pathophysiology of GD. On chromosome 11q11, the BTEB-1 gene encoding basic transcription element binding protein 1, which functions as a transcription factor, could represent a candidate gene conferring susceptibility to GD. Interestingly, the expression of BTEB-1 is regulated by the thyroid hormone [368].

Ban et al. [138] reported finding of the region on chromosome 3q37, which showed linkage to AITD in the subset of 34 US Caucasian AITD families with HLA-DR3 positive probands. For D3S1580 on chromosome 3q27, a maximum two-point LOD score of 2.1 was shown [138]. Thus, this locus could contain an AITD susceptibility gene, the genetic effect of which is modulated by the HLA-DR3 allele. However, due to the relatively small size of the the dataset analysed (34 families), the power to detect linked loci was reduced, especially, for the dominant model and therefore needs to be increased through the analysis of additional number of affected families.

A second whole-genome scan in the US Caucasian AITD family dataset (102 families) found a new GD-specific susceptibility locus on chromosome 7q [131]. A maximum LOD score (2.3) was obtained for D7S502, a marker located on chromosome 7q11.1 close to the centromere. The new GD susceptibility locus overlaps with regions showing linkage with allergy [369] and imflammatory bowel disease [370], suggesting an evidence for the presence of a common susceptibility gene. No candidate genes on chromosome 7q11-q21 were tested yet. The suggested set of positional candidate genes includes a Kruppel-type zinc finger gene claster encoding various transcription factors. For one of them, ZNF92, a higher expression in T lymphoid cells was shown [371]. There are two chemokine genes, CCL24 and CCL26, which could be also considered as a likely candidate for susceptibility to GD. These genes encode proteins responsible for cell trafficking of eosinophils and probably involved in the development of allergy and asthma [372].

Common Genetic Background of GD and other Autoimmune Pathologies

Coexistence of GD with other Autoimmune Disorders

It is well recognized that both GD and HT are frequently found in the members of the same family, implying a shared genetic predisposition. Strieder et al. [322] reported 33% of Dutch AITD families, having documented cases of both Graves' disease and Hashimoto's thyroiditis. Approximately 8% of familial GD patients from Japan are found to have HT in their first-degree relatives [10]. Graves' disease is shown to coexist frequently with nonthyroid autoimmune pathologies. According to the data of the Japanese Nationwide Epidemiologic Survey 2001, a total of 12% of familial GD is accomplished with nonthyroid autoimmune and allergic disorders, including T1D (3% of cases), atopic dermatitis (3%), asthma (1%), RA (1%) and allergic dermatitis (1%) as the most common coexisting diseases [10]. The association between different autoimmune diseases could suggest for their common pathogenic mechanisms and shared susceptibility genes [373,374]. Although many putative disease associations have been suggested for AITD, the validity of these associations is not clear in all cases. Significance and reason between the disease associations are considered in the reviews of Jenkins & Weetman [375] and Szyper-Kravitz et al. [374]. It seems that cojunction between GD and other autoimmune diseases as a part of autoimmune polyglandular sydromes type 2 and 3 is not occasional but could be explained by common genetic background and similar etiological features. Among non-thyroid diseases, type 1 diabetes most often accompanies GD.

Shared Genetic Susceptibility between GD and T1D

Graves' disease and type 1 diabetes represent two of the most common autoimmune endocrinopathies. Both are organ-specific autoimmune diseases. These disorders often occur together. The prevalence of TAb in type 1 diabetic patients usually ranges between 20-30% [376-379]. Around a half of T1D patients with thyroid abnormalities further develop AITD [378,380,381]. On the other hand, 5-10% GD patients have anti-islet antibodies [382,383]. Since both pathologies demonstrate similar mechanisms of Tcell-mediated immune response through the infiltration of T lympocytes into the target organ (thyroid gland in GD and pancreatic islets in T1D) the etiology of T1D and GD (or AITD) may involve common genetic backgrounds. This could be also supported by the increased segregation of thyroid autoimmunity in diabetic families. Up to 36% of T1D probands were shown to have AITD (27% had HT and 9% had GD) [384]. The increased frequency of coexistent thyroid disease has been reported to present in 15.9% of parents with diabetes, and only 6.1% of parents without diabetes [385].

Common genetic markers for T1D and thyroid autoimmunity are extensively considered in several reviews [88,386] (see also Table 3). The role of the HLA region as a common susceptibility locus for a variety of autoimmune diseases is well established [387]. For T1D, the most common risk markers are the HLA-DR3 and HLA-DR4 alleles. Their frequency in diabetic Caucasians is up to 95% compared to 50% in controls, with RR of 9.8 and 8.3 for the DR3/DR3 and DR3/DR4 genotypes, respectively [388]. For GD, the predisposing allele is also DR3 but its contribution to genetic susceptibility for Graves' disease is much weaker than that for type 1 diabetes, providing RR of up to 5.7 [88]. In T1D, the etiological variant of HLA is the absence of aspartic acid at position 57 (non-Asp-57) of the DQβ chain [389]. The relative risk of T1D for individuals, who is homozygous for non-Asp-57, is 107. Later, the significance of the position 52 of the DQα chain for T1D susceptibility was also shown. The presence of arginine at this position (Arg-52) confers the increased risk to diabetes, but this risk is additive with the increased risk resulted from the absence of aspartate in codon 57 of the DQβ chain [390]. Thus, in Caucasians, the presence of non-Asp-57 in the DQβ chain and Arg-52 in the DQα chain permits a self-antigen to fit in the antigen-binding pocket inside the HLA molecule and to be recognized by the TcR. In GD, an importance of the position 74 of the DRB1β chain was recently shown, with the protective role of Gln-74 and predisposing effect of Arg-74 for development of the disease [153,154]. As in T1D, the presense of arginine-74 allows a self-antigen peptide to fit in the antigen-binding groove of the HLA class II molecule and initiate thyroid-specific autoimmune response [153].

Table 3. Inventory of susceptibility loci for GD and T1D.

Type 1 diabetes	Chromosome	Graves' disease
IDDM1/HLA (DR3)	6p21	HLA (DR3/DR4)
IDDM2/INS-VNTR	11p15.5	
IDDM3	15q26	
IDDM4/LRP5	11q13	
IDDM5/TAB2?	6q23-q24	
IDDM6	18q21	IDDM6 (D18S487)
IDDM7/BETA2/NeuroD1?	2q31	
IDDM8/PDCD2? IGF2R?	6q27-qter	
IDDM9	3q21-q11.2	
IDDM10	10p11.2-q11.2	
IDDM11	14q24.3-q31	
IDDM12/CTLA-4	2q33	CTLA-4
IDDM13/IGFBP5?	2q33-q36	
IDDM15	6q21	AITD-1
IDDM16/IgH?	14q32.3	
IDDMX	Xp11-p13	IDDMX (DXS8083)
PTNP22	1p13	PTNP22
VDR	12q12-q14	VDR
	1q21-q23	FCRL3?
CD25	10p15.1	
D16S520	16q22-q24	
D14S70	14q12-q21	
D19S247-D19S226	19p13-q13	
	14q31	GD-1/TSHR?
	20q11.2	GD-2/CD40
	Xq21	GD-3
IDDM18/IL12B 3'UTR	5q31-q33	D5S436/IL gene cluster?
	8q23-q24	Tg

Putative susceptibility genes are marked with a sign question.

Abberviations: AITD-1, autoimmune thyroid disease susceptibilty locus-1; BETA2/NeuroD1, basic helix–loop–helix transcription factor; CTLA-4, cytotoxic T lymphocyte associated antigen-4; FCRL3, Fc receptor-like 3; GD, Graves' disease susceptibility locus, HLA, Human Leucocyte Antigens; IDDM, type 1 diabetes susceptibility locus; IGFBP5, insulin-like growth factor binding protein-5; IGF2R, insulin-like growth factor II receptor; IgH, immunoglobulin heavy chain gene cluster; INS-VNTR, insulin variable number of tandem repeats; IL, interleukin; IL12B 3'UTR, 3'untranslated region of the interleukin-12B gene; LRP5, low-density lipoprotein receptor-related protein 5; PDCD2, programmed cell death 2; PTNP22, lymphoid protein tyrosine phosphatase; TAB2, TAK1-binding protein 2; Tg, thyroglobulin, TSHR, thyrotropin receptor; VDR, vitamin D receptor.

There are several population-based studies presenting results on the evaluation of a role of HLA in conferring susceptibility to both type 1 diabetes and AITD. In Germany, Tabs were more prevalent in the subset of patients with the predisposing DR3/DR4 genotype compared to other HLA allele variants [377]. In Czech Republic, elevated levels of Tabs were detected in T1D patients carrying the HLA-DQB1*0302 allele [391]. Studies in France and Japan found no differences in the distribution of HLA class II alleles between diabetic patients with and without AITD [392,393]. However, another study in Japanese population showed a higher prevalence of HLA-DR9, DQA1*0301 and DPB1*0501 in T1D subjects complicated with GD [394]. In Taiwanese, who had both diabetes and AITD, the DRB1*0405/DQA1*301/ DQB1*0401 haplotype was reported to be increased [395]. In Korea, a predisposive role of the HLA-DQB1*0401 allele for the development of thyroid autoimmunity was shown in patients with T1D [396].

Family-based genetic analyses provided more consistent results in determining common HLA markers for susceptibility for both T1D and AITD. Santamaria et al. [397] showed that diabetic subjects with the DQB1*0302 allele have a higher risk to develop GD. The susceptible role of the DR3 and DR4 allele was confirmed in other studies [84,398,399,400]. Levin et al. [400] dissected a role of these alleles showing that DR3 is the major HLA allele, contributing to the joint genetic susceptibility to T1D and AITD, whereas other alleles (e.g., DR4) are phenotype-specific. A subsequent study in the enlarged family dataset (55 families with AITD and T1D from the US) revealed that DR3-DQB1*0201 is the major HLA haplotype contributing to the shared susceptibility, with DR3 conferring most of the shared risk [401]. In the study of Golden et al. [401], the LOD score for HLA was highest for T1D alone, and when the AITD-affected individuals were added to the analysis, the LOD score decreased from 7.57 to 2.2. This decrease in LOD score shows that HLA contributes significantly less to the inherited susceptibility to AITD in T1D families. Therefore, other non-HLA genes must contribute to the strong familial clustering of T1D and AITD.

One of the non-HLA genes, sharing genetic susceptibility for diabetes and thyroid autoimmunity, is CTLA-4 [85,86]. In T1D, CTLA-4 represents a susceptibility gene within IDDM12 locus [74,402]. The association of the G(+49) allele of CTLA-4 with the increased risk of AITD in diabetic individuals was shown by several studies [111,403,404]. The CTLA-4 locus showed suggestive linkage with disease in the subset of US Caucasian families affected with both AITD and T1D (e.g., affected with APS2 - autoimmune polyglandular syndrome type 2), then providing an evidence for the contribution of CTLA-4 to both diabetes and AITD in the same individual [401]. Kemp et al. [405] reported an association between CTLA-4 and APS variant, in which the main components were vitiligo with AITD or T1D. A number of investigations reported an association between CTLA-4 and APS variant, containing Addison's disease in combination with T1D and/or AITD [83]. Therefore, it is likely that the CTLA-4 gene contributes to the expression of only certain APS variants.

As mentioned above, the main susceptibility region for GD in the CTLA-4 locus was mapped to the 6.1-kb region 3' of the CTLA-4 gene [68]. The G allele of the A/G +6230 CTLA-4 SNP was associated with a higher risk of the development of both GD and T1D, but the assocation of this allele with GD (OR = 1.45) was much stronger than that for T1D (OR = 1.15). Therefore, the influence of other etiological variants of CTLA-4, including polymorphisms on the 5'region of this gene, should be included into consideration in T1D [103]. The contribution of the CTLA-4 is estimated to explain 30-35% of family segregation of AITD that is significantly greater than its role in family clastering of T1D. In contrast, the

HLA region represents a major susceptibility locus for T1D, accounting for up to 45% of the family clustering of this disorder, while the genetic effect of HLA in the pathogenesis AITD is much weaker explaining only up to 15% of the family segregation of thyroid autoimmunity [88,406].

Evaluation of the variable number of tandem repeats (which is located 5' upstream of the insulin gene (INS-VNTR) and represents IDDM2 susceptibility locus for T1D) in 55 families of US Caucasians, in which AITD and T1D clustered, showed that, in addition to HLA, the INS-VNTR or a nearby gene in linkage disequilibrium may also contributes to the familial clustering of T1D and AITD [401]. However, IDDM2 locus showed no association with GD in UK Caucasians [407]. Lack of association analysis between the INS-VNTR and GD or MS was later confirmed in the analysis of a large population dataset of UK Caucasians (823 families with GD and MS, 1433 patients with GD and MS and 837 healthy controls) failed to show association, suggesting that this locus acts as a T1D-specific susceptibility gene rather than influences general autoimmunity [408].

Other IDDM loci, such as IDDM4 (chromosome 11q), IDDM5 (6q25) and IDDM8 (6q27), have been tested but showed no evidence for linkage or association with AITD [83,209]. IDDM6 locus (18q21) was found to be linked to GD in the UK population [353]. The 18q21 region also showed linkage to SLE and RA, suggesting that this locus can play a role in several forms of autoimmunity. AITD-1 locus located near but distinct from the HLA region could also contain a general autoimminity gene, because it overlaps with the susceptibility locus for T1D (IDDM15) [409] and SLE [410].

Thus, suggestive evidence for linkage was obtained only for the HLA region and likely for the CTLA-4 gene as loci, contributing to the shared genetic susceptibility to GD (and AITD) and type 1 diabetes. Association studies supported evidence for the CTLA-4 and HLA genes as common susceptibility genes for both diseases and, in addition, suggested a role in shared susceptibility for the vitamin D receptor (VDR) [411] and lymphoid thyrosine phoshatase (PTPN22) genes [412]. To date, more then 20 predisposing loci have been mapped for T1D in the human genome [413], whereas around 15 loci have been identified for GD and AITD [72] (Table 3). It is likely that some of these loci can be simultaneously involved in the pathogenesis of AITD and diabetes, such as IDDM6, IDDM15 and IDDMX, but remain undefined. This provides new perspectives for further discovery of common susceptibility loci for both diseases as well as search for genes responsible for general autoimmunity. Several recent findings enlarged a list of common susceptibility markers in autoimmunity and will be discussed below.

GD as a Part of Autoimmune Polyglandular Syndromes

Autoimmune polyglandular syndromes characterize by the coexistence of at least two endocrine gland insufficiencies that are based on autoimmune mechanisms. Associations with non-endocrine immune diseases may occur. Two major subtypes of APS, types I and 2, are distinguished according to age of presentation, characteristic patterns of disease combinations and different modes of inheritance [375]. APS1 includes coexistence of hypoparathyroidism (frequency 80-85%) with mucocutaneous candidiasis (frequency 70-80%), Addison's disease

(60-70%), T1D (less than 20%), hypogonadism (12%), AITD (10%) and non-endocrine autoimmune pathology, such as vitiligo, Sjogren's syndrome, myasthenia gravis, autoimmune hepatitis, autoimmune gastritis and some others [414]. APS2 contains combinations between thyroid disease (70-75%), T1D (50-60%), Addison's disease (40-50%) and hypoparathyroidism (less than 5%), with absence of candidasiasis and non-endocrine disorders [415]. A third subtype, APS3, was described in adults and, contrary to types 1 and 2, does not involve the adrenal cortex [416]. Besides the absence of adrenal failure, no clinical differences between types 2 and 3 were found. For genetics of polyglandular autoimmunity, see recent reviews by Robles et al. [417], Betterle et al. [418] and Simmonds & Gough [419].

Compared to APS2 and APS3, APS type 1 (or APECED – autoimmune polyendocrinopathy-candidiasis-ectodermal dystrophy) shows no association with the HLA region [420]. The gene for autoimmune regulator 1 (AIRE1) responsible for APS1 was mapped to chromosome 21q22.3 [421]. The AIRE1 gene is widely expressed in lymphoid tissues, adrenal cortex and thyroid [421]. A 13-bp deletion at nucleotide 964 in exon 8 is a common mutation that accounts for more than 70% of APECED alleles in a British population [422]. However, of 302 UK patients with GD tested, only one, who was heterozygous for this mutation, has been found [423]. In addition, a total of 139 Germans affected with GD was screened, and no of them were shown to contain this deletion [424]. It seems highly likely therefore the 13-bp deletion polymorphism of AIRE1 leads specifically to the development of APECED.

Since thyroid disease is the most frequent component of both APS2 and APS3, it is possible to expect that GD genetic markers can also contribute to the susceptibility to these polyendocrinopathies. Studies on HLA showed an association of the GD-predisposing DR3 and DR4 alleles with APS type 2 and type 3 [425-428]. The association of the DR4 allele with these syndromes could be attributed to its major role in conferring susceptibility to T1D, which is a significant component of both APS2 and APS3 [427,429]. However, a study in Norway reported the association between APS2 and DR3/DR4 independently from the presence of type 1 diabetes [430]. A role of another general susceptibility gene for autoimmunity, CTLA-4, in polyglandular autoimmunity is briefly discussed above, suggesting that this gene is likey to be important in the development of certain APS variants, such as combinations between Addison's disease with either GD or T1D [82,83], vitiligo with either AITD or T1D [405] and between AITD and diabetes [84].

The Vitamin D Receptor Gene as a Susceptibility Gene for General Autoimmunity

The VDR gene could be considered as another good candidate conferring general susceptibility to a variety of autoimmune diseases. The receptor plays a delivery role for vitamin D, which is crucial in regulation of multiple vital mechanisms, including inhibition of the proliferation of activated T lymphocytes, suppression of the expression of IL-2 and IFN-γ, induction of regulatory T cells, stimulation of the phagocytosis by macrophages and interference with apoptosis [431]. The administration of low dose of vitamin D significantly decreased the incidence of Tg-induced EAT in rats [432]. Contrary, vitamin D deficiency in early developmental stages was shown to accelerate experimental diabetes in NOD mice [433]. These observations therefore suggest a protective role of vitamin D in preventing autoimmunity against thyroid and pancreatic islets.

The VDR gene was mapped to chromosome 12q12-q14 [434]. Vitamin D receptor is expressed in a variety of tissues, including immune cells, and its expression in macrophages and activated CD4+ and CD8+ T lymphocytes is greatly stimulated by vitamin D [435], suggesting for significant influence of this vitamin on the function of the immune cells. Five common polymorphic markers have been previously described in the VDR gene: the FokI restriction fragment length polymorphism (RFLP) at the start codon of exon 2 (T/C2), BsmI- and ApaI-RFLPs (both in intron 8), TaqI-RFLP (T/C1055, exon 9) and a poly(A) polymorphism in the 3'UTR. To date, a high dense SNP map of the VDR gene, comprising 98 nucleotide substitutions, is available [436]. The reconstruction of haplotypes from the subset of 55 common SNPs revealed three blocks of LD. FokI-RFLP was not in LD with any other common SNP and, therefore, was not informative for capturing information from those SNPs. The three other SNPs (BsmI, ApaI and TaqI) were localized to block B and did not capture any information about SNPs in other blocks [436]. These common SNPs failed to show association with T1D in the recent study, using a large family and population datasets from UK, USA, Norway, Finland and Romania [436]. This conflicts with results of the study in German diabetic patients showing the association between the BsmI/ApaI/TaqI haplotype and disease [437]. In the study of Nejentsev et al. [436], a weak association with diabetes (OR = 1.07-1.14) was shown for three another SNPs, rs4303288, rs12721366 and rs2544043 located in introns 2 and 6 and the 3'UTR, respectively.

Poon et al. [438] measured LD between 12 SNP within the VDR gene, including common FokI, TaqI, BsmI and ApaI polymorphisms, and found two LD blocks. Block 1 was 5.8-kb long and located toward the 3' end of VDR, consisting TaqI, ApaI and BsmI SNPs, whereas the 8.4-kb block 2 was situated toward the 5' end of VDR. The two blocks were separated by 10.8 kb [438]. The block 1 corresponds to the block B, while the block 2 is roughly corresponds to the block C identified by Nejentsev et al. [436]. LD patterns indicated that associations between certain VDR variants, comprising extended haplotypes, and asthma/atopy occured across the two blocks within a 28-kb region of the VDR gene in the asthma family-based cohort from Canadian province of Quebec. The disease-associated haplotypes included alleles of TaqI, ApaI and BsmI markers [438]. Thus, haplotypes rather than individual SNPs could be responsible for the association of the VDR gene with different autommune disorders. Multiple associations described earlier on for particular SNPs of VDR, including those for GD [439,440,441] and Addison's disease [442], could be altered by environmental factor(s), influencing vitamin D levels and specific to certain groups of affected patients [443].

Among the disease-associated polymorphisms of the VDR gene, a functional relevance is described only for the polymorphic FokI site. The C allele of the FokI-RFLP abolishes the start codon, and translation starts further downstream. This results in producing of the more active VDR variant, which consists of 424 amino acids and is shorter of the T-allele encoded variant by 3 amino acids [444]. The FokI-site alters binding of the transcription factor IIB and therefore affects the transcription of the VDR gene. The altered VDR variant is found to modulate biological effects of vitamin D, such as inhibition of the cell growth of peripheral blood monocytes [445] and regulation of the intrabody calcium level [446]. Durrin et al. [447] failed to find functional polymorphisms at the 3'UTR of the VDR influencing stability of the mRNA transcript. Hence, additional studies are required to detect more functionally active variations within the VDR gene that should help to explain a role of this gene in conferring genetic susceptibility as well as to find etiological VDR variants responsible for certain autoimmune pathology.

The Lymphoid Protein Thyrosine Phospatase Gene, a Recently Discovered Susceptibility Gene for General Autoimmunity

The PTPN22 gene encoding lymphoid protein tyrosine phosphatase (LYP), a suppressor of T-cell activation, is likely to represent another gene involved in the control of general autoimmunity [448]. The role of the PTPN22 gene in the pathogenesis of autoimmune disease was recently discovered. The gene is located on chromosome 1p13, spans a genomic distance of 57 kb and consists of 21 exons [449]. LYP is expressed in lymphocytes. The enzyme contains a phophorylase domain on its N-terminus and through its most N-terminal proline-rich motif physically associates with the SH3 domain of the Csk kinase, an important suppressor of the Src family kinases Lck and Fyn, which mediate TCR signaling [450] (Fig. 3). LYP is among the most powerful inhibitors of T-cell activation. The suppressing effect is accomplished by dephosphorylation of TCR-associated kinases, like Lck, Fyn and ZAP-70 [450,451]. Dephosphorylation of ZAP-70 may be connected to the negative regulatory function of the c-Cbl proto-oncogene, as LYP forms a complex with c-Cbl [449].

A functional SNP, representing a cytosine-to-thymine substitution at nucleotide 1858 of the PTPN22 gene, was found [452]. This changes an arginine (CGC) to tryptophane (TGG) in codon 620. Bottini et al. [452] reported an association between the Trp620 variant with higher risk of T1D in the independent datasets from USA (OR = 1.83) and Sardinia (OR = 2.31). Functional analysis showed that LYP with tryptophane-620 is not able to bind to Csk, a protein substrate to be dephosphorylated, because the replacement of an arginine to tryptophane at position 620 disrupts its interaction with a tryptophane (Trp47) of Csk [452]. The finding of Bottini et al. [452] on the association between the PTPN22 R620W polymorphism and T1D was rapidly replicated in several studies [46,412,453-455].

The chromosomal region 11p13 showed evidence for linkage with SLE and RA in early genome-wide scans [410,456]. The evaluation of the PTPN22 gene found strong association between the codon 620 SNP and both autoimmune diseases [457-459], suggesting that this gene represents a SLE and RA susceptibility gene on chromosome 11p13. In addition, the PTN22 gene showed association with several other autoimmune disorders, such as GD [412,460,461], vitiligo [462] (Canton et al. in press), Addison's disease [460] and juvenile idiopathic arthritis [459,463]. Wu et al. [464] observed the increased frequency of the predisposing Trp620 allele in SLE patients with AITD, supporting evidence for the ability of this allele to modulate risk of the development of thyroid autoimmunity in individuals affected with SLE. Finally, recent investigations in the collection of 265 US families affected with various diseases, such as T1D, RA, SLE, HT, GD, juvenile RA, inflammatory bowel disease, MS, psoriasis and primary Sjogren syndrome, showed association of the W620 allele with the higher risk of first four of nine above disorders [465].

The above data strongly suggest that the PTN22 gene represents another, in addition to CTLA-4, non-HLA gene, which showed consistent association with various autoimmune diseases. Compared to CTLA-4, the genetic effect of PTPN22 seems to be stronger, since the W620 allele demonstrates OR values, ranging between 1.45 and 2.49 for different autoimmune diseases, while OR values for predisposing variants of CTLA-4 are usually less than 1.5 [465]. Since the PTPN22 gene shows association with both organ-specific and systemic autoimmune dieases, it clearly matches the suggestion on the general autoimmune disease susceptibility gene.

The R620W SNP of LYP is not likely to be the universal etiological variant fully explaining the association of the PTN22 locus with an autoimmune disorder. Carlton et al. [466] constructed a high dense map of 37 SNPs for this gene and derived extended haplotypes responsible for the association with RA in a cohort of 475 US patients and in the additional dataset of 661 individuals with RA. The Trp620 allele was a part of the extended haplotype and provided an OR value of 1.67, which was the highest among other polymorphic variants of PTPN22 [466]. When stratified for R620W, the association between RA and two new SNPs (rs1310182 and rs3789604), both located within putative transcription factor binding sites (PTFB), remained, suggesting for the potential predisposing role of these polymorphic markers independent of R620W. Further analysis revealed that these SNPs are not mutually independent risk factors and W620 and the rs3789604 risk allele together can explain the association observed between these three SNPs and RA, contributing into two major risk PTN22 haplotypes [466]. The rs3789604 SNP represents a cytosine-to-adenine substitution that lies 1496 bp downstream of PTPN22 in the PTFB at the 5' end of the round spermatid basic protein 1 (RSBN1) gene with unknown function. The minor risk allele of this SNP alters sequence of the PTFB for Pax-4, Pax-5, Nrf-1 and c-Myb transcrition factors. Among them, Pax-5 is shown to regulate translation specifically in B cells, and its deficiency leads to the convertion of B cells to other types of leukocytes, such as T cells, macrophages, granulocytes and natural killer cells [467]. The PTPN22 gene is a part the extended 300-kb LD block, which includes six other genes [466]. In addition, another causative SNP (rs3789604) associated with RA is actually located outside of PTPN22, in the promoter region of the RSBN1 gene. So, a possibility of the existence of other disease-associated SNPs, which are in LD with the above SNPs and could reside in PTPN22 or in other genes of the same haplotype block, cannot be excluded. Further dissection of the relationship between PTPN22 and susceptibility to autoimmune disease is required.

The Fc Receptor-Like 3 Gene as a Potential Candidate for a Common Autoimmunity Predisposing Gene

Recently, Kochi et al. [468] described a functional variant of the Fc receptor-like 3 (FCRL3) gene associated with several autoimmune pathologies, such as GD, HT, RA and SLE, in Japanese. The gene is located on chromosome 1q21-q23, a region, which harbors susceptibility loci for psoriasis [469] and MS [470], within a gene cluster of five functional genes, encoding Fc-like receptors 1-5, and a pseudogene for Fc-like receptor 4 [471]. FCRLs have high structural homologies with classical Fcγ receptors, binding the Fc portion of the immunoglobulin G [471]. However, ligands and function of FCRLs are not yet known.

Kochi et al. [468] found that all members of the FCRL gene family cluster on chromosome 11q23 lie in the 220-kb LD haplotype block and selected 41 common SNPs within the gene cluster. Case-control association test in 830 affected individuals and 658 controls showed strong association for four SNPs located at the promoter region (T/C(-169) and G/A(-110) markers), exon 2 (G/C+358 SNP) and intron 3 (G/A+1381 SNP) of the FCRL3 gene with RA. Minor alleles of these polymorphic sites were related to higher risk of the development of RA (OR 2.02 – 3.01) and constituted a common susceptible haplotype CACA. Among these SNPs, the FCRL3 (-169) promoter variant showed the most significant association with disease and, in addition, demonstrated functional activity in the luciferase gene reporter asssay [468]. The C(-169) variant was associated with higher promoter activity. The nucleotide variation at position –169 was shown to affect the predicted binding site for nuclear factor-kB (NF-kB), with higher matrix similarity for the disease-susceptible C(-169) variant. Further immunochemical experiments showed the ability of the FCRL promoter region to bind with NF-kB from nuclear extracts of Raji cells. Additionally, the carriage of the C/C genotype correlated with higher levels of RA-specific autoantibodies. Histochemical studies demonstrated that the expression of FCRL3 is higher in individuals with the disease-susceptible haplotype CACA [468]. The SNP at position –169 also showed strong association with other autoimmune diseases (GD, HT and SLE) in a Japanese population, with a total OR of 1.52 for all four forms of autoimminity. This polymorphism was associated with titers of SLE-specific Abs that were increased in patients homozygous for the predisposing C/C allele. Thus, higher expression of FCRL3 in B cells could be one of the pathogenic mechanisms, leading to RA, and the functional C/T(-169) SNP in the promoter of the FCRL3 gene can represent an etiological variant associated with autoimmunity [468].

Importance of B-cell hyperreactivity in autoimmunity and significance of B-cell blocking therapy was highlighted in the recent review by Hansen et al. [472]. Higher expression of FCRL3 in B lymphocytes under pathogenic conditions, associated with the contribution of the FCRL3 T/C(-169) molecular variant, might therefore provide a genetic basis for B-cell abnormality in autoimmunity. Although the precise function of FCRL3 is unknown, the higher expression of its mRNA was shown in the light zone of the human tonsil, where centrocytes undergo clonal selection and affinity maturation under control of positive or negative signal from antigen receptors and coreceptors [473,474]. The expression of FCRL3 in B cells is upregulated by CD40 [468]. This observation together with a recent finding of the functional GD-associated CD40 polymorphism, modulating translation of this antigen [291,292], provides new understanding of mechanisms of possible interaction between these regulatory proteins that can lead to autoimmunity. High expression of FCRL3 and augmented autoantibody production in individuals with the disease-predisposing genotype is consistent with the idea that FCRL3 influences the fate of B cells and augments the emergence of self-reactive cells in the germinal center of the tonsil [468]. However, to clarify this hypothesis, the knowledge on the precise function of FCRL3 is necessary. In addition, the exciting findings mentioned above were obtained only in Japanese and hence should be replicated in other populations.

Conclusion

The data presented above suggested that multiple genes confer susceptibility to Graves' disease (Fig.1). Some of these genes, such as CTLA-4, HLA, PTPN22, VDR and likely FCRL3, contrubute to general autoimmunity. Other genes, such as Tg, could underline thyroid specificity of AITD. Finally, CD40 and probably TSHR could be responsible for GD phenotype in thyroid autoimmunity. All genes, generally contributing to GD pathogenesis, function as important immune modulators, whereas genes, which determine the organ specificity of this disease, encode thyroid-specific proteins.

The evidence for a general role of most immune modulatory genes, implicating in GD susceptibility, in thyroid autoimmunity suggests that a breakdown in the mechanisms, maintaining peripheral tolerance, is a primary pathway that leads to the development GD, T1D and other autoimmune disorders [475]. Central tolerance to self-antigens results in thymic clonal deletion of self-reactive T cell [476]. However, some autoreactive T cells may escape this process, recognize peripheral autoantigens and subsequently provoke autoimmunity. Autoreactive T cells are normally present in all individuals, while autoimmune diseases affect only around 5% of the human population. This therefore suggests that peripheral tolerance must exist to control potentially pathogenic T lymphocytes [477]. Peripheral tolerance mechanisms include passive or activation-induced T and B cell apoptosis, anergy, ignorance, and suppression of autoreactivity by regulatory lymphocytes. Failure in immunoregulation is a key feature of autoimmune desease like AITD or T1D and hence highlights a role of the immune suppression, in which regulatory T cells (Treg) downregulate the activation and function of autoreactive T cells that escape other mechanisms of tolerance induction [478].

The general role CTLA-4 in conferring susceptibility to autoimmune diseases was finally established in 2003, when results of a large-scale population study of Ueda et al. [68] have been reported. The role of certain molecular variants of CTLA-4 in the breakage of peripheral tolerance, an initial stage of an autoimmune process, was suggested to be associated with CD4+ CD25+ Treg cells, which represent 5-10% of the CD4+ T lymphocytes in human and are able to express CTLA-4 constitutively [479,480]. In transgenic mouse models, these cells are generated in response to both systemic and tissue-specific self-antigens, but the induction is much stronger with the tissue antigen, suggesting for the exclusive role of Treg cells in maintaining peripheral tolerance to organ-specific cell antigens [481]. The accelerating autoimmunity status is often associated with decrease in the population of Treg cells. For example, depletion of CD4(+)CD25(+) Treg cells with anti-CD25 antibodies was shown to result in the increased susceptibility to thyroiditis [482] and arthritis severity in mice [483]. However, CTLA-4 and Treg are likely to act supplementary in the regulation of responses to self-antigen [484]. This suggestion is supported, for example, by observations showing the possibility to induce colitis in normal Balb/c mice only when CD25+ Treg were depleted and CTLA-4 was blocked but not either Treg depletion or CTLA-4 blockage alone [480]. It seems that a role of CTLA-4 in maintaining the tissue-restricted peripheral tolerance could be focused on the anergy-related mechanisms, e.g. increasing the activation threshold of T cells and preventing responses to the self-antigen [485,486].

HLA class II genes could contrubute to the pathogenesis of GD and AITD on the stage of the antigen presentation by APC and subsequent recognition of the complex between self-antigen and class II molecule by T lymphocytes (Fig. 6). A role of Tg and probably TSHR on this stage is likely to be sufficient, since both genes are thyroid-specific and encode major targets for binding autoantibodies in thyroid autoimmunity. Putative mechanism of the envolvement of predisposing HLA alleles in the development of GD is already discussed above and demonstrates many similarities with the way, by which the susceptibility HLA variants contribute into the pathogenesis of T1D.

The exciting role of a LYP molecular variant, a product of the PTPN22 gene, as a common risk factor for multiple autoimmune disorders was very recently shown, only in 2004 [448]. The contribution of PTPN22 could be crucial on the stage of the activation of self-reactive T lymphocytes, when a stimulating signal schedules through TcR-mediated signaling pathways into the cell (Fig. 3). The current information on human LYP is mainly based on our knowledge of its murine orthologue PEST-domain enriched thyrosine phospatase (PEP). The expression of both regulatory protein phospatases is obligatory to leukocytes, including T lymphocytes [487]. Within the cell, PEP is distributed near the plasma membrane, in the nucleus and other intracellular structures [488]. PEP plays a role in the negative regulation of signal delivery from TcR by dephosporylation of the activation loops of LCK, FYN and ZAP70 protein kinases [489]. PEP is more potent negative regulator for TcR signaling than SHP domain-containing protein phosphatase 1 (SHP-1) [451]. When associated with the SH3 domain of CSK protein kinase, REP is shown to phosphorylate the positive-regulatory Y394 and Y417 residues of LCK and FYN, respectively [451,489]. The association between LYP and CBL could mediate phosphorylation of ZAP-70 [449]. A negative role for PEP in TcR signaling was recently supported by studies in PEP-deficient mice, which showed the increased expansion and function of the effector/memory T cell pool associated with elevated serum antibody levels. The effector/memory T cells demonstrated enhanced activation of Lck [490]. The inactivation of the PTPN22 gene in Jurkat T cells using RNA interference, resulted in two-fold increase of the NF-kB-reporter response, confirming a suppressing function of LYP in TcR signaling [457]. The R620W amino acid change in LYP prevents LYP-mediated negative regulation of TcR signaling, which could be associated with non-controlled expansion and hyperactivity of self-reactive T lymphocytes [448].

In GD, the role of predisposing variants of CD40 and FCRL3 could be crucial in autoimmunity mediated by B cells after stimulation by T lymphocytes. Both CD40 and FCRL3 are shown to be among the regulatory factors, overexpression of which in B lymphocytes is associated with the breakdown of peripheral B-cell tolerance and induction of B cell hyperreactivity [468,491]. Activated CD4+ T helper cells are shown to prevent apoptosis of B cells via CD40 after interaction with CD40L present on the activated T cells [492-494]. Abnormalities in the CD40/CD40L signaling mechanism caused by overexpression of CD40 or CD40L could therefore help autoreactive B cells to escape from deletion in the thymus, bone marrow and periphery and induce clonal expansion and self-antibody production [495]. The finding of disease-associated functional polymorphisms within the CD40 and CD40L gene and in the FCRL3 gene (expression of which is regulated through the CD40/CD40L pathway), influencing expression of these genes, could explain pathogenic mechanisms, by which these genes contribute in autoimmunity [55,291,292,468].

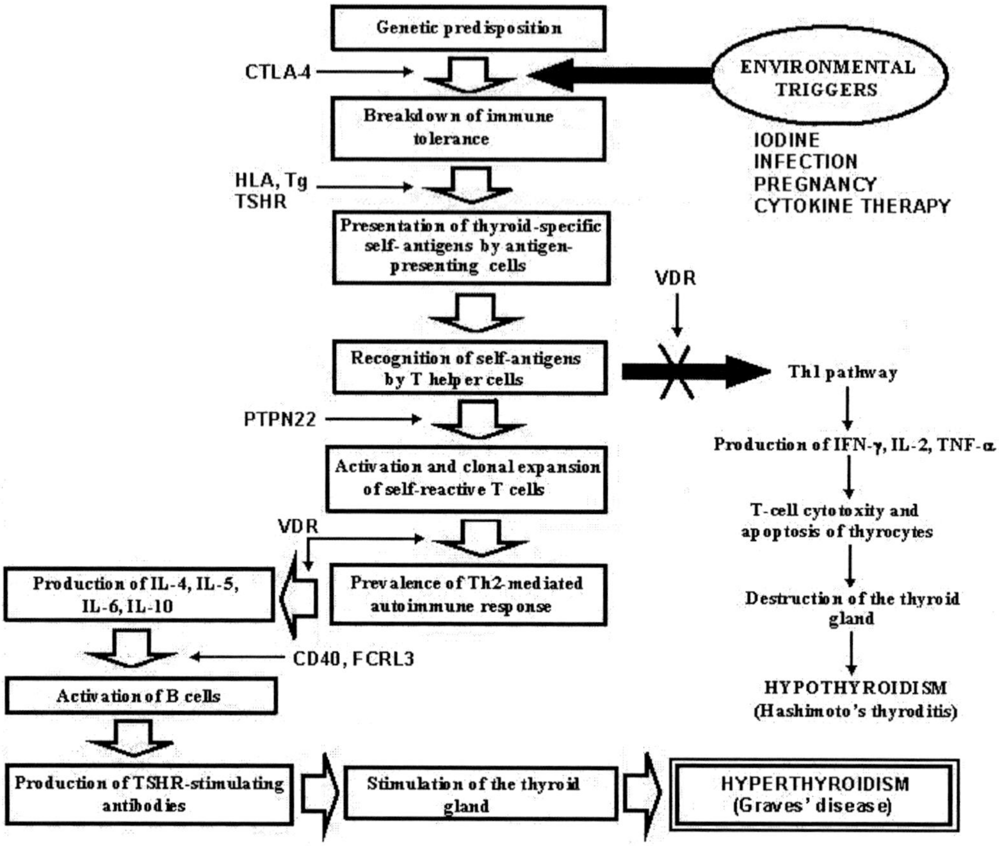

Fig. 6. Simplified scheme of Th1 and Th2-mediated pathways of the development of thyroid autoimmunity. Th1 pathway leads to clinical hyperthyroidism, e.g. to Graves' disease (GD), whereas Th2 pathway supports the development of hypothyroidism, e.g. Hashimoto's thyroiditis (HT). When the clinical presentation of autoimmune thyroid disease is switched toward GD, the alternative way, leading to HT, is suppressed through antiapoptotic mechanisms by activated T cells, cytokines and thyroid-stimulating antibodies, promoting thyrocyte survival. Predisposing variants of the susceptibility genes could contribute on different stages of the pathogenesis of GD. Putative sites of their implication in the pathogenic mechanism of GD are marked by narrow arrows. Abbreviations: CTLA-4, cytotoxic T lymphocyte associated antigen-4; FCRL3, Fc receptor-like 3; HLA, Human Leucocyte Antigens; IFN, interferon; IL, interleukin, PTPN22, lymphoid protein thyrosine phosphatase; Tg, thyroglobulin; TNF, tumour necrosis factor; TSHR, thyroid-stimulating hormone receptor; VDR, vitamin D receptor.

The CD40/CD40L signaling mediates B-cell differentiation and antibody production. The majority of antibodies in GD patients is shown to lie in IgG subclass [496]. CD40 initiates in B cells process of immunoglobulin isotype switching, but for which the specificity of the isotype is determined by cytokines. The cooperation between CD40/CD40L pathway and IL4/IL13 induce switch to IgE and IgG4, whereas IL-10 induces switch to IgG1 and IgG3 [497]. However, the presence of cis-acting response element(s) for CD40 ligation in γ1 heavy chain transgenes in mice suggest for possibility of direct effects of CD40 to the expression of immunoglobulines, which are rather modest but could be strengthened by synergic action of IL-4 [498]. The CD40/CD40L interaction is not only cooperates with Th2 type cytokines but causes their production in B lymphocytes, which may act as autocrine and paracrine growth and differentiation factors [497,499]. The envolvement of CD40 in the regulation of production of the Th2 panel of cytokines and interaction with their biological effects therefore explains, why this gene specifically contributes to GD susceptibility and suggests for a significant role of CD40 in switching thyroid autoimmunity to GD phenotype.

A metabolically active form of vitamin D, 1,25-dihydroxyvitamin D_3 (1,25-$(OH)_2D_3$), was shown to stimulate transforming growth factor TGFβ-1 and IL-4, both of which are anti-inflammatory Th2 type cytokines, and therefore support Th2 immune response with simultaneous suppression of Th1 proinflammatory response [500,501]. Additionally, vitamin D is able to prevent or markedly suppress such Th1-mediated autoimmune diseases as T1D, SLE, RA, both experimental autoimmune encephalomyelitis and thyroiditis and inflammatory bowel disease [501]. These findings suggest that vitamin D could also contribute in determining GD phenotype through stimulation of Th2 cytokine panel and direct suppression of the production of Th1 cytokines and cell apoptosis (Fig.6). This therefore could explain the most suitable role of the VDR gene, which mediates biological effects of vitamin D, in GD pathology. However, assuming a variety of biological effects of vitamin D, its involment (and therefore, contribution of its receptor) could be also sufficient in other stages of thyroid autoimmunity.

To date, a significant progress in the identification of susceptibility genes for GD was achieved. A total of 15 loci responsible for pathogenesis of GD and AITD have been mapped in different populations and a part of them was independently replicated (Fig. 1). Several susceptibility genes have been found and disease-associated functional variations within them were characterized, explaining contribution of these genes in the pathogenesis of thyroid autoimmunity. Although most of the susceptibility loci (about 10) remained undefined, it is possible to identify a susceptibility gene in each of them in the nearest future, due to the availability of the human whole genome sequence and visible progress in SNP discovery and haplotype structure analysis of the human genome in frames of the HapMap project [502]. The application of high dence SNP panels will help to found true disease-associated polymorphic functional variants of susceptibility genes and further characterize them using advanced molecular tools for functional analyses, including microarrays, RNA interference and others. This provides selection of new potential targets and determinants for early diagnostics of disease as well as for pharmaceutical and immunosuppressive therapy according to the principals of pharmacogenomics, the art of providing tailored pharmacological therapy with the highest therapeutic index based on the genomic composition of the individual [503]. Particularly, the discovery of predisposing genes, contributing in several autoimmune disorders, and detection of their molecular variants responsible for shared genetic susceptibility should help in the design of more universal approaches applicable to the prevention and treatment of a variety of autoimmune diseases.

REFERENCES

[1] Bradley, E.A. (2001). Graves ophthalmopathy. *Current Opinion in Ophthalmology, 12*, 347-351.

[2] Hollowell, J.G., Staehling, N.W., Flanders, W.D., Hannon, W.H., Gunter, E.W., Spencer, C.A. & Braverman, L.E. (2002). Serum TSH, T(4), and thyroid antibodies in the United States population (1988 to 1994): National Health and Nutrition Examination Survey (NHANES III). *Journal of Clinical Endocrinology and Metabolism, 87*, 489-499.

[3] Ai, J., Leonhardt, J.M. & Heymann, W.R. (2003). Autoimmune thyroid diseases: etiology, pathogenesis, and dermatologic manifestations. *Journal of American Academy of Dermatology, 48*, 641-662.

[4] Biondi, B., Palmieri, F.A., Klain, M., Schlumberger, M., Filetti, S. & Lombardi, G. (2005). Subclinical hyperthyroidism: clinical features and treatment options. *European Journal of Endocrinology, 152*, 1-9.

[5] Surks, M.I., Ortiz, E., Daniels, G.H., Sawin, C.T., Col, N.F., Cobin, R.H., Franklyn, J.A., Burman, K.D., Denke, M.A., Cooper, R.S. & Weissman, N.J. (2004). Subclinical thyroid disease. Scientific review and gidelines for diagnosis and management. *Journal of American Medical Association, 29*1, 228-238.

[6] Canaris, G.J., Manowitz, N.R., Mayor, G. & Ridgway, E.C. (2000). The Colorado thyroid disease prevalence study. *Archives of Internal Medicine, 160*, 526-534.

[7] Li, Y., Li., C. & Yin, H. (2000). A large scale epidemiological survey of Graves' disease in Daqing area. *Chinese Medical Journal, 113*, 31-34.

[8] Vanderpump, M.P., Tunbrigge, W.M., French, J.M., Appleton, D., Bates, D., Clark, F., Grimley Evans J., Hasan, D.M., Rodgers, H. & Tunbridge, F. (1995). The incidence of thyroid disorders in the community: a twenty-year follow-up of the Whickham Survey. *Clinical Endocrinology (Oxford), 43*, 55-68.

[9] Brownlie, B.E. & Wells, J.E. (1990). The epidemiology of thyrotoxicosis in New Zealand: incidence and geographical distribution in north Canterbury, 1983-1985. *Clinical Endocrinology (Oxford), 33*, 249-259.

[10] Akamizu, T., Nakamura, Y., Tamaoki, A., Inaba, Y., Amino, N. & Seino, Y. (2003). Prevalence and clinico-epidemiology of familial Graves' disease in Japan based on nationwide epidemiologic survey in 2001. *Endocrine Journal, 50*, 429-436.

[11] Yang, F., Teng, W., Shan, Z., Guan, H., Li, Y., Jin, Y., Hu, F., Shi, X., Tong, Y., Chen, W., Yuan, B., Wang, Z., Cui, B. & Yang, S. (2002). Epidemiological survey on the relationship between diffent iodine intakes and the prevalence of hyperthyroidism. *European Journal of Endocrinology, 146*, 613-618.

[12] Laurberg, P., Pedersen, K.M., Vestergaard, H. & Sigurdsson, G. (1991). High incidence of multinodular toxic goitre in the elderly population in a low iodine intake area vs. high incidence of Graves' disease in the young in a high iodine intake area: comparative surveys of thyrotoxicosis epidemiology in East-Jutland Denmark and Iceland. *Journal of Internal Medicine, 229*, 415-420.

[13] Stanbury, J.B., Ermans, A.E., Bourdoux, P., Todd, C., Oken, E., Tonglet, R., Vidor, G., Braverman, L.E. & Medeiros-Neto, G. (1998). Iodine-induced hyperthyroidism: occurrence and epidemiology. *Thyroid, 8*, 83-100.

[14] Berglund, J., Ericsson, U.B. & Hallengren, B. (1996). Increased incidence of thyrotoxicosis in Malmo during the years 1988-1990 as compared to the years 1970-1974. *Journal of Internal Medicine, 239*, 57-62.

[15] Wong, G.W. & Cheng. P.S. (2001). Increasing incidence of childhood Graves' disease in Hong Kong: a follow-up study. *Clinical Endocrinology, 54*, 547-550.

[16] Todd, C.H., Allain, T., Gomo, Z.A., Hasler, J.A., Ndiweni, M. & Oken, E. (1995). Increase in thyrotoxicosis associated with iodine supplements in Zimbabwe. *Lancet, 346*, 1563-1564.

[17] Mostbeck, A., Galvan, G., Baurer, P., Eber, O., Atefie, K., Dam, K., feichtinger, H., Fritzsche H., Haydl, H., Kohn, H., Konig, B., Koriska, K., Kroiss, A., Lind, P., Markt, B., Maschek, W., Pesl, H., Ramschak-Schwarzer, S., Riccabona, G., Stockhammer, M. & Zechmann, W. (1998). The incidence of hyperthyroidism in Austria from 1987 to 1995 before and after an increase in salt iodization in 1990. *European Journal of Nuclear Medicine, 25*, 367-374.

[18] Chopra, I.J., Solomon, D.H., Chopra, U., Yodhihara, E., Tersaki, P.L. & Smith, F. (1977). Abnormalities in thyroid function in relatives of patients with Graves' disease and Hashimoto's thyroiditis; lack of correlation with inheritance of HLA-B8. *Journal of Clinical Endocrinology and Metabolism, 45*, 45-54.

[19] Carey, C., Skosey, C., Pinnamaneni, K.M., Barsano, C.P. & DeGroot L.J. (1980). Thyroid abnormalities in children of parents who have Graves' disease: possible pre-Graves' disease. *Metabolism, 29*, 369-376.

[20] Burek, C.L., Hoffman, W.H. & Rose, N.R. (1982). The presence of thyroid autoantibodies in children and adolescens with AITD and their sublings and parents. *Clinical Immunology and Immunopathology, 25*, 395-404.

[21] Risch, N. (1990). Linkage strategies for genetically complex traits. II. The power of affected relative pairs. *American Journal of Human Genetics, 46*, 229-241.

[22] Stenszky, V., Kozma, L., Balasz, C., Rochlitz, S., Bear, J.C. & Farid, N.R. (1985). The genetics of Graves' disease: HLA and disease susceptibility. *Journal of Clinical Endocrinology and Metabolism, 61*, 735-740.

[23] Brix, T.H., Kyvik, K.O. & Hegelus, L. (1998). What is the evidence of genetic factors in the etiology of Graves' disease? A brief review. *Thyroid, 8*, 727-734.

[24] Villanueva, R., Greenberg, D.A., Davies, T.F. & Tomer, Y. (2003). Sibling recurrence risk in autoimmune thyroid disease. *Thyroid, 13*, 761-764.

[25] Brix, T.H., Christensen, K., Holm, N.V., Harvald, B. & Hegedus, L. (1998). A population-based study of Graves' diseases in Danish twins. *Clinical Endocrinology (Oxford), 48*, 397-400.

[26] Brix, T.H., Kyvik, K.O., Christensen, K., Hedegus, L. (2001). Evidence for a major role of heredity in Graves disease: a population-based study of two Danish twin cohorts. *Journal of Clinical Endocrinology and Metabolism, 86*, 930-934.

[27] Ringold, D.A., Nicoloff, J.T., Kesler, M., Davis, H., Hamilton, A. & Mack, T. (2002). Further evidence for a strong genetic influence on the development of autoimmune thyroid disease: the California twin study. *Thyroid, 12*, 647-653.

[28] Mikozami, T., Wu, L.A., El-Kaissi, S. & Wall, J.R. (2004). Stress and thyroid autoimmunity. *Thyroid, 14*, 1047-1055.

[29] Oppenheim, Y., Ban, Y. & Tomer, Y. (2004). Interferon induced autoimmune thyroid disease (AITD): a model for human autoimmunity. *Autoimmunity Reviews, 3*, 388-393.

[30] Prummel, M.F., Strieder, T. & Wiersinga, W.M. (2004). The environment and autoimmune thyroid diseases. *European Journal of Endocrinology, 150*, 605-618.

[31] Lazarus, J.H. (2005). Thyroid disorders associated with pregnancy: etiology, diagnosis, and management. *Treatments in Endocrinology, 4*, 31-41.

[32] Risch, N. (1990). Linkage strategies for genetically complex traits. I. Multilocus models. *American Journal of Human Genetics*, *46*, 222–228.

[33] Kruglyak, L. & Lander, E.S. (1995). High-resolution genetic mapping of complex traits. *American Journal of Human Genetics, 56*, 1212–1223.

[34] Falk, T. & Rubinstein, P. (1987). Haplotype relative risks: an easy reliable way to construct a proper control sample for risk calculations. *Annals of Human Genetics, 51*, 227–233.

[35] Terwilliger, J.D. & Ott, J. (1992). A haplotype-based "haplotype relative risk" approach to detecting allelic associations. *Human Heredity, 42*, 337–346.

[36] Spielman, R.S., McGinnis, R.E. & Ewens, W.J. (1993). Transmission test for linkage disequilibrium: The insulin gene region and insulin-dependent diabetes mellitus (IDDM). *American Journal of Human Genetics, 52*, 506–516.

[37] Risch, N. & Teng, J. (1998). The relative power of family-based and case-control designs for linkage disequilibrium studies of complex human diseases I. DNA pooling. *Genome Research, 8*, 1273–1288.

[38] Morton, N.E. (1955). Sequential tests for the detection of linkage. *American Journal of Human Genetics, 7*, 277–318.

[39] Durner, M., Vieland, V.J. & Greenberg, D.A. (1999). Further evidence for the increased power of LOD scores compared with nonparametric methods. *American Journal of Human Genetics, 64*, 281–289.

[40] Terwilliger, J.D. & Ott, J. (1994). Handbook of Human Genetic Linkage. Baltimore: Johns Hopkins University Press.

[41] McCarthy, M.I., Kruglyak, L. & Lander, E.S. (1998). Sib-pair collection strategies for complex diseases. *Genetic Epidemiology, 15*, 317–340.

[42] Bishop, D.T. & Williamson, J.A. (1990). The power of identity-by-state methods for linkage analysis. *American Journal of Human Genetics, 46*, 254–265.

[43] Kruglyak, L. & Lander, E.S. (1995) Complete multipoint sib-pair analysis of qualitative and quantitative traits. *American Journal of Human Genetics, 57*, 439–454.

[44] Lander, E. & Kruglyak, L. (1995). Genetic dissection of complex traits: guidelines for interpreting and reporting linkage results. *Nature Genetics, 11*, 241–247.

[45] Kruglyak, L., Daly, M.J., Reeve Daly, M.P. & Lander, E.S. (1996). Parametric and nonparametric linkage analysis: a unified multipoint approach. *American Journal of Human Genetics, 58*, 1347–1363.

[46] Onengut-Gumuscu, S., Ewens, K.G., Spielman, R.S. & Concannon, P. (2004). A functional polymorphism (1858C/T) in the PTPN22 gene is linked and associated with type I diabetes in multiplex families. *Genes and Immunity, 5*, 678-680.

[47] Brookes, A.J. (1999). The essense of SNPs. *Gene, 234*, 177-186.

[48] Hodge, S.E. (1994). What association analysis can and cannot tell us about the genetic of complex disease. *American Journal of Medical Genetics, 54*, 318-323.

[49] Wall, J.D. & Pritchard, J.K. (2003). Haplotype blocks and linkage disequilibrium in the human genome. *Nature Reviews Genetics, 4*, 587-597.

[50] Deloukas, P. & Bentley, D. (2004). The HapMap project and its application to genetic studies of drug response. *Pharmacogenomics Journal, 4*, 88-90.

[51] Johnson, G.C., Esposito, L., Barratt, B.J., Heward, J., Di Genova, G., Ueda, H., Cordell, H.J., Eaves, I.A., Dudbridge, F., Twells, R.C., Payne, F., Hughes, W., Nutland, S., Stevens, H., Carr, P., Tuomilehto-Wolf, E., Tuomilehto, J., Gough, S.C., Clayton, D.G. & Todd, J.A. (2001). Haplotype tagging for the identification of common disease genes. *Nature Genetics, 29*, 233-237.

[52] Cardon, L.R. & Abecasis, G.R. (2003). Using haplotype blocks to map human complex trait loci. *Trends in Genetics, 19*, 135-140.

[53] Clark, A.G. (2004). The role of haplotypes in candidate gene studies. *Genetic Epidemiology, 27*, 321-333.

[54] Martin, E.R., Lai, E.H., Gilbert, J.R., Rogala, A.R., Afshari, A.J., Riley, J., Finch, K.L., Stevens, J.F., Livak, K.J., Slotteebeck, B.D., Slifter, S.H., Warren, L.L., Conneally, P.M., Schmechel, D.E., Purvis, I., Pericak-Vance, M.A., Roses, A.D. & Vance, J.M. (2001). SNPing away at complex diseases: analysis of single-nucleotide polymorphisms around APOE in Alzheimer disease. *Nature Genetics, 29*, 233-237.

[55] Citores, M.J., Rua-Figueroa, I., Rodriguez-Gallego, C., Durantez, A., Garcia-Laorden, M.I., Rodriguez-Lozano, C., Rogriguez-Perez, J.C., Vargas, J.A. & Perez-Aciego, P. (2004). The dinucleotide repeat polymorphism in the 3'UTR of the CD154 gene has a functional role on protein expression and is associated with systemic lupus erythematosus. *Annals of Rheumatic Diseases, 63*, 310-317.

[56] Ogura, Y., Bonen, D.K., Inohara, N., Nicolae, D.L., Chen, F.F., Ramos, R., Britton, H., Moran, T., Karaliuskas, R., Duerr, R.H., Achkar, J.P., Brant, S.R., Bayless, T.M., Kirschner, B.S., Hanaurer, S.B., Nunez, G. & Cho, J.H. (2001). A frameshift mutation in NOD2 associated with susceptibility to Crohn's disease. *Nature, 411*, 603-606.

[57] Ross, J.S., Schenkein, D.P., Kashala, O., Linette, G.P., Stec, J., Symmans, W.F., Pusztai L. & Hortobagyj G.N. (2004). Pharmacogenomics. *Advances in Anatomic Pathology, 11*, 211-220.

[58] Weetman, A.P. & McGregor, A.M. (1994) Autoimmune thyroid disease: further developments in our understanding. *Endocrine Reviews, 15*, 788-830.

[59] Kinjo, Y., Takasu, N., Komiya, I., Tomoyose, T., Takara, M., Kouki, T., Shimajiri, Y., Yabiku, K. & Yoshimura, H. (2002). Remission of Graves' hyperthyroidism and A/G polymorphism at position 49 in exon 1 of cytotoxic T lymphocyte-associated molecule-4 gene. *Journal of Clinical Endocrinology and Metabolism, 87*, 2593-2596.

[60] Bernardczuk, T. Placha, G. Jazdewski, K., Kurylowicz, A., Kloza, M., Makowska, U., Hiromatsu, Y. & Nauman, J (2003). Interleukin-13 gene polymorphisms in patients with Graves' disease. *Clinical Endocrinology (Oxford), 59*, 519-525.

[61] Fukutani, T., Horomatsu, Y., Kaku, H., Miyake, I., Mikai, T., Imammura, Y., Kohno, S., Takane, N., Shoji, S., Otabe, S. & Yamada, K. (2004). A polymorphism of interferon-gamma gene associated with changes of anti-thyrotropin receptor antibodies induced by antithyroid drug treatment for Graves' disease in Japanese patients. *Thyroid, 14*, 93-97.

[62] Wang, P.W., Liu, R.T., Juo, S.H., Wang, S.T., Hu, Y.H., Hsieh, C.J., Chen, M.H., Chen, I.Y. Wu, C.L. (2004). Cytotoxic T lymphocyte-associated molecule-4 polymorphism and relapse of Graves' hyperthyroidism after antithyroid withdrawal. *Journal of Clinical Endocrinology and Metabolism, 89*, 169-173.

[63] Pauli-Magnus, C. & Kroetz, D.L. (2004). Functional implications of genetic polymorphisms in the multidrug resistance gene MDR1 (ABCB1). *Pharmaceutical Research, 21*, 904-913.

[64] Vaidya, B., Imrie, H., Perros, P., Young, E.T., Kelly, W.F., Carr, D., Large, D.M., Toft, A.D., McCarty, M.I., Kendall-Taylor, P. & Pearce, S.H. (1999). The cytotoxic T lymphocyte antigen-4 is a major Graves' disease locus. *Human Molecular Genetics, 8*, 1195-1199.

[65] Tomer, Y., Greenberg, D.A., Barbesino, G., Concepcion, E. & Davies, T.F. (2001) CTLA-4 and not CD28 is a susceptibility gene for thyroid autoantibody production. *Journal of Clinical Endocrinology and Metabolism, 86*, 1687-1693.

[66] Ling, V., Wu, P.W., Finnerty, H.F., Agostino, M.J., Graham, J.R., Chen, S., Jussiff, J.M., Fisk, G.J., Miller, C.P. & Collins, M. (2001) Assembly and annoptation of human chromosome 2q33 sequence containing the CD28, CTLA4, and ICOS gene cluster: analaysis by computational, comparative, and microarray approaches. *Genomics, 78*, 155-168.

[67] Ban, Y., Davies, T.F., Greenberg, D.A., Kissin, A., Marder, B., Murphy, B., Concepcion, E.S., Villanueva, R.B., Barbesino, G., Ling, V. & Tomer, Y. (2003). Analysis of the CTLA-4, CD28, and inducible costimulator (ICOS) genes in autoimmune thyroid disease. *Genes and Immunity, 4*, 586-593.

[68] Ueda, H., Howson, J.M., Esposito, L.,Heward, J., Snook, H., Chamberlain, G., Rainbow, D.B., Hunter, K.M., Smith, A.N., Di Genova, G., Herr, M.H., Dahlman, I., Payne, F., Smyth, D., Lowe, C., Twells, R.C., Howlett, S., Healy, B., Nutland, S., Rance, H.E., Everett, V., Smink, L.J., Lam, A.C., Cordell, H.J., Walker, N.M., Bordin, C., Hulme, J., Motzo, C., Cucca, F., Hess, J.F., Metzker, M.L., Rogers, J., Gregory, S., Allahabadia, A., Nithiyananthan, R., Tuomilehto-Wolf, E., Tuomilehto, J., Bingley, P., Gillespie, K.M., Undlien, D.E., Roningen, K.S., Guja, C., Ionescu-Tirgoviste, C., Savage, D.A., Maxwell, A.P., Carson D.J., Patterson, C.C., Franklyn, J.A., Clayton, D.G., Peterson, L.B., Wicker, L.S., Todd, J.A. & Gough, S.C. (2003). Association of the T-cell regulatory gene CTLA4 with susceptibility to autoimmune disease. *Nature, 423*, 506-511.

[69] Chistiakov, D.A. & Turakulov. R.I. (2003). CTLA-4 and its role in autoimmune thyroid disease. *Journal of Molecular Endocrinology, 31*, 21-36.

[70] Tomer, Y. & Davies, T.F. (2003). Searching for the autoimmune thyroid disease susceptibility genes: from gene mapping to gene function. *Endocrine Reviews, 24*, 694-717.

[71] Simmonds, M.J. & Gough, S.C.L. (2004). Unravelling the genetic complexity of autoimmune thyroid disease: HLA, CTLA-4 and beyond. *Clinical and Experimental Immunology, 136*, 1-10.

[72] Ban, Y. & Tomer, Y. (2005) Susceptibility genes in thyroid autoimmunity. *Clinical and Developmental Immunology. 12*, 47-58.

[73] Ban, Y., Concepcion, E.S., Villanueva, R., Greenberg, D.A., Davies, T.F. & Tomer, Y. (2004) Analysis of immune regulatory genes in familial and sporadic Graves' disease. *Journal of Clinical Endocrinology and Metabolism, 89*, 4562-4568.

[74] Marron, M.P., Raffel, L.J., Garchon, H.J., Jacob, C.O., Serrano-Rios, M., Martinez Larrad, M.T., Teng, W.P., Park, Y., Zhang, Z.X., Goldstein, D.R., Tao, Y.W., Baaurain, G., Bach, J.F., Huang, H.S., Luo, D.F., Zeidler, A., Rotter, J.I., Yang, M.C., Modilevsky, T., Maclaren, N.K. & She, J.X. (1997). Insulin-dependent diabetes mellitus (IDDM) is associated with CTLA4 polymorphisms in multiple ethnic groups. *Human Molecular Genetics, 6*, 1275-1282.

[75] Djilali-Saiah I, Schmitz J., Harfouch-Hammond E., Mougenot, J.F., Bach, J.F. & Caillat-Zucman, S. (1998). CTLA-4 gene polymorphism is associated with predisposition to coeliac disease. *Gut, 43*, 187-189.

[76] Harbo, H.F., Celius, E.G., Vartdal, F. & Spurkland, A. (1999). CTLA-4 promoter and exon 1 dimorphisms in multiple sclerosis. *Tissue Antigens,* 1999, 53, 106-110.

[77] Lee, Y.H., Harley, J.B. & Nath, S.K. (2005). CTLA-4 polymorphisms and systemic lupus erythematosus (SLE): a meta-analysis. *Human Genetics, 116*, 361-367.

[78] Seidl, C., Donner, H., Fischer, B., Usadel, K.H., Seifried, E., Kaltwasser, J.P. & Badenhoop, K. (1998). CTLA4 codon 17 dimorphism in patients with rheumatoid arthritis. *Tissue Antigens, 51*, 62-66.

[79] Vaidya, B., Pearce, S.H., Charlton, S., Marshall, N., Rowan, A.D., Griffiths, I.D., Kendall-Taylor, P., Cawston, T.E. & Young-Min, S. (2002). An association between the CTLA4 exon 1 polymorphism and early rheumatoid arthritis with autoimmune endocrinopathies. *Rheumatology (Oxford), 41*, 180-183.

[80] Agarwal, K., Jones, A.K., Daly, A.K., James, O.F., Vaidya, B., Pearce, S. & Bassendine, M.F. (2000). CTLA-4 gene polymorphism confers susceptibility to primary biliary cirrhosis. *Journal of Hepatology, 32*, 538-541.

[81] Donner, H., Braun, J., Seidl, C., Rau, H., Finke, R., Ventz, M., Walfish, P.G., Usadel, K.H. & Badenhoop, K. (1997a). Codon 17 polymorphism of the cytotoxic T lymphocyte antigen 4 gene in Hashimoto's thyroiditis and Addison's disease. *Journal of Clinical Endocrinology and Metabolism, 82*, 4130-4132.

[82] Kemp, E.H., Ajjan, R.A., Husebye, E.S., Peterson, P., Uibo, R., Imrie, H., Pearce, S.H., Watson, P.F. & Weetman, A.P. (1998) A cytotoxic T lymphocyte antigen-4 (CTLA-4) gene polymorphism is associated with autoimmune Addison's disease in English patients. *Clinical Endocrinology (Oxford), 49*, 609-613.

[83] Vaidya, B., Imrie, H., Geatch, D.R., Perros, P., Ball, S.G., Baylis, P.H., Carr, D., Hurel, S.J., James, R.A., Kelly, W.F., Kemp, E.H., Young, E.T., Weetman, A.P., Kendall-

Taylor, P. & Pearce, S.H. (2000) Association analysis of the cytotoxic T lymphocyte antigen-4 (CTLA-4) and autoimmune regulator-1 (AIRE-1) genes in sporadic autoimmune Addison's disease. *Journal of Clinical Endocrinology and Metabolism, 85*, 688-689.

[84] Einarsdottir, E., Soderstrom, I., Logfren-Burstrom, A., Haraldsson, S., Nillson-Qrdnor, S., Penha-Goncalves, C., Lind, L., Holmgren, G., Holmsberg, M., Asplund, K. & Holmsberg, D. (2003). The CTLA4 region as a general autoimmunity factor: an extended pedigree provides evidence for synergy with the HLA locus in the etiology of type 1 diabetes mellitus, Hashimoto's thyroiditis and Graves' disease. *European Journal of Human Genetics, 11*, 81-84.

[85] Kristiansen, O.P., Larsen, Z.M. & Pociot, F. (2000). CTLA-4 in autoimmune diseases - a general susceptibility gene to autoimmunity? *Genes and Immunity, 1*, 170-184.

[86] Vaidya, B. & Pearce, S. (2004). The emerging role of the CTLA-4 gene in autoimmune endocrinopathies. *European Journal of Endocrinology, 1*50, 619-626.

[87] Holmberg, D., Cilio, C.M., Lindholm, M. & Motta, V. (2005). CTLA-4 (CD-152) and its involvement in autoimmune disease. *Autoimmunity, 38*, 225-233.

[88] Levin, L. & Tomer, Y. (2003). The etiology of autoimmune diabetes and thyroiditis: evidence for common genetic susceptibility. *Autoimmunity Reviews, 2*, 377-386.

[89] Oaks, M.K. & Hallett, K.M. (2000). Cutting edge: a soluble form of CTLA-4 in patients with autoimmune thyroid disease. *Journal of Immunology, 164*, 568-572.

[90] Liu, M.F., Wang, C.R., Chen, P.C. & Fung, L.L. (2003). Increased expression of soluble cytotoxic T-lymphocyte-associated antigen-4 molecule in patients with systemic lupus erythematosus. *Scandinavian Journal of Immunology, 57*, 568-572.

[91] Wong, C.K., Lit, L.C., Tam, L.S., Li, E.K. & Lam, C.W. (2005). Aberrant production of soluble costimulatory molecules CTLA-4, CD28, CD80 and CD86 in patients with systemic lupus erythematosus. *Rheumatology (Oxford), 44*, 989-994.

[92] Sato, S., Fujimoto, M., Hasegawa, M., Komura, K., Yanaba, K., Hayakawa, I., Matsushita, T. & Takehara, K. (2004). Serum soluble CTLA-4 levels are increased in diffuse cutaneous systemic sclerosis. *Rheumatology (Oxford), 43*, 1261-1266.

[93] Ip, W.K., Wong, C.K., Leung, T.F. & Lam, C.W. (2005). Elevation of plasma soluble T cell costimulatory molecules CTLA-4, CD28 and CD80 in children with allergic asthma. *International Archives of Allergy and Immunology, 137*, 45-52.

[94] Holopainen, P.M. & Partanen, J.A. (2001). Technical note: linkage disequilibrium and disease-associated CTLA4 polymorphisms. *Jounal of Immunology, 167*, 2457-2458.

[95] Kouki, T., Sawai, Y., Gardine, C.A., Fisfalen, M.E., Alegre, M.L. & Degroot, L.J. (2000). CTLA-4 gene polymorphism at position 49 in exon 1 reduces the inhibotory function of CTLAS-4 and contributes to the pathogenesis of Graves' disease. *Journal of Immunology, 165,* 6606-6611.

[96] Maurer, M., Loserth, S., Kolb-Maurer, A., Ponath,. A., Wiese, S., Kruse, N. & Rieckmann, P. (2002). A polymorphism in the human cytotoxic T-lymphocyte antigen 4 (CTLA4) gene (exon 1 +49) alters T-cell activation. *Immunogenetics, 54*, 1-8.

[97] Zaletel, K., Krhin, B., Gaberscek, S., Pirnat, E. & Hojker, S. (2002). The influence of the exon 1 polymorphism of the cytotoxic T lymphocyte antigen 4 gene on thyroid

antibody production in patients with newly diagnosed Graves' disease. *Thyroid, 12*, 373-376.

[98] Anjos, S., Nguyen, A., Ounissi-Benhalha, H., Tessier, M.H. & Polychronakos, C. (2002). A common autoimmunity predisposing signal peptide variant of the cytotoxic T-lymphocyte antigen 4 results in inefficient glycosylation of the susceptibility allele. *Journal of Biological Chemistry, 277*, 46478-46486.

[99] Badenhoop, K. & Seidl, C. (2003). Fine-tuning of T lymphocytes in autoimmunity: genetic association of CTLA-4 variants and Graves disease revisited. *Clinical Endocrinology (Oxford), 59*, 555-557.

[100] Anjos, S. & Polychronakos, C. (2004). Mechanisms of genetic susceptibility to type I diabetes: beyond HLA. *Molecular Genetics and Metabolism, 81*, 187-195.

[101] Ligers, A., Teleshova, N. , Masterman, T., Huang, W.X. & Hillert J. (2001). CTLA-4 gene expression is influenced by promoter and exon 1 polymorphisms. *Genes and Immunity, 2*, 145-152.

[102] Wang, X.B., Zhao, X., Giscombe, R. & Lefvert, A.K. (2002). A CTLA-4 gene polymorphism at position -318 in the promoter region affects the expression of protein. *Genes and Immunity, 3*, 233-234.

[103] Anjos, S.M., Tessier, M.C. & Polychronakos, C. (2004). Association of the cytotoxic T lymphocyte-associated antigen 4 gene with type 1 diabetes: evidence for independent effects of two polymorphisms on the same haplotype block. *Journal of Clinical Endocrinology and Metabolism, 89*, 6257-6265.

[104] Perkins, D., Wang, Z., Donovan, C., He, H., Mark, D., Guan, G., Wang, Y., Walunas, T., Bluestone, J., Listman, J. & Finn, P.W. (1996). Regulation of CTLA-4 expression during T cell activation. *Journal of Immunology, 156*, 4154-4159.

[105] Ling, V., Wu, P.W., Finnerty, H.F., Sharpe, A.H., Gray, G.S. & Collins, M. (1999). Complete sequence determination of the mouse and human CTLA4 gene loci: cross-species DNA sequence similarity beyond exon borders. *Genomics, 60*, 341–355.

[106] Lindsten, T., Lee, K.P., Harris, E.S., Petryniak, B., Craighead, N., Reynolds, P.J., Lombard, D.B., Freeman, G.J., Nadler, L.M. & Gray, G.S. (1993). Characterization of CTLA-4 structure and expression on human T cells. *Journal of Immunology, 151*, 3489–3499

[107] Chen, C.Y. & Shyu, A.B. (1995). AU-rich elements: characterization and importance in mRNA degradation. *Trends in Biochemical Sciences, 20*, 465-470.

[108] Finn, P.W., He, H., Wang, Y., Wang, Z., Guan, G., Listman, J. & Perkins, D.L (1997). Synergistic induction of CTLA-4 expression by costimulation with TCR plus CD28 signals mediated by increased transcription and messenger ribonucleic acid stability. *Journal of Immunology, 158*, 4074-4081.

[109] Wang, X.B., Kakoulidou, M., Giscombe, R., Qiu, Q., Huang, D., Pirskanen, R., Lefvert, A.K. (2002). Abnormal expression of CTLA-4 by T cells from patients with myasthenia gravis: effect of an AT-rich gene sequence. *Journal of Neuroimmunology, 130*, 224-232.

[110] Huang, D., Giscombe, R., Zhou, Y., Pirskanen, R., Lefvert, A.K. (2000). Dinucleotide repeat expansion in the CTLA-4 gene leads to T cell hyper-reactivity via the CD28 pathway in myasthenia gravis. *Journal of Neuroimmunology, 105*, 69-77.

[111] Takara, M., Kouki, T. & De Groot, L.J. (2003). CTLA-4 AT-repeat polymorphism reduces the inhibitory function of CTLA-4 in Graves' disease. *Thyroid, 13*, 1083-1089.
[112] Anjos, S.M., Shao, W., Marchand, L. & Polychronakos, C. (2005). Allelic effects on gene regulation at the autoimmunity-predisposing CTLA4 locus: a re-evaluation of the 3' +6230G>A polymorphism. *Genes and Immunity, 6*, 305-311.
[113] Magistrelli, G., Jeannin, P., Herbault, N., Benoit De Coignac, A., Bonnefoy, J.Y. & Delneste, Y. (1999). A soluble form of CTLA-4 generated by alternative splicing is expressed by nonstimulated human T cells. *European Journal of Immunology, 29*, 3596-3602.
[114] Oaks, M.K., Hallett, K.M., Penwell, R.T., Stauber, E.C., Warren, S.J. & Tector, A.J. (2000). A native soluble form of CTLA-4. *Cell Immunology, 201*, 144-153.
[115] Appleman, L.J. & Boussiotis, V.A. (2003). T cell anergy and costimulation. *Immunology Reviews, 192*, 161-180.
[116] Carreno, B.M. & Collins, M. (2002). The B7 family of ligands and its receptors: new pathways for costimulation and inhibition of immune responses. *Annual Reviews in Immunology, 20*, 29-53.
[117] Waterhouse, P., Penninger, J.M., Timms, E., Wakeham, A., Shahinian, A., Lee, K.P., Thompson, C.B., Griesser, H. & Mak, T.W. (1995). Lymphoproliferative disorders with early lethality in mice deficient in CTLA-4. *Science, 270*, 985 988.
[118] Chambers, C.A., Cado, D., Truong, T. & Allison J.P. (1997). Thymocyte differentiation occurs normally in the absence of CTLA-4. *Proceedings of the National Academy Sciences of the USA 94*, 9296 9301.
[119] Luhder, F., Hoglund, P., Allison, J.P., Benoist, C. & Mathis, D. (1997). CTLA-4 regulates unfolding of autoimmune diabetes. *Journal of Experimental Medicine, 187*, 427-432.
[120] Rao, S., Vasu, C., Martinez, O., Kaithamana, S., Prabhakar, B.S. & Hotterman, M.J. (2001). Targeted delivery of anti-CTLA4-antibody downregulates T cell function in vitro and in vivo. *Clinical Immunology, 101*, 136-145.
[121] Goldrath, A.W. & Bevan, M.J. (1999). Low-affinity ligands for the TCR drive proliferation of mature CD8+ T cells in lymphopenic hosts. *Immunity, 11*, 183-190.
[122] Chambers, C.A., Sullivan, T.J. & Allison, J.P. (1997). Lymphoproliferation in CTLA-4-deficient mice is mediated by costimulation-dependent activation of CD4+ T cells. *Immunity, 7*, 885-895.
[123] Crane, I.J. & Forrester, J.V. (2005). Th1 and Th2 lymphocytes in autoimmune disease. *Critical Reviews in Immunology, 25*, 75-102.
[124] Oosterwegel, M.A., Mandelbrot, D.A., Boyd, S.D., Lorsbach, R.B., Jarrett, D.Y., Abbas, A.K. & Sharpe, A.H. (1999). The role of CTLA-4 in regulating Th2 differentiation. *Journal of Immunology, 163*, 2634-2639.
[125] Roura-Mir, C., Catalfamo, M., Sospedra, M., Alcalde, L., Pujol-Borrell, R. & Jaraquemada, D. (1997). Single-cell analysis of intrathyroidal lymphocytes shows differential cytokine expression in Hashimoto's and Graves' disease. *European Journal of Immunology, 27*, 3290-3302.
[126] Vasu C., Gorla, S.R., Prabhakar, B.S. & Holterman, M.J. (2003). Targeted engagement of CTLA-4 prevents autoimmune thyroiditis. *International Immunology, 15*, 641-654.

[127] Chen, W., Jin, W. & Wahl, S.M. (1998). Engagement of cytotoxic T lymphocyte-associated antigen 4 (CTLA-4) induces transforming growth factor beta (TNF-beta) production by murine CD4(+) T cells. *Journal of Experimental Medicine, 188*, 1849-1857.

[128] Gomez, N.A., Gattass C.R., Barreto-de-Souza, V., Wilson, M.E. & DosReis, G.A. (2000). TGF-β mediates suppression of cellular immunity in murine kalaazar. *Journal of Immunology, 164*, 2001-2008.

[129] Dai, Z. & Lakkis, F.G. (1999). The role of cytokines, CTLA-4 and costimulation in transplant tolerance and rejection. *Current Opinion in Immunology, 11*, 504-548.

[130] Tomer, Y., Barbesino, G., Greenberg, D.A., Concepcion, E. & Davies, T.F. (1999). Mapping the major susceptibility loci for familial Graves' and Hashimoto's diseases: evidence for genetic heterogeneity and gene interactions. *Journal of Clinical Endocrinology and Metabolism, 84*, 4656-4664.

[131] Tomer, Y., Ban, Y., Concepcion, E., Villanueva, R., Greenberg, D.A. & Davies, T.F. (2003) Common and unique susceptibility loci in Graves and Hashimoto diseases: results of whole-genome screening in a data set of 102 multiplex families. *American Journal of Human Genetics, 73*, 736-747.

[132] Shiina, T., Inoko, H. & Kulski, J.K. (2004). An update of the HLA genomic region, locus information and disease associations: 2004. *Tissue Antigens, 64*, 631-649.

[133] Bode, H.H., Dorf, M.E. & Forbes, A.P. (1973). Familial lymphocytic thyroiditis: analysis of linkage with histocompatibility and blood groups. *Journal of Clinical Endocrinology and Metabolism, 37*, 692-697.

[134] Hawkins, B.R., Ma, J.T., Lam, K.S., Wang, C.C. & Yeung, R.T. (1985). Analysis of linkage between HLA haplotype and susceptibility to Graves' disease in multiple-case Chinese families in Hong Kong. *Acta Endocrinologica (Copenhagen), 110*, 66-69.

[135] Roman, S.H., Greenberg, D., Rubinstein, P., Wallenstein, S. & Davies, T.F. (1992). Genetics of autoimmune thyroid disease: lack of evidence for linkage to HLA within families. *Journal of Clinical Endocrinology and Metabolism, 74*, 496-503.

[136] Barbesino, G., Tomer, Y., Concepsion, E., Davies, T.F. & Greenberg, D.A. (1998). Linkage analysis of candidate genes in autoimmune thyroid disease: 1. Selected immunoregulatory genes. International Consortium for the Genetics of Autoimmune Thyroid Disease. *Journal of Clinical Endocrinology and Metabolism,* 83, 1580-1584.

[137] Sakai, K., Shirasawa, S., Ishikawa, N., Ito, K., Tamai, H., Kuma, K., Akamizu, T., Tanimura, M., Furugaki, K., Yamamoto, K. & Sasazuki T. (2001). Identification of susceptibility loci for autoimmune thyroid disease to 5q31-q33 and Hashimoto's thyroiditis to 8q23-q24 by multipoint affected sib-pair linkage analysis in Japanese. *Human Molecular Genetics, 10*, 1379-1386.

[138] Ban, Y., Davies, T.F., Greenberg, D.A., Concepcion, E.S. & Tomer, Y. (2002). The influence of human leucocyte antigen (HLA) genes on autoimmune thyroid disease (AITD): results of studies in HLA-DR3 positive AITD families. *Clinical Endocrinology (Oxford), 57*, 661-667.

[139] Shields, D.C., Ratanachaiyavong, S., McGregor, A.M., Collins, A. & Morton, N.E. (1994) Combined segregation and linkage analysis of Graves disease with a thyroid autoantibody diathesis. *American Journal of Human Genetics, 55*, 540-554.

[140] Ayadi, H., Kacem, H.H., Rebai, A., & Farid, N.R. (2004). The genetics of autoimmune thyroid disease.*Trends in Endocrinology and Metabolism, 15*, 233-239.

[141] Farid, N.R., Stone, E. & Johnson, G. (1980). Graves disease and HLA: clinical and epidemiological associations. *Clinical Endcorinology (Oxford) 13*, 535-544.

[142] Volpe, R. (1990). Immunology of human thyroid disease. In R. Volpe (Ed.), *Autoimmunity in endocrine disease* (p. 73). Boca Raton, FL: CRC Press.

[143] Maciel, L.M., Rodrigues, S.S., Dibbern, R.S., Navarro, P.A. & Donadi, E.A. (2001). The HLA-DRB1*0301 and HLA-DQA1*0501 alleles with Graves' disease in a population representing the gene contribution from several ethnic backgrounds. *Thyroid, 11*, 31-35.

[144] Hawkins, B.R., Ma, J.T., Lam, K.S., Wang, C.C. & Yeung, R.T. (1985b) Association of HLA antigens with thyrotoxic Graves' disease and periodic paralysis in Hong Kong Chinese. *Clinical Endocrinology (Oxford) 23*, 245-252.

[145] Tandon, N., Mehra, N.K., Taneja, V., Vaidya, M.C. & Kochupillai, N. (1990). HLA antigens in Asian Indian patients with Graves' disease. *Clinical Endocrinology (Oxford), 33*, 21-26.

[146] Chen, Q.Y., Nadell, D., Zhang, X.Y., Kukreja, A., Huang, Y.J., Wise, J., Svec, F. Richards, R., Friday, K.E., Vargas, A., Gomez, R., Chalew, S., Lan, M.S., Tomer, Y. & Maclaren, N.K. (2000). The human leukocyte antigen HLA DRB3*020/DQA1*0501 haplotype is associated with Graves' disease in African Americans. *Journal of Clinical Endocrinology and Metabolism, 85*, 1545-1549.

[147] Yanagawa, T., Mangklabruks, A. & De Groot, L.J. (1994). Strong association between HLA-DQA1*0501 and Graves' disease in a male Caucasian population. *Journal of Clinical Endocrinology and Metabolism, 79*, 227-229.

[148] Barlow, A.B., Wheatcroft, N., Watson, P. & Weetman, A.P. (1996). Association of HLA-DQA1*0501 with Graves' disease in English Caucasian men and women. *Clinical Endocrinology (Oxford), 44*, 73-77.

[149] Badenhoop, K., Donner, H., Braun, J., Siegmund, T., Rau H. & Usadel, K.H. (1996). Genetic markers in diagnosis and prediction of relapse in Graves' disease. *Experimental and Clinical Endocrinology and Diabetes, 104*, 98-100.

[150] Philippou, G., Krimitzas, A., Kaltzas, G., Anastasiou, E., Souvatzoglou, A. & Alevizaki, M. (2001). HLA DQA1*0501 and DRB1*0301 antigens do not independently convey susceptibility to Graves' disease. *Journal of Endocrinological Investigations, 24*, 88-91.

[151] Zamani, M., Spaepen, M., Bex, M., Bouillon, R. & Cassiman, J.J. (2000). Primary role of the HLA class II DRB1*0301 allele in Graves disease. *American Journal of Medical Genetics, 95*, 432-437.

[152] Marsh, S.G., Albert, E.D., Bodmer, W.F., Bontrop, R.E., Dupont, B., Erlich, H.A., Geraghty, D.E., Hansen, J.A., Hurley, C.K., Mach, B., Mayr, W.R., Parham, P., Petersdorf, E.W., Sasazuki, T., Schreuder, G.M., Strominger, J.L., Svejgaard, A., Terasaki, P.I. & Trowsdale, J. (2005). Nomenclature for factors of the HLA system, 2004. *Tissue Antigens, 65*, 301-369.

[153] Ban, Y., Davies, T.F., Greenberg, D.A., Concepcion, E.S., Osman, R., Oashi, T. & Tomer, Y. (2004). Arginine at position 74 of the HLA-DR β1 chain is associated with Graves' disease. *Genes and Immunity, 5*, 203-208.

[154] Simmonds, M.J., Howson, J.M.M., Heward, J.M., Cordell, H.J., Foxall, H., Carr-Smith, J., Gibson, S.M., Walker, N., Tomer, Y., Franklyn, J.A., Todd, J.A. & Gough, S.C.L. (2005). Regression mapping of association between the Human Leukocyte Antigen region and Graves disease. *American Journal of Human Genetics, 76*, 157-163.

[155] Orhan, Y., Azezli, A., Carin, M., Aral, F., Sencer, E. & Molvalivar, S. (1993). Human lymphocyte antigens (HLA) and Graves' disease in Turkey. *Journal of Clinical Immunology, 13*, 339-343.

[156] Chen, Q.Y., Huang, W., She, J.X., Baxter, F., Volpe, R. & Maclaren, N.K. (1999). HLA-DRB1*08, DRB1*03/DRB3*0101, and DRB3*0202 are susceptibility genes for Graves' disease in North American Caucasians, whereas DRB1*07 is protective. *Journal of Clinical Endocrinology and Metabolism, 84*, 3182-3186.

[157] Trucco, M. (1992). To be or not to be Asp 57, that is the question. *Diabetes Care, 15*, 705-715.

[158] Lee, K.H., Wucherpfennig, K.W. (2001). Structure of a human insulin peptide-HLA-DQ8 complex and susceptibility to type 1 diabetes. *Nature Immunology, 2*, 501-507.

[159] Doebele, R.C., Pashine, A., Liu, W., Zaller, D.M., Belmares, M., Busch, R. & Mellins, E.D. (2003). Point mutations in or near the antigen-binding groove of HLA-DR3 implicate class II-associated invariant chain peptide affinity as a constraint on MHC class II polymorphism. *Journal of Immunology, 170*, 4683-4692.

[160] Chelvanayagam, G., Apostoloupos, V. & McKenzie, I.F. (1997). Milestones in the molecular structure of the major histocompatibility complex. *Protein Engineering, 10*, 471-474.

[161] Kong, Y.C., Lomo, L.C., Motte, R.W., Giraldo, A.A., Baisch, J., Strauss, G., Hammerling, C.J. & David, C.S. (1996). HLA-DRB1 polymorphism determines susceptibility to autoimmune thyroiditis in transgenic mice: definitive association with HLA-DRB1*0301 (DR3) gene. *Journal of Experimental Medicine, 184*, 1167-172.

[162] Wan, Q., Shah, R., Panos, J.C., Giraldo, A.A., David, C.S. & Kong Y.M. (2002). HLA-DR and HLA-DQ polymorphism in human thyroglobulin-induced autoimmune thyroiditis: DR3 and DQ8 transgenic mice are susceptible. *Human Immunology, 63*, 301-310.

[163] Pichurin, P., Chen, C.R., Pichurina, O., David, C., Rapoport, B. & McLachlan, S.M. (2003). Thyrotropin receptor-DNA vaccination of transgenic mice expressing HLA-DR3 or HLA-DQ6b. *Thyroid, 13*, 911-917.

[164] Flynn, J.C., Wan, Q., Panos, J.C., McCormick, D.J., Giraldo, A.A., David, C.S. & Kong, Y.C. (2002). Coexpression of susceptible and resistant HLA class II transgenes in murine experimental autoimmune thyroiditis: DQ8 molecules downregulate DR3-mediated thyroiditis. *Journal of Autoimmunity, 18*, 213-220.

[165] Sawai Y. & DeGroot, D.J. (2000). Binding of human thyrotropin receptor peptides to Graves' disease-predisposinh human leukocyte antigen class II molecule. *Journal of Clinical Endocrinology and Metabolism, 85*, 1176-1179.

[166] Hanazusa, T., Pujol Boreell, R., Chiovato, L., Russell, R.C., Doniach, D. and Bottazzo, G.F. (1983). Aberrant expression of HLA-DR antigen on thyrocytes in Graves' disease: relevance for autoimmunity. *Lancet, 2*, 1115-1119.

[167] Khoury, E.L. (1987). Aberrant expression of class II HLA antigens by the target cell: cause or consequence of the autoimmune aggression? *Acta Endocrinologica (Copenhagen), 281*, 35-41.

[168] Montani, V., Taniguchi, S.I., Shong, M., Suzuki, M., Ohmori, M., Guiliani, C., Napolitano, G., Saji, M., Fiorentino, B., Reimold, A.M., Ting, J.P., Kohn, L.D. & Singer, D.S. (1998). Major histocompatibility class II HLA-DR alpha gene expression in thyrocytes: counter regulation by the class II transactivator and the thyroid Y box protein. *Endocrinology, 139*, 280-289.

[169] Khoury, E.L., Pereira, L. & Greenspan, F.S. (1991). Induction of HLA-DR expression on thyroid follicular cells by cytomegalovirus infection in vitro. Evidence for a dual mechanism of induction. *American Journal of Pathology, 138*, 1209-1223.

[170] Jaspan, J.B., Sullivan, K., Garry, R.F., Lopez, M., Wolfe, M., Clejan, S., Yan, C., Tenenbaum, S., Dander, D.M., Ahmed, B. & Bryer-Ash, M. (1996). The interaction of a type A retroviral particle and class II human leukocyte antigen susceptibility genes in the pathogenesis of Graves' disease. *Journal of Clinical Endocrinology and Metabolism, 81*, 2271-2279.

[171] Pichert, G., Jost, L.M., Zobeli, I., Odermatt, B., Pedia, G. & Stahel, R.A. (1990). Thyroiditis after treatment with interleukin-2 and interferon alpha-2a. *British Journal of Cancer, 62*, 100-104.

[172] Migita, K., Eguchi, K., Otsubo, T., Kawakami, A., Nakao, H., Ueki, Y., Shimomura, C., Kurata, A., Fukuda, T., Matsunaga, M., Ishikawa, N., Ito, K. & Nagataki, S. (1990). Cytokine regulation of HLA on thyroid epithelial cells. *Clinical and Experimental Immunology, 82*, 548-552.

[173] Kraiem, Z., Sobel, E., Sadeh, O., Kinarty, A. & Lahat, N. (1990). Effects of gamma-interferon on DR antigen expression, growth, 3,5,3'-triiodothyronine secretion, iodide uptake, and cyclic adenosine 3',5'-monophosphate accumulation in cultured human thyroid cells. *Journal of Clinical Endocrinology and Metabolism, 71*, 817-824.

[174] Fierabracci, A., Hammond, L., Lowdell, M., Chiovato, L., Goode, A.W., Botazzo, G.F & Mirakian, R. (1999). The effect of staphylococcal enterotoxin B on thyrocyte HLA molecule expression. *Journal of Autoimmunity, 12*, 305-314.

[175] Rose, N.R., Saboori, A.M., Bresler, H.S. & Burek, C.L. (1997). The role of iodine in autoimmune thyroiditis. *Critical Reviews in Immunology, 17*, 511-517.

[176] Shimojo, N., Kohno Y., Yamaguschi, K., Kikuoka, S., Hoshioka, A., Niimi, H., Hirai, A., Tamura, Y., Sajto, Y., Kohn, L.D. & Tahara, K. (1996). Induction of Graves-like disease in mice by immunization with fibroblasts transfected with the thyrotropin receptor and a class II molecule. *Proceedings of the National Academy of Sciences of the USA, 93*, 11074-11079.

[177] Shimojo, N., Arima, T., Yamaguchi, K., Kikuoka, S., Kohn, L.D. & Kohno, Y. (2000). A novel mouse model of Graves' disease: implications for a role of aberrant MHC class II expression in its pathogenesis. *International Reviews in Immunology, 19*, 619-631.

[178] Tomer, Y., Greenberg, D.A., Concepcion, E., Ban, Y. & Davies, T.F. (2002) Thyroglobulin is a thyroid specific gene for the familial autoimmune thyroid diseases. *Journal of Clinical Endocrinology and Metabolism, 87*, 404-407.

[179] Collins, J.E., Heward, J.M., Carr-Smith, J., Daykin, J., Franklyn, J.A. & Gough, S.C. (2003). Association of a rare thyroglobulin gene microsatellite variant with autoimmune thyroid disease. *Journal of Clinical Endocrinology and Metabolism, 88*, 5039-5042.

[180] Ban, Y., Greenberg, D.A., Concepcion, E., Skrabanek, L., Villanueva, R. & Tomer, Y. (2003b). Amino acid substitutions in the thyroglobulin gene are associated with susceptibility to human and murine autoimmune thyroid disease. *Proceedings of the National Academy of Sciences of the USA, 100*, 15119-15124.

[181] Collins, J.E., Heward, J.M., Howson, J.M., Foxall, H., Carr-Smith, J., Franklyn, J.A. & Gough, S.C. (2004). Common allelic variants of exons 10, 12, and 33 of the thyroglobulin gene are not associated with autoimmune thyroid disease in the United Kingdom. *Journal of Clinical Endocrinology and Metabolism, 89*, 6336-6339.

[182] Ban, Y., Tozaki, T., Taniyama, M., Tomiza, M. & Ban, Y. (2004c). Association of a thyroglobulin gene polymorphism with Hashimoto's thyroiditis in the Japanese population. *Clinical Endocrinology (Oxford), 61,* 263-268.

[183] Tomer, Y. & Greenberg, D. (2004). The thyroglobulin gene as the first thyroid-specific susceptibility gene for autoimmune thyroid disease. *Trends in Molecular Medicine, 10*, 306-308.

[184] Shirasawa, S., Harada, H., Furugaki, K., Akamizu, T., Ishikawa, N., Ito, K., Tamai, H., Kuma, K., Kubota, S., Hiratani, H., Tsuchiya, T., Baba, I., Ishikawa, M., Tanaka, M., Sakai, K., Aoki, M., Yamamoto, K. & Sasazuki, T. (2004). SNPs in the promoter of a B-cell-specific antisense transcript, SAS-ZFAT, determine susceptibility to autoimmune thyroid disease. *Human Molecular Genetics, 13*, 2221-2231.

[185] Van de Graaf, S.A.R., Ris-Stalpers, C., Pauws, E., Mendive, F.M., Targovnik, H.M., de Vijlder, J.J.M. (2001). Up to date with human thyroglobulin. *Journal of Endocrinology, 170*, 307-321.

[186] Dupuy, C., Ohayon, R., Val;ent, A., Noel-Hudson, M.-S., Deme, D. & Vrion, A. (1999). Purification and of a novel flavoprotein involved in the thyroid NADPH oxidase. *Journal of Biological Chemistry, 274*, 37265-37269.

[187] Rasooly, L., Rose, N.R., Saboori, N.M., Ladenson, P.W. & Burek, C.L. (1998). Iodine is essential for human T cell recognition of human thyroglobulin. *Autoimmunity, 27*, 213-219.

[188] Rose, N.R. & Burek, C.L. (2000). Autoantibodies to thyroglobulin in health and disease. *Applied Biochemistry and Biotechnology, 83*, 245-251

[189] McLachlan, S.M. & Rapoport, B. (2004). Why measure thyroglobulin autoantibodies rather than thyroid peroxidase antibodies? *Thyroid, 14*, 510-520.

[190] Tomer, Y. (1997). Anti-thyroglobulin autoantibodies in autoimmune thyroid diseases: cross-reactive or pathogenic? *Clinical Immunology and Immunopathology, 82*, 3-11.

[191] Taneja,V. & David, C.S. (1998). HLA transgenic mice as humanized mouse models of disease and immunity. *Journal of Clinical Investigations, 101*, 921–926.

[192] Cihakova, D., Sharma, R.B., Fairweather, D., Afanasyeva, M. & Rose, N.R. (2004). Animal models for autoimmune myocarditis and autoimmune thyroiditis. *Methods in Molecular Medicine, 102*, 175-193.

[193] Kong, Y.M., David, C.S., Lomo, L.C., Fuller, B.E., Motte, R.W. & Giraldo, A.A. (1997). Role of mouse and human class II transgenes in susceptibility to and protection against mouse autoimmune thyroiditis. *Immunogenetics, 46*, 312-317.

[194] Kong, Y.C., Flynn, J.C., Wan, Q. & David, C.S. (2003). HLA and H2 class II transgenic mouse models to study susceptibility and protection in autoimmune thyroid disease. *Autoimmunity, 36*, 397-404.

[195] Sigihara, S., Fujiwara, H. & Shearer, G.M. (1993). Autoimmune thyroiditis induced in mice depleted of particular T cell subsets. Characterization of thyroiditis-inducing T cell lines and clones derived from thyroid lesions. *Journal of Immunology, 150*, 683-694.

[196] Matsuoka, N., Unger, P., Ben-Nun, A., Graves, P. & Davies, T.F. (1994). Thyroglobulin-induced murine thyroiditis assessed by intrathyroidal T cell receptor sequencing. *Journal of Immunology, 152*, 2562-2568.

[197] Dawe, K.I., Hutchings, P.R., Geysen, M., Champion, B.R., Cooke, A. & Roitt, I.M. (1996). Unique role of thyroxine in T cell recognition of a pathogenic peptide in experimental autoimmune thyroiditis. *European Journal of Immunology, 26*, 768-772.

[198] Ruwhof, C. & Drexhage, H.A. (2001). Iodine and thyroid autoimmune disease in animal models. *Thyroid. 11*, 427-436.

[199] Dawe, K.I., Hutchings, P.R., Geysen, M., Champion, B.R., Cooke, A. & Roitt, I.M. (1996). Unique role of thyroxine in T cell recognition of a pathogenic peptide in experimental autoimmune thyroiditis. *European Journal of Immunology, 26*, 768-772.

[200] Flynn, J.C., McCormick, D.J., Brusic, V., Wan, Q., Panos, J.C., Giraldo, A.A., David, C.S. & Kong, Y.C. (2004). Pathogenic human thyroglobulin peptides in HLA-DR3 transgenic mouse model of autoimmune thyroiditis. *Cell Immunology, 229*, 79-85.

[201] Volpe, R. (1995). The pathogenesis of Graves' disease. Endocrine Practice, 1, 103-115.

[202] Rose N.R., Bonita, R. & Burek, C.L. (2002). Iodine: an environmental trigger of thyroiditis. *Autoimmunity Reviews, 1*, 97-103.

[203] Dai, Y.D., Rao, V.P. & Carayanniotis, G. (2002). Enhanced iodination of thyroglobulin facilitates processing and presentation of a cryptic pathogenic peptide. *Journal Immunology, 168*, 5907-5911.

[204] Carayanniotis, G. (2003). The cryptic self in thyroid autoimmunity: the paradigm of thyroglobulin. *Autoimmunity, 36*, 423-428.

[205] Mahmoud, I., Colin, I., Many, M.C. & Denef, J.F. (1986). Direct toxic effect of iodide in excess on iodine-deficient thyroid glands: epithelial necrosis and inflammation associated with lipofuscin accumulation. *Experimental and Molecular Pathology*, 1986, 4, 259-271.

[206] Corvilain, B., Collyn, L., van Sande, J. & Dumont, J.E. (2000). Stimulation by iodide of H(2)O(2) generation in thyroid slices from several species. *American Journal of Physiology, Endocrinology and Metabolism, 278*, E692-E699.

[207] Lafrofa, F., Phillips, M., Rapoport, B. & McLachlan, S.M. (2004). Human monoclonal thyroglobulin autoantibodies: epitopes and immunoglobulin genes. *Journal of Clinical Endocrinology and Metabolism, 89*, 5116-5123.

[208] Saboori A.M., Rose N.R., Bresler H.S., Vladut-Talor M. & Burek, C.L. (1998). Iodination of human thyroglobulin (Tg) alters its immunoreactivity. I. Iodination alters multiple epitopes of human Tg. *Clinical and Experimental Immunology, 113*, 297-302.

[209] Tomer, Y., Barbesino, G., Keddache, M., Greenberg, D.A. & Davies, T.F. (1997). Mapping of a major susceptibility locus for Graves' disease (GD-1) to chromosome 14q31. *Journal of Clinical Endocrinology and Metabolism, 82*, 1645-1648.

[210] Tomer, Y., Barbesino, G., Greenberg, D.A., Concepcion, E. & Davies, T.F. (1998). Linkage analysis of candidate genes in autoimmune thyroid disease. III. Detailed analysis of chromosome 14 localizes Graves' disease-1 (GD-1) close to multinodular goiter-1 (MNG-1). International Consortium for the Genetics of Autoimmune Thyroid Disease. *Journal of Clinical Endocrinology and Metabolism, 83*, 4321-4327.

[211] Imrie, H., Vaidya, B., Kelly W.F., Toft, A.D., Young, E.T., Kendall-Taylor, P. & Pierce, S.H. (2001). Evidence for a Graves' disease susceptibility locus at chromosome Xp11 in a United Kingdom population. *Journal of Clinical Endocrinology and Metabolism, 86*, 626-630.

[212] Chistiakov, D.A. (2003). Thyroid-stimulating hormone receptor and its role in Graves' disease. *Molecular Genetics and Metabolism, 80*, 377-388.

[213] de Roix, N., Shields, D.C., Misrahi, M., Ratanachaivoyavong, S., McGregor, A.M. & Milgrom, E. (1996). Analysis of the thyrotropin receptor as a candidate gene in familial Graves' disease. *Journal of Clinical Endocrinology and Metabolism, 81*, 3483-3486.

[214] Tonacchera, M. & Pinchera, A. (2000). Thyrotropin receptor polymorphisms and thyroid diseases. *Journal of Clinical Endocrinology and Metabolism, 85*, 2637-2639.

[215] Cuddihy, R.M., Dutton, C.M. & Bahn, R.S. (1995). A polymorphism in the extracellular domain of the thyrotropin receptor is highly associated with autoimmune thyroid disease in females. *Thyroid, 5*, 89-95.

[216] Chistiakov, D.A., Savost'anov, K.V., Turakulov, R.I., Petunina, N., Balabolkin, M.I. & Nosikov, V.V. (2002). Further studies of genetic susceptibility to Graves' disease in a Russian population. *Medical Science Monitor, 8*, CR180-184.

[217] Ban, Y., Greenberg, D.A., Concepcion, E.S. & Tomer, Y (2002b). A germline single nucleotide polymorphism at the intracellular domain of the human thyrotropin receptor does not have a major effect on the development of Graves' disease. *Thyroid, 12*, 1079-1083.

[218] Sale, M.M., Akamizu, T., Howard, T.D., Yokota, T., Nakao, K., Mori, T., Iwasaki, H., Rich, S.S., Jennings-Gee, J.E., Yamada, M. & Bowden, D.W. (1997). Association of autoimmune thyroid disease with a microsatellite marker for the thyrotropin receptor gene and CTLA-4 in a Japanese population. *Proceedings of the Association of American Physicians, 109*, 453-461.

[219] Akamizu, T., Sale, M.M., Rich, S.S., Hiratani, H., Noh, J.Y., Kanamoto, N., Saijo, M., Miyamoto, Y., Saito, Y., Nakao, K. & Bowden, D.W. (2000). Association of autoimmune thyroid disease with microsatellite markers for the thyrotropin receptor gene and CTLA-4 in Japanese patients. *Thyroid, 10*, 851-858.

[220] Hiratani, H., Bowden, D.W., Ikegami, S., Shirasawa, S., Shimizu, A., Iwatani, Y. & Akamizu, T. (2005). Multiple SNPs in intron 7 of thyrotropin receptor are associated with Graves' disease. *Journal of Clinical Endocrinology and Metabolism, 90*, 2898-2903.

[221] Ban, Y., Taniyama, M., Tozaki, T., Yanagawa, T., Tomita, M. & Ban, Y. (2001). SEL1L microsatellite polymorphism in Japanese patients with autoimmune thyroid diseases. *Thyroid, 11*, 335-338.

[222] Chistiakov, D.A., Savost'anov, K.V. & Turakulov, R.I. (2004). Screening of SNPs at 18 positional candidate genes, located within the GD-1 locus on chromosome 14q23-q32, for susceptibility to Graves' disease: a TDT study. *Molecular Genetics and Metabolism, 83*, 264-270.

[223] Bianco, A.C., Salvatore, D., Geberen, B., Berry M.J. & Larsen, P.R. (2002). Biochemistry, cellular and molecular biology, and physiological roles of the iodothyronine selenodeiodinases, *Endocrine Reviews, 23*, 38–89.

[224] Peeters, R.P., van Toor, H., Klootwijk, W., de Rijke, Y.B., Kuiper, G.G.J.M., Uitterlinden, A.G. & Visser, T.J. (2003). Polymorphisms in thyroid hormone pathway genes are associated with plasma TSH and iodothyronine levels in healthy subjects, *Journal of Clinical Endocrinology and Metabolism, 88*, 2880-2888.

[225] Peeters, R.P., van den Beld, A.W., Attalki, H., Toor, H., de Rijke, Y.B., Kuiper, G.G., Lamberts, S.W., Janssen, J.A., Uitterlinden, A.G. & Visser, T.J. (2005). A new polymorphism in the type II deiodinase gene is associated with circulating thyroid hormone parameters. *American Journal of Physiology. Endocrinology and Metabolism, 289*, E75-E81.

[226] Rapoport, B., Chazenbalk, G.D., Jaume, J.C. & Mclahlan, S.M. (1998). The thyrotropin (TSH) receptor: interaction with TSH and autoantibodies. *Endocrine Reviews, 19*, 673-716.

[227] Tanaka, K., Chazebalk, G.D., McLachlan, S.M. & Rapoport, B. (1999). Subunit structure of thyrotropin receptors expressed on the cell surface. *Jounal of Biological Chemistry, 274*, 33979-22784

[228] de Bernard, S., Misrahi, M., Huet, J.C., Beau, I., Desroches, A., Loosfelt, H., Pichon, S., Pernollet, J.C. & Millgrom, E. (1999). Sequential cleavage and excision of a segment of the thyrotropin receptor ectodomain. *Journal of Biological Chemistry, 274*, 101-107.

[229] Smits, G., Campillo, M., Govaerts, C., Janssens, V., Richter, C., Vassart, G., Pardo, L. & Costagliola, S. (2003). Glycoprotein hormone receptors: determinants in leucine-rich repeats responsible for ligand specificity. *EMBO Journal, 22*, 2692-2703.

[230] Loosfelt, H., Pichon, C., Jolivet, A., Misrahi, M., Jamous, M., Vannier, B. & Milgrom, E. (1992). Two-subunit structure of the human thyrotropin receptor. *Proceedings of the National Academy Sciences of the USA, 89*, 3765-3769.

[231] Couet, J., de Bernard, S., Loosfelt, H., Saunier, B., Milgrom, E. & Misrahi, M. (1996). Cell surface protein disulfide-isomerase is involved in the shedding of human thyrotropin receptor ectodomain. *Biochemistry, 35*, 14800–14805.

[232] Kohn, L.D. & Harii, N. (2003). Thyrotropin receptor autoantibodies (TSHRAbs): epitopes, origins and clinical significance. *Autoimmunity, 36*, 331-337.

[233] Orgiazzi, J., Madec, A.M., Ducottet, X. (2003). The role of stimulating, function-blocking and growth-blocking anti-TSH receptor antibodies (TRAbs) in GD, Hashimoto's disease and in atrophic thyroiditis. *Annales d' Endocrinologie (Paris), 64*, 31-36.

[234] Ando, T., Latif, R. & Davies, T.F. (2005). Thyrotropin receptor antibodies: new insights into their actions and clinical relevance. *Best Practice and Research Clinical Endocrinology and Metabolism, 19*, 33-52.

[235] Davies, T.F., Ando, T., Lin, R.-Y., Tomer, Y. & Latif, R. (2005). Thyrotropin receptor-associated diseases: from adenomata to Graves disease. *Journal of Clinical Investigations, 115*, 1972-1983.

[236] Seetharamaiah, G.S. (2003). Animal models of Graves' hyperthyroidism. *Autoimmunity, 36*, 381-387.

[237] Yamaguchi, K., Shimojo, N., Kikuoka, S., Hoshioka, A., Hirai, A., Tahara, K., Kohn, L.D., Kohno, Y. & Niimi, H. (1997). Genetic control of anti-thyrotropin receptor antibody generation in H-2K mice immunized with thyrotropin receptor-transfected fibroblasts. *Journal of Clinical Endocrinology and Metabolism, 82*, 4266-4269.

[238] Costagliola, S., Rodien, P., Many, M.C., Ludgate, M. & Vassart, G. (1998). Genetic immunization against the human thyrotropin receptor causes thyroiditis and allows production of monoclonal antibodies recognizing the native receptor. *Journal of Immunology, 160*, 1458-1465.

[239] Nagayama, Y., Kita-Furuyama, Ando, T., Nakao, K., Mizugichi, H., Hayakawa, T., Eguchi, K. & Niwa M. (2002). A novel murine model of Graves' hyperthyroidism with intramuscular injection of adenovirus expressing the thyrotropin receptor. *Journal of Immunology, 168*, 2789-2794.

[240] Kikuoka, S., Shimojo, N., Yamaguchi, K.I., Watanabe, Y., Hoshioka, A., Hirai, A., Sajto, Y., Tahara, K., Kohn, L.D., Maruyama, N., Kohno, Y. & Niimi, H. (1998). The formation of thyrotropin receptor (TSHR) antibodies in a Graves' animal model requires the N-terminal segment of the TSHR extracellular domain. *Endocrinology, 139*, 1891-1898.

[241] Chen, C.R., Pichurin, P., Nagayama, Y., Lafrofa, F., Rapoport, B. & McLachlan, S.M. (2003). The thyrotropin receptor autoantigen in Graves disease is the culprit as well as the victim. *Journal of Clinical Investigations, 111*, 1897-1904.

[242] Ando, T., Latif, R., Pritsker, A., Moran, T., Nagayama, Y. & Davies, T.F. (2002). A monoclonal thyroid-stimulating antibody. *Journal of Clinical Investigations, 110*, 1667-1674.

[243] Sanders, J., Jeffreys., J., Depraetere, H., Richards, T., Kiddie, A., Brereton, K., Groenen, M., Oda, Y., Furmaniak, J. & Rees Smith, B. (2002). Thyroid-stimulating monoclonal antibodies. *Thyroid, 12*, 1043-1050.

[244] Sanders, J., Evans, M., Premawardhana, L.D., Depraetere, H., Jeffreys, J., Richards, T., Furmaniak, J., Rees Smith, B. (2003). Human monoclonal thyroid stimulating autoantibody. *Lancet, 362*, 126-128.

[245] Chazenbalk, G.D., Jaume, J.C., McLachlan, S.M., Rapoport, B. (1997). Engineering the human thyrotropin receptor ectodomain from a non-secreted form to a secreted, highly

immunoreactive glycoprotein that neutralizes autoantibodies in Graves' patients' sera. *Journal of Biological Chemistry, 272*, 18959-18965.

[246] Chazenbalk, G.D., Pichurin, P., Chen, C.R., Latrofa, F., Johnstone, A.P., McLachlan, S.M. & Rapoport B. (2002). Thyroid-stimulating autoantibodies in Graves disease preferentially recognize the free A subunit, not the thyrotropin holoreceptor. *Journal of Clinical Investigations, 110*, 209–217

[247] Nagayama, Y., Wardsworth, H.L., Russo, D., Chazenbalk, G.D. & Rapoport, B. (1991). Binding domains of stimulatory and inhibitory thyrotropin (TSH) receptor autoantibodies determined with chimeric TSH-lutropin/chorionic gonadotropin receptors. *Journal of Clinical Investigations, 88*, 336-340.

[248] Ando, T., Latif, R., Daniel, S., Eguchi, K. & Davies,T.F. (2004). Dissecting linear and conformational epitopes on the native thyrotropin receptor. *Endocrinology, 145*, 5185-5193.

[249] McLachlan, S.M. & Rapoport, B. (1996). Monoclonal, human autoantibodies to the TSH receptor--the Holy Grail and why are we looking for it? *Journal of Clinical Endocrinology and Metabolism, 81*, 3152-3154.

[250] Davies, T.F., Bobovnikova, Y., Weiss, M., Vlase, H., Moran T. & Graves, P.N. (1998). Development and characterization of monoclonal antibodies specific for the murine thyrotropin receptor. *Thyroid, 8*, 693–701.

[251] Costagliola, S., Franssen, J.D., Bonomi, M., Urizar, E., Willnich, M., Bergmann, A. & Vassart, G. (2002). Generation of a mouse monoclonal TSH receptor antibody with stimulating activity. *Biochemical and Biophysical Research Communications, 299*, 891-896.

[252] Costagliola, S., Bonomi, M., Morgenthaler, N.G., Van Durme, J., Panneels, V., Refetoff, S. & Vassart, G. (2004). Delineation of the discontinuous-conformational epitope of a monoclonal antibody displaying full in vitro and in vivo thyrotropin activity. *Molecular Endocrinology, 1*8, 3020-3034.

[253] Jeffreys, J., Depraetere, H., Sanders, J., Oda, Y., Evans, M., Kiddie A., Richards, T., Furmaniak, J. & Rees Smith, B. (2002). Characterization of the thyrotropin binding pocket. *Thyroid, 12*, 1051–1061.

[254] Sanders, J., Jeffreys, J., Depraetere, H., Evans, M., Richards, T., Kiddie, A., Brereton, K., Premawardhana, L.D., Chirgadze, D.Y., Nunez Miguel, R., Blundell, T.L., Furmaniak, J. & Rees Smith, B. (2004). Characteristics of a human monoclonal autoantibody to the thyrotropin receptor: sequence structure and function. *Thyroid, 14*, 560-570.

[255] Feldt-Rasmussen, U., Schleusener, H., Carayon, P. (1994). Meta-analysis evaluation of the impact of thyrotropin receptor antibodies on long term remission after medical therapy of Graves' disease. *Journal of Clinical Endocrinology and Metabolism 78*, 98-102.

[256] Davies, T.F., Roti, E., Braverman, L.E. & DeGroot , L.J. (1998). Thyroid controversy-stimulating antibodies. *Journal of Clinical Endocrinology and Metabolism, 83*, 3777-3785.

[257] Schott, M., Morgenthaller, N.G., Fritzen, R., Feldkamp, J., Willenberg, H.S., Scherbaum, W.A. & Seissler, J. (2004). Levels of autoantibodies against human TSH

receptor predict relapse of hyperthyroidism in Graves' disease. *Hormone and Metabolic Research, 36*, 92-96.

[258] Ando, T. & Davies, T.F. (2005). Monoclonal antibodies to the thyrotropin receptor. *Clinical and Developmental Immunology, 12*, 137-143.

[259] Weetman, A.P., Yateman, M.E., Ealey, P.A., Black, C.M., Reimer, C.B., Williams, R.C., Jr, Shine, B. & Marshall, N.J. (1990). Thyroid-stimulating antibody activity between different immunoglobulin G subclasses. *Journal of Clinical Investigations, 86*, 723-727.

[260] Kraiem, Z., Cho, B.Y., Sadeh, O., Shong, M.H., Pickerill, P. & Weetman, A.P. (1992). The IgG subclass distribution of TSH receptor blocking antibodies in primary hypothyroidism. *Clinical Endocrinology (Oxford), 37*, 135-140.

[261] Li, H., Akamizu, T., Okuda, J., Sugawa, H., Matsuda, F., Tsubata, T. & Mori, T. (1995). Isolation of Epstein–Barr-virus-transformed lymphocytes producing IgG class monoclonal antibodies using a magnetic cell separator (MACS): preparation of thyroid-stimulating IgG antibodies from patients with Graves' disease. *Biochemical and Biophysical Research Communications, 207*, 985–993.

[262] Morgenthaler, N.G., Kim, M.R., Tremble, J., Huang, G.C., Richter, W., Gupta, M., Scherbaum, W.A., McGregor, A.M. & Banga, J.P. (1996). Human immunoglobulin G autoantibodies to the thyrotropin receptor from Epstein–Barr virus-transformed B lymphocytes: characterization by immunoprecipitation with recombinant antigen and biological activity. *Journal of Clinical Endocrinology and Metabolism, 81*, 3155–3161.

[263] Akamizu T., Matsuda, F., Okuda, J., Li, H., Kanda, H., Watanabe, T., Honjo T. & Mori T. (1996). Molecular analysis of stimulatory anti-thyrotropin receptor antibodies (TSAbs) involved in Graves' disease. Isolation and reconstruction of antibody genes, and production of monoclonal TSAbs. *Journal of Immunology, 157*, 3148–3152.

[264] Shin, E.K., Akamizu, T., Matsuda, F., Sugawa, H., Fujikura, J., Mori, T. & Honjo, T. (1994). Variable regions of Ig heavy chain genes encoding antithyrotropin receptor antibodies of patients with Graves' disease. *Journal of Immunology, 152*, 1485-1492.

[265] Mullins, R.J., Chernajovsky, Y., Dayan, C., Londei, M. & Feldman, M. (1994). Transfection of thyroid autoantigens into EBV-transformed B cell lines. Recognition by Graves' disease thyroid T cells. *Journal of Immunology, 152*, 5572-5580.

[266] Molteni, M., Zulian, C., Scrofani, S., Della Bella, S., Bonara, P., Kohn, L.D. & Scorza, R. (1998). High frequency of T-cell lines responsive to immunodominant epitopes of thyrotropin receptor in healthy subjects. *Thyroid, 8*, 241–247.

[267] Murakami M., Miyashita K., Yamada, M., Iriuchijima, T. & Mori, M. (1992). Characterization of human thyrotropin receptor-related peptide-like immunoreactivity in peripheral blood of Graves' disease. *Biochemical and Biophysical Research Communications, 186*, 1074–1080.

[268] Stadlmyr, W., Spitzweg, C., Bichlmair, A.M. & Heufelder, A.E. (1997). TSH receptor transcripts and TSH receptor-like immunoreactivity in orbital and pretibial fibroblasts of patients with Graves' ophthalmopathy and pretibial myxedema. *Thyroid, 7*, 3-12.

[269] Martin, A., Matsuoka, N., Concepcion, E.S. & Davies, T.F. (1995). Endogenous antigen presentation by autoantigen-transfected Epstein-Barr virus-lymphoblastoid

cells: T cell receptor N-region hydrophobicity relates to thyroid antigen recognition. *Autoimmunity, 21*, 223-230.

[270] Martin, A., Barbesino, G. & Davies, T.F. (1999). T-cell receptors and autoimmune thyroid disease-signposts for T-cell-antigen driven diseases. *International Reviews in Immunology, 18*, 111-140.

[271] Soliman, M., Kaplan, E., Yanagawa, T., Hidaka, Y., Fisfalen, M.E. & DeGroot, L.J. (1995). T-cells recognize multiple epitopes in the human thyrotropin receptor extra-cellular domain. *Journal of Clinical Endocrinology and Metabolism, 80*, 905–914.

[272] Geluk, A., van Meijgaarden, K.E., Southwood, S., Oseroff, C., Drijfhout, J.W., de Vries, R.R., Ottenhoff, T.H. & Sette, A. (1994). HLA-DR3 molecules can bind peptides carrying two alternative specific submotifs. *Journal of Immunology, 152*, 5742–5748.

[273] Geluk, A., van Meijgaarden, K.E., Schloot, N.C., Drijfhout, J.W., Ottenhoff, T.H. & Roep, B.O. (1998) HLA-DR binding analysis of peptides from islet antigens in IDDM. *Diabetes, 47*, 1594-1601.

[274] Muraro, P.A., Vergelli, M., Kalbus, M., Banks, D.E., Nagle, J.W., Tranquill, L.R., Nepom, G.T., Biddison, W.E., McFarland, H.F. & Martin, R. (1997). Immunodominance of a low-affinity major histocompatibility complex-binding myelin basic protein epitope (residues 111-129) in HLA-DR4 (B1*0401) subjects is associated with a restricted T cell receptor repertoire. *Journal of Clinical Investigations, 100*, 339-349

[275] Liu, G.Y., Fairchild, P.J., Smith, R.M., Prowle, J.R., Kioussis, D. & Wraith, D.C. (1995). Low avidity recognition of self-antigen by T cells permits escape from central tolerance. *Immunity, 3,* 407–415.

[276] Pichurin, P., Chen, C.R., Pichurina, O., David, C., Rapoport, B. & Mclachlan, S.M. (2003). Thyrotropin receptor-DNA vaccination of transgenic mice expressing HLA-DR3 or HLA-DQ6b. *Thyroid, 13*, 911-917.

[277] Gustavsson, B., Eklof, C., Westermark, K., Westermark B. & Heldin, N.E. (1995). Functional analysis of a variant of the thyrotropin receptor gene in a family with Graves' disease. *Molecular and Cell Endocrinology, 111*, 167–173.

[278] Loos, U., Hagner, S., Bohr, U.R., Bogatkewitsch, G.S., Jakobs, K.H. & Van Koppen, C.J. (1995). Enhanced cAMP accumulation by the human thyrotropin receptor variant with the Pro52Thr substitution in the extracellular domain. *European Journal of Biochemistry, 232*, 62–65.

[279] Duprez, L., Parma, J. & Van Sande, J. (1998). TSH receptor mutations and thyroid disease. *Trends in Endocrinology and Metabolism, 9*, 133–140.

[280] Cuddihy, R.M., Bryant, W.P. & Bahn, R.S. (1995). Normal function in vivo of a homozygotic polymorphism in the human thyrotropin receptor. *Thyroid, 5*, 255–257.

[281] Gabriel, E.M., Bergert, E.R., Grant, C.S., van Heerden, J.A., Thompson, G.B. & Morris, G.C. (1999). Germline polymorphism of codon 727 of human thyroid-stimulating hormone receptor is associated with toxic multinodular goiter. *Journal of Clinical Endocrinology and Metabolism, 84*, 3328–3335.

[282] Nogueira, C.R., Kopp, P., Arseven, O.K., Santos, C.L., Jameson, J.L. & Medeiros-Neto, G. (1999). Thyrotropin receptor mutations in hyperfunctioning thyroid adenomas from Brazil. *Thyroid, 9*, 1063–1068.

[283] Sykiotis, G.P., Neumann, S., Georgopoulos, N.A., Sgourou, A., Papachatzopoulou, A., Markou, K.B., Kyriazopoulou, V., Paschke, R., Vagenakis, A.G. & Papavassiliou, A.G. (2003). Functional significance of the thyrotropin receptor germline polymorphism D727E. *Biochemical and Biophysical Research Communications, 301*, 1051–1056.

[284] Tomer, Y., Barbesino, G., Greenberg, D.A., Concepcion, E. & Davies, T.F. (1998). A new Graves disease-susceptibility locus maps to chromosome 20q11.2. International Consortium for the Genetics of Autoimmune Thyroid Disease. *American Journal of Human Genetics, 63*, 1749-1756.

[285] Pearce, S.H., Vaidya, B., Imrie, H., Perros, P., Kelly, W.F., Toft, A.D., McCarthy, M.I., Young, E.T. & Kendall-Taylor, P. (1999). Further evidence for a susceptibility locus on chromosome 20q13.11 in families with dominant transmission of Graves disease. *American Journal of Human Genetics, 65*, 1462-1465.

[286] Tomer, Y., Concepcion, E. & Greenberg, D.A. (2002). A C/T single-nucleotide polymorphism in the region of the CD40 gene is associated with Graves' disease. *Thyroid, 12*,1129-1135.

[287] Lafage-Pochitaloff, M., Herman, P., Birg, F., Galizzi, J.P., Simonetti, J., Mannoni, P. & Banchereau, J. (1994). Localization of the human CD40 gene to chromosome 20, bands q12-q13.2. *Leukemia, 8*, 1172-1175.

[288] Kim, T.Y., Park, Y.J., Hwang, J.K., Park, K.S., Cho, B.Y. & Park, D.J. (2003). A C/T polymorphism in the 5'-untranslated region of the CD40 gene is associated with Graves' disease in Koreans. *Thyroid, 13*, 919-925.

[289] Heward, J.M., Simmonds, M.J., Carr-Smith, J., Foxall, H., Franklyn, J.A. & Gough, S.C.L. (2004). A single nucleotide polymorphism in the CD40 gene on chromosome 20q (GD-2) provides no evidence for susceptibility to Graves' disease in UK Caucasians. *Clinical Endocrinology (Oxford), 61*, 269-272.

[290] Houston, F.A., Wilson, V., Jennings, C.E., Owen, C.J., Donaldson, P., Perros, P. & Pearce, S.H. (2004). Role of the CD40 locus in Graves' disease. *Thyroid,* 14, 506-509.

[291] Tomer, Y., Davies, T.F. & Greenberg, D.A. (2005). What is the contributuon of a Kozak SNP in the CD40 gene to Graves' disease? *Clinical Endocrinology (Oxford), 62*, 258.

[292] Jakobson, E.M., Concepcion, E., Oashi, T. & Tomer, Y (2005). A Graves' disease-associated Kozak sequence single-nucleotide polymorphism enchances the effeciency of CD40 gene translation: a case for translational pathophysiology. *Endocrinology, 146*, 2684-2691.

[293] Banchereau, J., Bazan, F., Blanchard, D., Brirere, F., Galizzi, J.P., van Kooten, C., Liu, Y.J., Rousset, F. & Saeland, S. (1994). The CD40 antigen and its ligand. *Annual Reviews in Immunology, 12*, 881-922.

[294] Metcalfe, R.A., McIntosh, R.S., Marelli-Berg, F., Lombardi, G., Lechler, R. & Weetman, A.P. (1998). Detection of CD40 in human thyroid follicular cells: analysis of expression and function. *Journal of Clinical Endocrinology and Metabolism, 83*, 1268-1274.

[295] Higuchi, T., Aiba, N., Nomura, T., Matsuda, J., Mochida, K., Suzuki, M., Kikutani, H., Honjo, T., Nishioka, K. & Tsubata, T. (2002). Cutting edge: ectopic expression of a

CD40 ligand on B cells induces lupus-like autoimmune disease. *Journal of Immunology, 168*, 9-12.

[296] Toubi, E. & Shoenfeld, Y. (2004). The role of CD40-CD154 interactions in autoimmunity and the benefit of disrupting this pathway. *Autoimmunity, 37*, 457-464.

[297] Liu, Z., Geboes, K., Colpaert, S., Overbergh, L., Mathieu, C., Heremans, H., de Boer, M., Boon, L., D'Haens, G., Rutgeerts, P. & Ceuppens, J.L. (2000). Prevention of experimental colitis in SCID mice reconstituted with CD45RBhigh CD4+ T cells by blocking the CD40-CD154 interactions. *Journal of Immunology, 164*, 6005-6014.

[298] Itoh, M., Uchimura, K., Makino, M., Kobayashi, T., Hayashi, R., Nagata, M., Kakizawa, H., Fujiwara, K. & Nagasaka, A. (2000). Production of IL-10 and IL-12 in CD40 and interleukin 4-activated mononulear cells from patients with Graves' disease. *Cytokine, 12*, 688-693.

[299] Uchimura, K., Itoh, M., Yamammoto, K., Imamura, S., Makino, M., Kato, T., Fijiwara, K. & Sawai, Y. (2002). The effects of CD40- and intereleukin (IL-4)-activated CD23+ cells on the production of IL-10 by mononuclear cells in Graves' disease; the role of CD8+ cells. *Clinical and Experimental Immunology, 128*, 308-312.

[300] Faure, G.C., Bensoussan-Lejzerowicz, D., Bene, M.C., Aubert, V. & Leclere. J. (1997). Coexpression of CD40 and class II antigen HLA-DR in Graves' disease thyroid epithelial cells. *Clinical Immunology and Immunopathology, 84*, 212-215.

[301] Kie, J.-H., Cho, M.-S. & Yang, W.-I. (2001). Expression of CD40 and apoptosis related molecules in autoimmune thyroid diseases. *Yonsei Medical Journal, 42*, 488-496.

[302] Salmaso, C., Olive, D., Pesce, G. & Bagnasco, M. (2002). Costimulatory molecules and autoimmune thyroid diseases. *Autoimmunity, 35*, 159-167.

[303] Wagner, D.H., Jr, Newell, E., Sanderson, R.J., Freed, J.H. & Newell, M.K. (1999) Increased expression of CD40 on thymocytes and peripheral T cells in autoimmunity: a mechanism for acquiring changes in the peripheral T cell receptor repertoire. *International Journal of Molecular Medicine, 4*, 231-242.

[304] Foy, T.M., Aruffo, A., Bajorath, J., Buhlmann, J.E. & Noelle, R.J. (1996). Immune regulation by CD40 and its ligand GP39. *Annual Reviews in Immunology, 14*, 591-617.

[305] Lind, P., Landsteger, W., Molnar, M., Gallowitsch, H.J., Mikosch, P. & Gomez, I. (1998). Epidemiology of thyroid diseases in iodine sufficiency. *Thyroid,* 1998, 8, 1179-1183.

[306] Barbesino, G., Tomer, Y., Concepsion, E., Davies, T.F. & Greenberg, D.A. (1998). Linkage analysis of candidate genes in autoimmune thyroid disease. II. Selected gender-related genes and the X-chromosome. International Consortium for the Genetics of Autoimmune Thyroid Disease. *Journal of Clinical Endocrinology and Metabolism, 83*, 3290-3295.

[307] Cucca, F., Goy, J.V., Kawaguchi, Y. , Esposito, L., Merriman, M.E., Wilson, A.J., Cordell, H.J., Bain, S.C. & Todd, J.A. (1998). A male-female bias in type 1 diabetes and linkage to chromosome Xp in MHC HLA-DR3-positive patients. *Nature Genetics, 19*, 301-312.

[308] Aruffo, A., Farrington, M., Hollenbaugh, D., Li, X., Milatovich, A., Nonoyama, S., Bajorath, J., Grosmaire, L. S., Stenkamp, R., Neubauer, M., Roberts, R. L., Noelle, R. J., Ledbetter, J. A., Francke, U. & Ochs, H. D. (1993). The CD40 ligand, gp39, is

defective in activated T cells from patients with X-linked hyper-IgM syndrome. *Cell,* 72, 291-300.

[309] Onouchi, Y., Onoue, S., Tamari, M., Wakui, K., Fukushima, Y., Yashiro, M., Nakamura, Y., Yanagawa, H., Kishi, F., Ouchi, K., Terai, M., Hamamoto, K., Kudo, F., Aotsuka, H., Sato, Y., Nariai, A., Kaburagi, Y., Miura, M., Saji, T., Kawasaki, T., Nakamura, Y. & Hata, A. (2004). CD40 ligand gene and Kawasaki disease. European *Journal of Human Genetics, 12,* 1062-1068.

[310] Cutolo, M., Sulli, A., Capellino, S., Villagio, B., Montagna, P., Seriolo, B. & Straub, R.H. (2004). Sex hormones influence on the immune system: basic and clinical aspects in autoimmunity. *Lupus, 13*, 635-638.

[311] Ban Y., Taniyama, M., Tozaki, T., Tomita, M. & Ban, Y. (2000). Estrogen receptor alpha dinucleotide repeat polymorphism in Japanese patients with autoimmune thyroid diseases. *BMC Medical Genetics*, 1:1.

[312] Ban, Y., Tozaki, T., Taniyama, M., Tomita, M. & Ban, Y. (2001). Lack of association between estrogen receptor beta dinucleotide repeat polymorphism and autoimmune thyroid diseases in Japanese patients. *BMC Medical Genetics*, 2:1

[313] Ansar Ahmed, S., Young, P.R. & Penhale, W.J. (1983). The effects of female sex steroids on the development of autoimmune thyroiditis in thymectomized and irradiated rats. *Clinical and Experimental Immunology, 54*, 351-358.

[314] Ansar Ahmed, S., Penhale, W.J. & Talal, N. (1985). Sex hormones, immune responses, and autoimmune diseases. Mechanisms of sex hormone action. *American Journal of Pathology, 121*, 531-551.

[315] Davies, T.F. (1999). The thyroid immunology of the postpartum period. *Thyroid, 9*, 675-684.

[316] Imaizumi, M., Pritsker, A., Under, P. & Davies, T.F. (2002). Intrathyroidal fetal microchimerism in pregnancy and postpartum. *Endocrinology, 143*, 247-253.

[317] Ando, T. & Davies, T.F. (2005). Monoclonal antibodies to the thyrotropin receptor. *Clinical and Developmental Immunology, 12*, 137-143.

[318] Sarkar, K. & Miller, F.W. (2004). Possible roles and determinants of microchimerism in autoimmune and other disorders. *Autoimmunity Reviews, 3*, 454-463.

[319] Renne, C., Ramos Lopez E., Steimle-Grauer, S.A., Ziolkowski, P., Pani, M.A., Luther, C., Holzer, C., Encke, A., Wahl, R.A., Bechstein, W.O., Usadel, K.H., Hansmann, M.L & Badenhoop, K. (2004). Thyroid fetal male microchimerisms in mothers with thyroid disorders: presence of Y-chromosomal immunofluorescence in thyroid-infiltrating lymphocytes is more prevalent in Hashimoto's thyroiditis and Graves' disease than in follicular adenomas. *Journal of Clinical Endocrinology and Metabolism,* 89, 5810-5814.

[320] Berry, S.M., Hassan, S.S., Russell, E., Kukuruga, D., Land, S., Kaplan, J. (2004). Association of maternal histocompatibility at class II HLA loci with maternal microchimerism in the fetus. *Pediatric Research, 56*, 73–78.

[321] Phillips, D.I., Lazarus, J.H. & Butland, B.K. (1990). The influence of pregnancy and reproductive span on the occurrence of autoimmune thyroiditis. *Clinical Endocrinology (Oxford), 32*, 301-316.

[322] Strieder, T.G., Prummel, M.F., Tijssen, J.G., Endert, E. & Wiersinga, W.M. (2003). Risk factors for and prevalence of thyroid disorders in a cross-sectional study among healthy female relatives of patients with autoimmune thyroid disease. *Clinical Endocrinology (Oxford), 59*, 396-401.

[323] Walsh, J.P., Bremner, A.P., Bulsara, M.K., O'Leary, P., Leedman, P.J., Feddema, P. & Michelangeli, V. (2006) Parity and the risk of autoimmune thyroid disease: a community-based study. *Journal of Clinical Endocrinology and Metabolism, 90*, 5309-5312.

[324] Stewart, J.J. (1998). The female X-inactivation mosaic in systemic lupus erythematosus. *Immunology Today, 19*, 352-357.

[325] Kast, R.E. (1977). Predominance of autoimmune and rheumatic diseases in females. *Journal of Rheumatology, 4*, 288-292.

[326] Invernizzi, P., Miozzo, M., Selmi, C., Persani, L., Batterzzati, P.M., Zuin, M., Lucchi, S., Meroni, P.L., Marasini, B., Zeni, S., Watnik, M., Grati, F.R., Simoni, G., Gershwin, M.E. & Podda, M. (2005). X chromosome monosomy: a common mechanism for autoimmune diseases. *Journal of Immunology, 175*, 575-578.

[327] Ozbalkan, Z., Bagislar, S., Kiraz, S., Akyerli, C.B., Ozer, H.T., Yavuz, S., Birlik, A.M., Calguneri, M. & Ozcelik, T. (2005). Skewed X chromosome inactivation in blood cells of women with scleroderma. *Arthritis and Rheumatism, 52*, 1564-1570.

[328] Martin-Villa, J.M., Corell, A., Ramos-Amador, J.T., Ruiz-Contreras, J. & Arnaiz-Villena, A. (1999). Higher incidence of autoantibodies in X-linked chronic granulomatous disease carriers: random X-chromosome inactivation may be related to autoimmunity. *Autoimmunity, 31*, 261-264.

[329] Ivarsson, S.A., Ericsson, U.B., Nilsson, K.O., Gustaffsson, J., Hagenas, L., Hager, A., Moell, C., Tuvem, T., Westphal, O & Albertsson-Wikland, K. (1995). Thyroid autoantibodies, Turner's syndrome and growth hormone therapy. *Acta Paediatrica, 84*, 63-65.

[330] Kelkar, R.L., Meherji, P.K., Kadam, S.S., Gupta, S.K. & Nandedkar, T.D. (2005). Circulating auto-antibodies against the zona pellucida and thyroid microsomal antigen in women with premature ovarian failure. *Journal of Reproductive Immunology*, 66, 53-67.

[331] Elsheikh, M., Wass, J.A. & Conway, G.S. (2001). Autoimmune thyroid syndrome in women with Turner's syndrome - the association with karyotype. *Clinical Endocrinology (Oxford), 55*, 223-226.

[332] Richardson, B. & Yung, R. (1999). Role of DNA methylation in the regulation of cell function. *Journal of Laboratory and Clinical Medicine, 134*, 333-340.

[333] Akamizu, T., Hiratani, H., Ikegami, S., Rich, S.S. & Bowden, D.W. (2003). Association study of autoimmune thyroid disease at 5q23-q33 in Japanese patients. *Journal of Human Genetics, 48*, 236-242.

[334] Jin, Y., Teng, W., Ben, S., Xiong, X., Zhang, J., Xu, S., Shugart, Y.Y., Jin, L., Chen, J. & Huang, W. (2003). Genome-wide scan of Graves' disease: evidence for linkage on chromosome 5q31 in Chinese Han pedigrees. *Journal of Clinical Endocrinology and Metabolism, 88*, 1798-1803.

[335] Sawcer, S., Ban, M., Maranian, M., Yeo, T.W., Compston, A., Kirby, A., Daly, M.J., De Jager, P.L., Walsh, E., Lander, E.S., Rioux, J.D., Hafler, D.A., Ivinson, A., Rimmler, J., Gregory, S.G., Scmidt, S., Pericak-Vance, M.A., Akesson, E., Hillert, J., Datta, P., Oturai, A., Ryder, L.P., Harbo, H.F., Spurkland, A., Myhr, K.M., Laaksonen, M., Booth, D., Heard, R., Steward, G., Lincoln, R., Barcellos, L.F., Hauser, S.L., Oksenberg, J.R., Kenealy, S.L. & Haines, J.L. (2005) A high-density screen for linkage in multiple sclerosis. *American Journal of Human Genetics, 77*, 454-467.

[336] Noguchi, E., Yokouchi, Y., Zhang, J., Shibuya, K., Shibuya, A., Bannai, M., Tokunaga, K., Doi, H., Tamari, M., Shimizu, M., Shirakawa, T., Shibasaki, M., Ichikawa, K. & Arinami, T. (2005). Positional identification of an asthma susceptibility gene on human chromosome 5q33. *American Journal of Respiratory and Critical Care Medicine, 172*, 183-188.

[337] Yokouchi, Y., Shibasaki, M., Noguchi, E., Nakayma, J., Ohtsuki, T., Kamioka, M., Yamakawa-Kobayashi, K., Ito, S., Takeda, K., Ichikawa, K., Nukaga, Y., Matsui, A., Hamaguchi, H. & Arinami, T. (2002). A genome-wide linkage analysis of orchard grass-sensitive childhood seasonal allergic rhinitis in Japanese families. *Genes and Immunity, 3*, 9-13.

[338] Ma, Y., Ohmen, J.D., Li, Z., Bentley, L.G., McElree, C., Pressman, S., Targan, S.R., Fischel-Ghodsian, N., Rotter, J.I. & Yang, H. (1999). A genome-wide search identifies potential new susceptibility loci for Crohn's disease. *Inflammatory Bowel Disease, 5*, 271-278.

[339] Kawashima, T., Noguchi, E., Arinami, T., Yamakawa, K., Obayashi, K., Nakagawa, H., Otsuka, F. & Hamaguchi, H. (1998). Linkage and association of an interleukin 4 gene polymorphism with atopic dermatitis in Japanese families. *Journal of Medical Genetics, 35*, 502–504.

[340] Zhong, F., McCombs, C.C., Olson, J.M., Elston, R.C., Stevens, F.M., McCarthy, C.F. & Michalski, J.P. (1996). An autosomal screen for genes that predispose to celiac disease in the western counties of Ireland. *Nature Genetics, 14*, 329-333.

[341] Ho, P., Bowes, J., Eyre, S., Bradburn, P., Newman, B., Bruce, I., Silman, A., Worthington, J. & Barton, A. (2004). Association of the organic cation transporter (OCTN) SLC22A4 and SLC22A5 genes with psoriatic arthritis. *Arthritis and Rheumatism, 50*, S258.

[342] Ferreira, A.C., Almeida, S., Tavares, M., Canedo, P., Pereira, F., Regalo, G., Figueiredo, C., Trindade, E., Seruca, R., Carneiro, F., Amil, J., Machado, J.C. & Tavarela-Veloso, F. (2005). NOD2/CARD15 and TNFA, but not IL1B and IL1RN, are associated with Crohn's disease. *Inflammatory Bowel Disease, 11*, 331-339.

[343] Brand, S., Staudinger, T., Schnitzler, F., Pfennig, S., Hofbauer, K., Dambacher, J., Seiderer, J., Tillack, C., Konrad, A., Crispin, A., Goke, B., Lohse, P., Ochsenkuhn, T. (2005). The role of Toll-like receptor 4 Asp299Gly and Thr399Ile polymorphisms and CARD15/NOD2 mutations in the susceptibility and phenotype of Crohn's disease. *Inflammatory Bowel Disease, 11*, 645-652.

[344] Weidinger, S., Klopp, N., Rummler, L., Wagenpfeil, S., Baurecht, H.J., Gauger, A., Darsow, U., Jakob, T., Novak, N., Schafer, T., Heinrich, J., Behrendt, H., Wichmann, H.E., Ring, J. & Illig, T. (2005). Association of CARD15 polymorphisms with atopy-

related traits in a population-based cohort of Caucasian adults. *Clinical and Experimental Allergy, 35*, 866-872.

[345] Rahman, P., Bartlett, S., Siannia, S., Pellett, F.J., Farewell, V.T., Peddle, L., Schentag, C.T., Alderdice, C.A., Hamilton, C., Kraishi, M., Tobin, Y., Hefferton, D. & Gladman, D.D. (2005). CARD15: a pleiotropic autoimmune gene that confers susceptibility to psoriatic arthritis. *American Journal of Human Genetics, 73*, 677-681.

[346] Peltekova, V.D., Wintle, R.F., Rubin, L.A., Amos, C.I., Huang, Q., Gu, X., Newman, B., van Oene, M., Cescon, D., Greenberg, G., Griffith, A.M., St George-Hyslop, P.H. & Siminovitch, K.A. (2004). Functional variants of OCTN cation transporter genes are associated with Grohn disease. *Nature Genetics, 36*, 471-475.

[347] Meyers, D.A., Postma, D.S., Panhuysen, C.I., Xu, J., Amelung, P.J., Levitt, R.C. & Bleecker, E.R. (1994). Evidence for a locus regulating total serum IgE levels mapping to chromosome 5. *Genomics, 23*, 464–470.

[348] Chistiakov, D.A. (2005). Immunogenetics of Hashimoto's thyroiditis. *Journal of Autoimmune Diseases*, 2:1.

[349] Mossmann, T.R. & Coffmann, R.L. (1989). TH1 and TH2 cells: different patterns of lymphokine secretion lead to different functional properties. *Annual Reviews in Immunology, 7*, 145-173.

[350] Hunt, P.J., Marshall, S.E., Weetman, A.P., Bell, J.L., Wass, J.A. & Welsh K.I. (2000) Cytokine gene polymorphisms in autoimmune thyroid disease. *Journal of Clinical Endocrinology and Metabolism, 85*, 1984-1988.

[351] Hiromatsu, Y., Fukutani, T., Ichimura, M., Mukai, T., Kaku, H., Nakyama, H., Miyake, I., Shoji, S., Koda, Y. & Bernarczuk, T. (2005). Interleukin-13 gene polymorphisms confer the susceptibility of Japanese populations to Graves' disease. *Journal of Clinical Endocrinology and Metablism, 90*, 296-301.

[352] Heward, J.M., Nithiyananthan, R., Allahabadia, A., Gibson, S., Franklyn, J.A. & Gough, S.C. (2001). No association of an interleukin 4 gene promoter polymorphism with Graves' disease in the United Kingdom. *Journal of Clinical Endocrinology and Metabolism, 86*, 3861-3863.

[353] Vaidya, B., Imrie, H., Perros, P., Young, E.T., Kelly, W.F., Carr, D., Large, D.M., Toft, A.D., Kendall-Taylor, P. & Pearce, S.H. (2000). Evidence for a new Graves disease susceptibility locus at chromosome 18q21. *American Journal of Human Genetics, 66*, 1710-1714.

[354] Merriman, T., Twells, R., Merriman, M., Eaves, I., Cox, R., Cucca, F., McKinney, P., Shield, J., Baum, J., Bosi, E., Pozzilli, P., Nistico, L., Buzzetti, R., Joner, G., Ronningen, K., Thorsby, E., Undlien, D., Pociot, F., Nerup, J., Bain, S., Barnett, A. & Todd, J. (1997). Evidence by allelic association-dependent methods for a type 1 diabetes polygene (IDDM6) on chromosome 18q21. *Human Molecular Genetics, 6*, 1003-1010.

[355] Cornelis, F., Faure, S., Martinez, M., Prud'homme, J.F., Fritz, P., Dib, C., Alves, H., Barrera, P., de Vries, N., Balsa, A., Pascual-Salcedo, D., Maenaut, K., Westhovens, R., Migliorini, P., Tran, T.H., Delaye, A., Prince, N., Lefevre, C., Thomas, G., Poirier, M., Soubigou, S., Alibert, O., Lasbleiz, S., Fouix, S., Bouchier, C., Liote, F., Loste, M.N., Lepage, V., Charron, D., Gyapay, G., Lopez-Vaz, A., Kuntz, D., Bardin, T. &

Weissenbach, J. (1998). New susceptibility locus for rheumatoid arthritis suggested by a genome-wide linkage study. *Proceedings of the National Academy of Sciences of the USA, 95*,10746–10750.

[356] Shai, R., Quismorio, F.P., Jr, Li, L., Kwon, O.J., Morrison, J., Wallace, D.J., Neuwelt, C.M., Brautbar, C., Gauderman, W.J. & Jacob, C.O. (1999). Genome-wide screen for systemic lupus erythematosus susceptibility genes in multiplex families. *Human Molecular Genetics, 8*, 639–644.

[357] Hsu, S.Y. & Hsueh, A.J. (2000). Tissue-specific Bcl-2 protein partners in apoptosis: An ovarian paradigm. *Physiological Reviews, 80*, 593-614.

[358] Labat-Moleur, F., Chabre, O., Guillermet, C., Chafanjon, P., Blummet-Rondeu, F., Bauchet, A., Franc, B., Brambilla, E., Bachelot, I., Dumont, J.E. & Negoescu, A. (1999). Graves-Basedow disease goiter: a model of Bax-Bcl2 regulated apoptosis. *Thyroid, 9*, 483-492.

[359] Giordano, C., Richiusa, P., Bagnasco, M., Pizzolanti, G., Di Blasti, F., Sbriglia, M.S., Mattina, A., Pesce, G., Montagna, P., Capone, F., Misiano, G., Scorsone, A., Pugliese, A., Galluzo, A. (2001). Differential regulation of Fas-mediated apoptosis in both thyrocyte and lymphocyte cellular compartments correlates with opposite phenotypic manifestations of autoimmune thyroid disease. *Thyroid, 11*, 233-244.

[360] Komaki, S., Kohno, M., Matsuura, N., Shimadzu, Adachi, N., Hoshide, R., Nishiyama, S. & Matsuda, I. (1998). The polymorphic 43Thr bcl-2 protein confers relative resistance to autoimmunity: an analytical evaluation. *Human Genetics, 103*, 435-440.

[361] Porter, A.G. & Dhakshinamoorthy, S. (2003). Apoptosis initiated by dependence receptors: a new paradigm for cell death? *Bioessays, 26*, 656-664.

[362] Hall, R.J., Merriman, M.E., Green, R.A., Markham, V.H., Smyth, D.J., Heward, J.M., Jennings, C.E., Braithwaite, A.W., Cundy, T., Darlow, B.A., Gow, P.J., Harrison, A.A., Highton, J., Hunt, P.J., Manning, P., Pokorny, V., Scott, R.S., Taylor, B.J., Willis, J.A., Yeoman, S., McLean, L., Gough, S.C., Pearce, S.H., Merriman, T.R. (2003) The deleted in colorectal carcinoma (DCC) gene 201R-->G polymorphism: no evidence for genetic association with autoimmune disease. *European Journal of Human Genetics, 11*,840-844.

[363] Henthorn, P., Kiledjian, M., & Kadesch, T. (1990). Two distinct transcription factors that bind the immunoglobulin enhancer microE5/kappa 2 motif. *Science, 247*, 467-470.

[364] Villanueva, R., Tomer, Y., Greenberg, D.A., Mao, C., Concepcion, E.S., Tucci, S., Estilo, G. & Davies, T.F. (2002). Autoimmune thyroid disease susceptibility loci in a large Chinese family. *Clinical Endocrinology (Oxford), 56*, 45-51.

[365] Padilla, O., Calvo, J., Vila, J.M., Arman, M., Gimferrer, I., Places, L., Arias, M.T., Pujana, M.A., Vives, J., Lozano, F. (2000). Genomic organization of the human CD5 gene. *Immunogenetics, 51*, 993-1001.

[366] Gimferrer, I., Farnos, M., Calvo, M., Mittelbrunn, M., Enrich, C., Sanchez-Madrid, F., Vives, J., Lozano, F. (2003). The accessory molecules CD5 and CD6 associate on the membrane of lymphoid T cells. *Journal of Biological Chemistry, 278*, 8564-8571.

[367] Iwatani, Y., Amino, N., Kaneda, T., Ichihara, K., Tamaki, H., Matsuzuka, F., Fukata, S., Kuma, K., Miyai, K. (1989). Marked increase of CD5 + B cells in hyperthyroid Graves' disease. *Clinical and Experimental Immunology, 78*, 196-200.

[368] Martel, J., Cayrou, C. & Puymirat, J. (2002). Identification of new thyroid hormone-regulated genes in rat brain neuronal cultures. *Neuroreport, 13*, 1849-1851.

[369] Koppelman, G.H., Stine, O.C., Xu, J., Howard, T.D., Zheng, S.L., Kauffman, H.F., Bleecker, E.R., Meyers, D.A. & Postma, D.S. (2002). Genome-wide search for atopy susceptibility genes in Dutch families with asthma. *Journal of Allergy and Clinical Immunology, 109*, 498-506.

[370] Van Heel, D.A., Fisher, S.A., Kirby, A., Daly, M.J., Rioux, J.D. & Lewis, C.M. (2004). Inflammatory bowel disease susceptibility loci defined by genome scan meta-analysis of 1952 affected relative pairs. *Human Molecular Genetics, 13*, 763-770.

[371] Bellefroid, E.J., Marine, J.C., Ried, T., Lecocq, P.J., Riviere, M., Amemiya, C., Poncelet, D.A., Coulie, P.G., de Jong. P. & Szpirer, C. (1993). Clustered organization of homologous KRAB zinc-finger genes with enhanced expression in human T lymphoid cells. *EMBO Journal, 12*, 1363-1374.

[372] Pease, J.E., Weller, C.L. & Williams, T.J. (2004) Regulation of eosinophil trafficking in asthma and allergy. *Ernst Schering Research Foundation Workshop, 45*, 85-100.

[373] Alarcon-Riquelme, M. (2005). The genetics of shared autoimmunity. *Autoimmunity, 38*, 205-208.

[374] Szyper-Kravitz, M., Marai, I. & Shoenfeld, Y. (2005). Coexistence of thyroid autoimmunity with other autoimmune diseases: friend or foe? Additional aspects of the mosaic of autoimmunity. *Autoimmunity, 38*, 247-255.

[375] Jenkins, R.C. & Weetman, A.P. (2002). Disease associations with autoimmune thyroid disease. *Thyroid, 12*, 977-988.

[376] Maclaren, N.K. & Riley, W.J. (1985). Thyroid, gastric, and adrenal autoimmunities associated with insulin-dependent diabetes mellitus. *Diabetes Care, 8*, 34-38.

[377] Holl, R.W., Bohm, B., Loos, U., Grabert, M., Heinze, E. & Homoki, J. (1999) Thyroid autoimmunity in children and adolescents with type 1 diabetes mellitus. Effect of age, gender and HLA type. *Hormone Research, 52*, 113-118.

[378] Kordonouri, O., Klinghammer, A., Lang, E.B., Gruters-Kieslich, A., Grabert, M. & Holl, R.W. (2002) Thyroid autoimmunity in children and adolescents with type 1 diabetes: a multicenter survey. *Diabetes Care, 25*, 1346-1350.

[379] Hansen, A., Lipsky, P.E. & Dorner, T. (2005). Immunopathogenesis of primary Sjogren's syndrome: implications for disease management and therapy. *Current Opinion in Rheumatology, 17*, 558-565.

[380] Burek, C.L., Rose, N.R., Guire, K.E. & Hoffman, W.H. (1990). Thyroid autoantibodies in black and in white children and adolescents with type 1 diabetes mellitus and their first-degree relatives. *Autoimmunity, 7*, 157-167.

[381] Dorman, J.S., McCarthy, B., McCanlies, E., Kramer, M.K., Vergona, R.J., Stone, R., Steenkiste, A.R., Kocova, M. & Trucco, M. (1996). Molecular IDDM epidemiology: international studies. WHO DiaMond Molecular Epidemiology Sub-Project Group. *Diabetes Research and Clinical Practice, 34*, S107-S116.

[382] Maugendre, D., Verite, F., Guilhem, I., Genetet, B., Allanic, H. & Delamaire, M. (1997). Anti-pancreatic autoimmunity and Graves' disease: study of a cohort of 600 Caucasian patients. *European Journal of Endocrinology. 137*, 503-510.

[383] Silva, R.C., Sallorenzo, C., Kater, C.E., Dib, S.A. & Falorni, A. (2003). Autoantibodies against glutamic acid decarboxylase and 21-hydroxylase in Brazilian patients with type 1 diabetes or autoimmune thyroid diseases. *Diabetes Nutrition and Metabolism,* 16, 160-168.

[384] McCanlies, E., O'Leary, L.A., Foley, T.P., Kramer, M.K., Burke, J.P., Libman, A., Swan, J.S., Steenkiste, A.R., Mccarthy, B.J., Trucco, M. & Dorman, J.S. (1998). Hashimoto's thyroiditis and insulin-dependent diabetes mellitus: differences among individuals with and without abnormal thyroid function. *Journal of Clinical Endocrinology and Metabolism, 83*, 1548-1551.

[385] Tait, K.F., Marshall, T., Berman, J., Carr-Smith, J., Rowe, B., Todd, J.A., Bain, S.C., Barnett, A.H. & Gough, S.C. (2004). Clustering of autoimmune disease in parents of siblings from the Type 1 diabetes Warren repository. *Diabetic Medicine, 21*, 358-362.

[386] Badenhoop, K. & Boehm, B.O. (2004). Genetic susceptibility and immunological synapse in type 1 diabetes and thyroid autoimmune disease. *Experimental and Clinical Endocrinology and Diabetes, 112*, 407-415.

[387] Devendra, D. & Eisenbarth, G.S. (2003). 17. Immunologic endocrine disorders. *Journal of Allergy and Clinical Immunology, 111*, S624-S636.

[388] Larsen, C.E. & Alper, C.A. (2004). The genetics of HLA-associated disease. *Current Opinion in Immunology, 16*, 660-667

[389] Todd, J.A., Bell, J.L. & McDevitt, H.O. (1987). HLA-DQ beta gene contributes to susceptibility and resistance to insulin-dependent diabetes mellitus. *Nature*, 1987, 329, 599-604.

[390] Deschamps, I., Beressi, J.P., Khalil, I., Robert, J.J. & Hors, J. (1991). The role of genetic predisposition to type I (insulin-dependent) diabetes mellitus. *Annals of Medicine, 23*, 427-435.

[391] Sumnik, Z., Drevinek, P., Snajderova, M., Kolouskova, S., Sedlakova, P., Pechova, M., Vavrinec, J. & Cinek, O. (2003). HLA-DQ polymorphisms modify the risk of thyroid autoimmunity in children with type 1 diabetes mellitus. *Journal of Pediatric Endocrinology and Metabolism, 16*, 851-858.

[392] Awata, T., Katsuren, E., Matsumoto, C., Nagayama, I., Uchigata, Y., Kuzuya, N. & Kanazawa, Y. (1995). Absence of shared HLA class II (DR, DQ)-linked genetic basis between IDDM and autoimmune thyroid disease in Japanese. *Diabetes Care, 18*, 582-583.

[393] Djilali-Saiah, I., Bertin, E., Larger, E., Timsit, J., Assan, R., Boitard, C., Bach, J.F. & Caillat-Zucman, S. (1998). Major histocompatibility class II genes polymorphism in insulin dependent diabetes mellitus with or without associated thyroid autoimmunity. *Human Immunology, 59*, 176-182.

[394] Chikuba, N., Akazawa, S., Yamaguchi, Y., Kawasaki, E., Takino, H., Yoshimoto, M., Ohe, N., Yamashita, K., Yano, A. & Nagataki, S. (1995). Immunogenetic heterogeneity in type 1 (insulin-dependent) diabetes among Japanese - class II antigen and autoimmune thyroid disease. *Diabetes Research and Clinical Practice, 27*, 31-37.

[395] Chuang, L.M., Wu, H.P., Chang, C.C., Tsai, W.Y., Chang, H.M., Tai, T.Y. & Lin, B.J. (1996). HLA DRB1/DQA1/DQB1 haplotype determines thyroid autoimmunity in

patients with insulin-dependent diabetes mellitus. *Clinical Endocrinology (Oxford), 45*, 631-636.

[396] Kim, E.Y., Shin, C.H. & Yang, S.W. (2003). Polymorphisms of HLA class II predispose children and adolescents with type 1 diabetes mellitus to autoimmune thyroid disease. *Autoimmunity, 36*, 177-181.

[397] Santamaria, P., Barbosa, J.J., Lindstrom, A.L., Lemke, T.A., Goetz, F.C. & Rich, S.S. (1994). HLA-DQB1-asociated susceptibility that distinguishes Hashimoto's thyroiditis from Graves' disease in type 1 diabetic patients. *Journal of Clinical Endocrinology and Metabolism*, 1994, 78, 878-883.

[398] Payami, H., Joe, S. & Thomson, G. (1989). Autoimmune thyroid disease in Type 1 diabetes. *Genetic Epidemiology, 6*, 137-141.

[399] Torfs, C.P., King M.-C., Bing, H., Malmgren, J. & Grumet, F.C. (1986). Genetic interrelationship between insulin-dependent diabetes mellitus, the autoimmune thyroid diseases and rheumatoid arthritis. *American Journal of Human Genetics, 38*, 170-187.

[400] Levin, L., Ban, Y., Concepcion, E., Davies, T.F., Greenberg, D.A. & Tomer, Y. (2004). Analysis of HLA genes in families with autoimmune diabetes and thyroiditis. *Human Immunology, 65*, 640-647.

[401] Golden, B., Levin, L., Ban, Y., Concepcion, E., Greenberg, D.A. & Tomer, Y. (2005). Genetic analysis of families with autoimmune disabetes and thyroiditis; evidence for common and unique genes. *Journal of Clinical Endocrinology and Metabolism, 90*, 4904-4911.

[402] Nistico, L., Buzzetti, R., Pritchard, L.E., Van der Auwera, B., Giovannini, C., Bosi, E., Larrad, M.T., Rios, M.S., Chow, C.C., Cockram, C.S., Jacobs, K., Mijovic, C., Bain, S.C., Barnett, A.H., Vandewalle, C.L., Schuit, F., Gorus, F.K., Tosi, R., Pozzilli, P. & Todd, J.A. (1996). The CTLA-4 gene region of chromosome 2q33 is linked to, and associated with, type 1 diabetes. Belgian Diabetes Registry. *Human Molecular Genetics, 5*, 1075-1080.

[403] Takara, M., Komiya, I., Kinio, Y., Tomoyose, T., Yamashiro, S., Akamine, H., Masuda, M. & Takasu, N. (2000) Association of CTLA-4 gene A/G polymorphism in Japanese type 1 diabetic patients with younger age of onset and autoimmune thyroid disease. *Diabetes Care, 23*, 975-978.

[404] Mochizuki, M., Amemiya, S., Kobayashi, K., Kobayashi, K., Shimura, Y., Ishihara, T., Nakagomi, Y., Onigata, K., Tamai, S., Kasuga, A. & Nanazawa, S. (2003). Association of the CTLA-4 gene 49 A/G polymorphism with type 1 diabetes and autoimmune thyroid disease in Japanese children. *Diabetes Care, 26*, 843-847.

[405] Kemp, E.H., Ajjan, R.A., Waterman, E.A., Gawkrodger, D.J., Cork, M.J., Watson, P.F. & Weetman, A.P. (1999). Analysis of a microsatellite polymorphism of the cytotoxic T-lymphocyte antigen-4 gene in patients with vitiligo. *British Journal of Dermatology, 140*, 73–78.

[406] Vaidya, B., Kendall-Taylor, P. & Pearce, S.H. (2002). The genetics of autoimmune thyroid disease. *Journal of Clinical Endocrinology Metabolism, 87*, 5385-5397.

[407] Allahabadia, A., Heward, J., Carr-Smith, J., Daykin, J., Barnett, A.H., Sheppard, M.C., Franklyn, J.A. & Gough, S.C. (1999). Sharing of susceptibility loci between

autoimmune diseases: lack of association of the insulin gene region with Graves' disease. *Thyroid, 9*, 317-318.

[408] Tait, K.F., Collins, J.F., Heward, J.M., Eaves, I., Snook, H., Franklyn, J.A., Barnett, A.H., Todd, J.A., Maranian, M., Compston, A., Sawcer, S. & Gough, S.C. (2004). Evidence for a Type 1 diabetes-specific mechanism for the insulin gene-associated IDDM2 locus rather than a general influence on autoimmunity. *Diabetic Medicine, 21*, 267-270.

[409] Concannon, P., Godolin-Ewens, K.J., Hinds, D.A., Wapelhorst, B., Morrison, V.A., Stirling, B., Mitra, M., Farmer, J., Williams, S.R., Cox, N.J., Bell, G.I., Risch, N. & Spielman, R.S. (1998). A second-generation screen of the human genome for susceptibility to insulin-dependent diabetes mellitus. *Nature Genetics, 19*, 292-296.

[410] Gaffney, P.M., Kearns, G.M., Shark, K.B., Ortmann, W.A., Selby, S.A., Malmgren, M.L., Rohlf, K.E., Ockenden, T.C., Messner, R.P., King, R.A., Rich, S.S. & Behrens, T.W. (1998). A genome-wide search for susceptibility genes in human systemic lupus erythematosus sib-pair families. *Proceedings of the National Academy of Sciences of the USA, 95*, 14875-14879.

[411] Mathieu, C. & Badenhoop, K. (2005). Vitamin D and type 1 diabetes mellitus: state of the art. *Trends in Endocrinology and Metabolism, 16*, 261-266.

[412] Smyth, D., Cooper, J.D., Collins, J.E., Heward, J.M., Franklyn, J.A., Howson, J.M., Vella, A., Nutland, S., Rance, H.E., Maier, L., Barratt, B.J., Guja, C., Ionescu-Tirgoviste, C., Savage, D.A., Dunger, D.B., Widmer, B., Strachan, D.P., Ring, S.M., Walker, N., Clayton, D.G., Twells, R.C., Gough, S.C. & Todd, J.A. (2004). Replication of an association between the lymphoid tyrosine phosphatase locus (LYP/PTPN22) with type 1 diabetes, and evidence for its role as a general autoimmunity locus. *Diabetes, 53*, 3020-3023.

[413] Pugliese, A. & Eisenbarth, G.S. (2004). Type 1 diabetes mellitus of man: genetic susceptibility and resistance. *Advances in Experimental Medicine and Biology, 552*, 170-203.

[414] Betterle, C., Greggio, N.A. & Volpato, M. (1998). Clinical review 93: autoimmune polyglandular syndrome type 1. *Journal of Clinical Endocrinology and Metabolism, 83*, 1049-1055.

[415] Betterle, C., Volpato, M., Greggio, A.N. & Presotto, F. (1996). Type 2 polyglandular autoimmune disease (Schmidt's syndrome). *Journal of Pediatric Endocrinology Metabolism, 9*, 113-123.

[416] Dittmar, M. & Kanaly, G.J. (2005). Polyglandular autoimmune syndromes: immunogenetics and long-term follow-up. *Journal of Clinical Endocrinology and Metabolism, 88*, 1983-2992.

[417] Robles, D.T., Fain, P.R., Gottlieb, P.A. & Eisenbarth, G.S. (2002). The genetics of autoimmune polyendocrine syndrome type II. *Endocrinology and Metabolism Clinics of North America, 31*, 353-368.

[418] Betterle, C., Lazzarotto, F. & Presotto, F. (2004). Autoimmune polyglandular syndrome Type 2: the tip of an iceberg? Clinical and Experimental Immunology, 137, 225-233.

[419] Simmonds, M.J. & Gough, S.C. (2005). Genetic insights into disease mechanisms of autoimmunity. *British Medical Bulletin, 71*, 93-113.

[420] Bjorses, P., Aaltonen, J., Horelli-Kuitunen, N., Yaspo, M.L. & Peltonen, L. (1998). Gene defect behind APECED: a new clue to autoimmunity. *Human Molecular Genetics, 7,* 1547-1553.

[421] Consortium (1997). An autoimmune disease, APECED, caused by mutations in a novel gene featuring two PHD-type zinc-finger domains. The Finnish-German APECED Consortium. Autoimmune Polyendocrinopathy-Candidiasis-Ectodermal Dystrophy. *Nature Genetics, 17*, 399-403.

[422] Pearce, S.H., Cheetham, T., Imrie, H., Vaidya, B., Barnes, N.D., Bilous, R.W., Carr, D., Meeran, K., Shaw, N.J., Smith, C.S., Toft, A.D. Williams, G. & Kendall-Taylor, P. (1998). A common and recurrent 13-bp deletion in the autoimmune regulator gene in British kindreds with autoimmune polyendocrinopathy type 1. *American Journal of Human Genetics, 63*, 1675-1684.

[423] Nithiyananthan, R., Heward, J.M., Allahabadia, A., Barnett, A.H., Franklyn, J.A. &Gough, S.C. (2000). A heterozygous deletion of the autoimmune regulator (AIRE1) gene, autoimmune thyroid disease, and type 1 diabetes: no evidence for association. *Journal of Clinical Endocrinology and Metabolism, 85*, 1320-1322.

[424] Meyer, G., Donner, H., Herwig, J., Bohles, H., Usadel, K.H. & Badenhoop, K. (2001). Screening for an AIRE-1 mutation in patients with Addison's disease, type 1 diabetes, Graves' disease and Hashimoto's thyroiditis as well as in APECED syndrome. *Clinical Endocrinology (Oxford), 54*, 335-338.

[425] Partanen, J., Peterson, P., Westman, P., Aranko, S. & Krohn, K. (1994). Major histocompatibility complex class II and III in Addison's disease. MHC alleles do not predict autoantibody specificity and 21-hydroxylase gene polymorphism has no independent role in disease susceptibility. *Human Immunology, 41*, 135-140.

[426] Cofie, D.Q., Rogers, R., Draelos, M.T., Olansky, L. & Scofield, R.H. (1995). Syndrome of type II polyglandular autoimmunity associated with HLA-DR4 in a large kindred, including HLA-DR3/DR4 heterozygosity in the probands, identical twins with identical manifestations. *Endocrine Practice, 1*, 395-398.

[427] Huang, W., Connor, E., Rosa, T.D., Muir, A., Schatz, D., Silverstein, J., Crockett, S., She, J.X. & Maclaren, N.K. (1996). Although DR3-DQB1*0201 may be associated with multiple component diseases of the autoimmune polyglandular syndromes, the human leukocyte antigen DR4-DQB1*0302 haplotype is implicated only in beta-cell autoimmunity. *Journal of Clinical Endocrinology and Metabolism, 81*, 2559-2563.

[428] Wallaschowski, H., Meyer, A., Tuschy, U. & Lohmann, T. (2003). HLA-DQA1*0301-associated susceptibility for autoimmune polyglandular syndrome type II and III. *Hormone and Metabolic Research, 35*, 120-124.

[429] Takamatsu, K., Nishiyama, T., Nakauchi, Y., Yamano, T. & Ohno, F. (1989). A case of insulin dependent diabetes mellitus associated with relapsing polychondritis, Hashimoto's thyroiditis and pituitary adrenocortical insufficiency in succession. *Japan Journal of Medicine, 28*, 232-236.

[430] Myhre, A.G., Undlien, D.E., Lovas, K., Uhlving, S., Nedrebo, B.G., Fougner, K.J., Trovik, T., Sorheim, J.L. & Husebye, E.S. (2002). Autoimmune adrenocortical failure in Norway autoantibodies and human leukocyte antigen class II associations related to clinical features. *Journal of Clinical Endocrinology and Metabolism, 87*, 618-823.

[431] May, E., Asadullah, K. & Zugel, U. (2004). Immunoregulation through 1,25-dihydroxyvitamin D3 and its analogs. Current Drug Targets. *Inflammation and Allergy, 3*, 377-393

[432] Chen, W., Lin, H. & Wang, M. (2002). Immune intervention effects on the induction of experimental autoimmune thyroiditis. Journal of Huazhong University of Science and Technology. *Medical Sciences, 22*, 343-354.

[433] Giulietti A., Gysemans, C., Stoffels, K., van Etten, E., Decallone, B., Overbergh, L., Boullion, R. & Mathieu, C. (2004). Vitamin D deficiency in early life accelerates Type 1 diabetes in non-obese diabetic mice. *Diabetologia, 47*, 451-462.

[434] Labuda, M., Fujiwara, T.M., Ross, M.V., Morgan, K., Garcia-Heras, J., Ledbetter, D.H., Hughes, M.R. & Glorieux, F.H. (1992). Two hereditary defects related to vitamin D metabolism map to the same region of human chromosome 12q13-14. *Journal of Bone and Mineral Research, 7*, 1447-1453.

[435] Veldman, C.M., Cantorna, M.T. & Deluca, H.F. (2000). Expression of 1,25-dihydroxyvitamin receptor in the immune system. *Archives of Biochemistry and Biophysics, 374*, 334-338.

[436] Nejentsev, S., Godfrey, L., Snook, H., Rance, H., Nutland, S., Walker, N.M., Lam, A.C., Guja, C., Ionescu-Tirgoviste, C., Undlien, T.E., Ronningen, K.S., Tuomilehto-Wolf, E., Tuomilehto, J., Newport, M.J., Clayton, D.G. & Todd, J.A. (2004). Comparative high-resolution analysis of linkage disequilibrium and tag single nucleotide polymorphisms between populations in the vitamin D receptor gene. *Human Molecular Genetics, 13*, 1633-1639.

[437] Pani, M.A., Knapp, M., Donner, H., Braun, J., Baur, M.P., Usadel, K.H. & Badenhoop, K. (2000) Vitamin D receptor allele combinations influence genetic susceptibility to type 1 diabetes in Germans. *Diabetes, 49*, 504 –507.

[438] Poon, A.H., Laprise, C., Lemire, M., Montpetit, A., Sinnett, D., Schurr, E. & Hudson, T.J. (2004). Association of vitamin D receptor genetic variants with susceptibility to asthma and atopy. *American Journal of Respiration and Critical Care Medicine, 170*, 967-973.

[439] Ban, Y., Taniyama, M. & Ban, Y. (2000). Vitamin D receptor gene polymorphism is associated with Graves' disease in the Japanese population. *Journal of Clinical Endocrinology and Metabolism, 85*, 4639-4643.

[440] Pani, M.A., Regulla, K., Segni, M., Hofmann, S., Hufner, M., Pasquino, A.M., Usadel, K.H. & Badenhoop, K. (2002). A polymorphism within the vitamin D-binding protein gene is associated with Graves' disease but not with Hashimoto's thyroiditis. *Journal of Clinical Endocrinology and Metabolism, 87*, 2564-2567.

[441] Stefanic, M., Karner, I., Glavas-Obrovac, L., Papic, S., Vrdoljak, D., Levak, G. & Krstonosic, B. (2005). Association of Vitamin D Receptor Gene polymorphism with susceptibility to Graves' disease in Eastern Croatian population: case-control Study. *Croatian Medical Journal, 46*, 639-646.

[442] Pani, M.A., Seissler, J., Usadel, K.H. & Badenhoop, K. (2002). Vitamin D receptor genotype is associated with Addison's disease. *European Journal of Endocrinology, 147*, 635-640.

[443] Zittermann, A. (2003). Vitamin D in preventive medicine: are we ignoring the evidence? *British Journal of Nutrition, 89*, 552-572.

[444] Jurutka, P.W., Remus, L.S., Whitefield, G.K., Thompson, P.D., Hsieh, J.C., Zitzer, H., Tavakkoli, P., Galligan, M.A., Dang, H.T., Haussler, C.A. & Haussler, M.R. (2000). The polymorphic N terminus in human vitamin D receptor isoforms influences transcriptional activity by modulating interaction with transcription factor IIB. *Molecular Endocrinology, 14*, 401-420.

[445] Colin, E.M., Weel, A.E., Uitterlinden, A.G., Buurman, C.J., Birkenhager, J.C., Pols, H.A. & van Leeuwen, J.P. (2000). Consequences of vitamin D receptor gene polymorphisms for growth inhibition of cultured human peripheral blood mononuclear cells by 1, 25-dihydroxyvitamin D3. *Clinical Endocrinology (Oxford), 52*, 211-216.

[446] Wong, H.L., Seow, A., Arakawa, K., Lee, H.P., Yu, M.C. & Ingles, S.A. (2003). Vitamin D receptor start codon polymorphism and colorectal cancer risk: effect modification by dietary calcium and fat in Singapore Chinese. *Carcinogenesis, 24*, 1091-1095.

[447] Durrin, L.K., Haile, R.W., Ingles, S.A. & Coetzee, G.A. (1999). Vitamin D receptor 3'-untranslated region polymorphisms: lack of effect on mRNA stability. *Biochimica et Biophysica Acta, 1453*, 311-320.

[448] Siminovitch, K.A. (2004). PTPN22 and autoimmune disease. *Nature Genetics, 36*, 1248-1249.

[449] Cohen, S., Dadi, H., Shaoul, N. & Roifman, C.M. (1999). Cloning and characterization of a lymphoid-specific, inducible human protein tyrosine phosphatase. *Lyp. Blood*, 1999, 93, 2013-2024.

[450] Cloutier, J.F. & Veillette, A. (1999). Cooperative inhibition of T-cell antigen receptor signaling by a complex between a kinase and a phosphatase. *Journal of Experimental Medicine, 189*, 111-121.

[451] Gjorloff-Wingren, A., Saxena, M., Williams, S., Hammi, D. & Mustelin, T. (1999). Characterization of TCR-induced receptor-proximal signaling events negatively regulated by the protein tyrosine phosphatase PEP. *European Journal of Immunology, 29*, 3845-3854.

[452] Bottini, N., Musumeci, L., Alonso, A., Rahmouni, S., Nika, K., Rostamkahani, M., MacMurray, J., Meloni, G.F., Lucarelli, P., Pellecchia, M., Eisenbarth, G.S., Comings, D. & Mustelin, T. (2004). A functional variant of lymphoid tyrosine phosphatase is associated with type I diabetes. *Nature Genetics, 36*, 337-338.

[453] Ladner, M.B., Bottini, N., Valdes, A.M. & Noble, J.A. (2005). Association of the single nucleotide polymorphism C1858T of the PTPN22 gene with type 1 diabetes. *Human Immunology, 66*, 60-64.

[454] Zheng, W. & She, J.X. (2005). Genetic association between a lymphoid tyrosine phosphatase (PTPN22) and type 1 diabetes. *Diabetes, 54*, 906-968.

[455] Qu, H., Tessier, M.C., Hudson, T.J. & Polychronakos, C. (2005). Confirmation of the association of the R620W polymorphism in the protein tyrosine phosphatase PTPN22 with type 1 diabetes in a family based study. *Journal of Medical Genetics, 42*, 266-270.

[456] Jawaheer, D., Seldin, M.F., Amos, C.I., Chen, W.Y., Shigeta, R., Etzel, C., Damle, A., Xiao, X., Chen, D., Lum, R.F., Monteiro, J., Kern, M., Criswill, L.A., Albani, S.,

Nelson, J.L., Clegg, D.O., Pope, R., Schroeder, H.W. Jr, Bridges, S.L. Jr, Pisetsky, D.S., Ward, R., Kastner, D.L., Wilder, R.L., Pincus, T., Callahan, L.F., Flemming, D., Wener, M.H. & Gregersen, P.K. (2003). Screening the genome for rheumatoid arthritis susceptibility genes: a replication study and combined analysis of 512 multicase families. *Arthritis and Rheumatism, 48*, 906-916

[457] Begovich, A.B., Carlton, V.E., Honigberg, L.A., Schrodi, S.J., Chokklingam, A.P., Alexander, H.C., Ardlie, K.G., Huang, Q., Smith, A.M., Spoerke, J.M., Conn, M.T., Chang, M., Chang, S.Y., Saiki, R.K., Catanese, J.J., leong, D.U., Garcia, V.E., McAllister, L.B., Jeffery, D.A., Lee, A.T., Baltiwalla, F., Remmers, E., Cristwell, L.A., Seldin, M.F., Kastner, D.L., Amos, C.I., Sninsky, J.J. & Gregersen, P.K. (2004). A missense single-nucleotide polymorphism in a gene encoding a protein tyrosine phosphatase (PTPN22) is associated with rheumatoid arthritis. *American Journal of Human Genetics, 75*, 330-337.

[458] Kyogoku, C., Langefeld, C.D., Ortmann, W.A., Lee, A., Selby, S., Carlton, V.E., Chang, M., Ramos, P., Baechler, E.C., Baltiwalla, F.M., Nivitzke, J., Williams, A.H., Gillett, C., Rodine, P., Graham, R.R., Ardlie, K.G., Galfney, P.M., Moser, K.L., Petri, M., Begovich, A.B., Gregersen, P.K. & Behrens, T.W. (2004). Genetic association of the R620W polymorphism of protein tyrosine phosphatase PTPN22 with human SLE. *American Journal of Human Genetics, 75*, 504-547.

[459] Hinks, A., Barton, A., John, S., Bruce, I., Hawkins, C., Griffiths, C.E., Donn, R., Thomson, W., Silman, A. & Worthingthon, J. (2005). Association between the PTPN22 gene and rheumatoid arthritis and juvenile idiopathic arthritis in a UK population: further support that PTPN22 is an autoimmunity gene. *Arthritis and Rheumatism, 52*, 1694-1699.

[460] Velaga, M.R., Wilson, V., Jennings, C.E., Owen, C.J., Herington, S., Donaldson, P.T., Ball, S.G., James, R.A., Quinton, R., Perros, P., Pearce, S.H. (2004). The codon 620 tryptophan allele of the lymphoid tyrosine phosphatase (LYP) gene is a major determinant of Graves' disease. *Journal of Clinical Endocrinology and Metabolism, 89*, 5862-5865.

[461] Skorka, A., Bernarczuk, T., Bar-Andziak, E., Nauman, J. & Ploski, R. (2005). Lymphoid tyrosine phosphatase (PTPN22/LYP) variant and Graves' disease in a Polish population: association and gene dose-dependent correlation with age of onset. *Clinical Endocrinology (Oxford), 62*, 679-682.

[462] Canton, I., Akhtar, S., Gavalas, N.G., Gawkrodger, D.J., Blomhoff, A., Watson, P.F., Weetman, A.P. & Kemp, E.H. (2005). A single-nucleotide polymorphism in the gene encoding lymphoid protein tyrosine phosphatase (PTPN22) confers susceptibility to generalised vitiligo. *Genes and Immunity, 6*, 584-587.

[463] Viken, M.K., Amundsen, S.S., Kvien, T.K., Boberg, K.M., Gilboe, I.M., Lilleby, V., Sollid, L.M., Forre, O.T., Thorsby, E., Smerdel, A. & Lie, B.A. (2005). Association analysis of the 1858C>T polymorphism in the PTPN22 gene in juvenile idiopathic arthritis and other autoimmune diseases. *Genes and Immunity, 6*, 271-273.

[464] Wu, H., Cantor, R.M., Graham, D.S., Lingren, C.M., Farwell, L., Jager, P.L., Bottini, N., Grossman, J.M., Wallace, D,J., Hahn, B.H., Julkunen, H., Hebert, L.A., Birmingham, D.J., Rioux, J.D., Yu, C.Y., Kere, J., Vyse, T.J. & Tsao, B.P. (2005).

Association analysis of the R620W polymorphism of protein tyrosine phosphatase PTPN22 in systemic lupus erythematosus families: Increased T allele frequency in systemic lupus erythematosus patients with autoimmune thyroid disease. *Arthritis and Rheumatism, 52*, 2396-2402.

[465] Criswell, L.A., Pfeiffer, K.A., Lum, R.F., Gonzales, B., Novitzke, J., Kern, M., Moser, K.L., Begovich, A.B., Carlton, V.E, Li, W., Lee, A.T., Ortmann, W., Behrens, T.W. & Gregersen, P.K. (2005). Analysis of families in the multiple autoimmune disease genetics consortium (MADGC) collection: the PTPN22 620W allele associates with multiple autoimmune phenotypes. *American Journal of Human Genetics, 76*, 561-571.

[466] Carlton, V.E., Hu, X., Chokkalingam, A.P., Schrodi, S.J., Brandon, R., Alexander, H.C., Chang, M., Catanese, J.J., Leong, D.U., Ardlie, K.G., Kastner, D.L., Seldin, M.F., Criswell, L.A., Gregersen, P.K., Beasley, E., Thomson, G., Amos, C.I. & Begovich, A.B. (2005). PTPN22 Genetic Variation: Evidence for Multiple Variants Associated with Rheumatoid Arthritis. *American Journal of Human Genetics, 77*, 567-581.

[467] Nutt, S.L., Heavey, B., Rolink, A.G. & Busslinger, M. (1999). Commintment to the B-lymphoid lineage dependens on the transcription factor Pax5. *Nature, 401*, 556-562.

[468] Kochi, Y., Yamada, R., Suzuki, A., Harley, J.B., Shirasawa, S., Sawada, T., Bae, S.C., Tokuhiro, S., Chang, X., Sekine, A., Takanashi, A., Tsunoda, T., Ohnishi, Y., Kaufman, K.M., Kang, C.P., Kang, C., Otsubo, S., Yumura, W., Mimori, A., Koike, T., Nakamura, Y., Sasazuki, T. & Yamamoto, K. (2005). A functional variant in FCRL3, encoding Fc receptor-like 3, is associated with rheumatoid arthritis and several autoimmunities. *Nature Genetics, 37*, 478-485.

[469] Capon, F., Sempirini, S., Chimenti, S., Fabrizi, G., Zambruno, G., Murgia, S., Carcassi, C., Fazio, M., Mingarelli, R., Dallapiccola, B. & Novelli, G. (2001). Fine mapping of the PSORS4 psoriasis susceptibility region on chromosome 1q21. *Journal of Investigative Dermatology, 116*, 728-730.

[470] Dai, K.Z., Harbo, H.F., Celius, E.G., Otirai, A., Sorensen, P.S., Ryder, L.P., Datta, P., Svejgaard, A., Hillert, J., Fredrikson, S., Sandberg-Wollheim, M., Laaksonen, M., Myhr, K.M., Nyland, H., Vartdal, F. & Spurkland, A. (2001). The T cell regulator gene SH2D2A contributes to the genetic susceptibility of multiple sclerosis. *Genes and Immunity, 2*, 263-268.

[471] Ravetch, J.V. & Bolland, S. (2001). IgG Fc receptors. *Annual Reviews in Immumology, 19*, 275-290.

[472] Hansen, A., Lipsky, P.E. & Dorner, T. (2005). Immunopathogenesis of primary Sjogren's syndrome: implications for disease management and therapy. *Current Opinion in Rheumatology, 17*, 558-565.

[473] Gray, D., Bergthorsdottir, S., van Essen, D., Wykes, M., Poudrier, J. & Siepmann, K. (1997). Observations on memory B-cell development. *Seminars in Immunology, 9*, 249-254.

[474] Miller, I., Hatzivassilou, G., Cattoretti, G., Mendelsohn, C. & Dalla-Favera, R. (2002). IRTAs: a new family of immunoglobulin-like receptors differentially expressed in B cells. *Blood, 99*, 2662-2669.

[475] Bach, J.F. & Chatenoud, L. (2001). Tolerance to islet autoantigens in type 1 diabetes. *Annual Reviews in Immunology, 19*, 131-161.
[476] Sakaguchi, S. (2000). Regulatory T cells: key controllers of immunologic self-tolerance. *Cell, 101*, 455-458.
[477] Ring, G.H. & Lakkis, F.G. (1999). Breakdown of self-tolerance and the pathogenesis of autoimmunity. *Seminares in Nephrology, 19*, 25-33.
[478] O'Garra, A. & Vieira, P. (2004). Regulatory T cells and mechanisms of immune system control. *Nature Medicine, 10*, 801-805.
[479] Read, S., Malstrom, V. & Powrie, F. (2000). Cytotoxic T lymphocyte-aasociated antigen 4 plays an essential role in the function of CD25(+)CD4(+) regulatory cells that control intestinal inflammation. *Journal of Experimental Medicine, 192*, 295-302.
[480] Takanashi, T., Tagami, T., Yamasaki, S., Uede, T., Shimizu, J., Sakaguchi, N. & Mak, T.W. (2000). Immunologic self-tolerance maintained by CD25(+)CD4(+) regulatory T cells constitutively expressing cytotoxic T lymphocyte-associated antigen 4. *Journal of Experimental Medicine, 192*, 303-310.
[481] Lohr, J., Knoechel, B., Nagabhushanam, V. & Abbas, A.K. (2005). T-cell tolerance and autoimmunity to systemic and tissue-restricted self-antigens. *Immunology Reviews*, 2005, 204, 116-127.
[482] Wei, W.Z., Morris, G.P. & Kong, Y.C. (2004) Anti-tumor immunity and autoimmunity: a balancing act of regulatory T cells. *Cancer Immunology and Immunotherapy, 53*, 73-78.
[483] Morgan, M.E., Witteveen, H.J., Sutmuller, R.P., de Vries, R.R. & Toes, R.E. (2004). CD25+ regulatory cells from HLA-DQ8 transgenic mice are capable of modulating collagen-induced arthritis. *Human Immunology, 65*, 1319-1327.
[484] Sutmuller, R.P., van Duivenvoorde, L.M., van Elsas, A., Schumacher, T.N., Wildenberg, M.E., Allison, J.P., Toes, R.E., Offringa, R. & Melief, C.J. (2001) Synergism of cytotoxic T lymphocyte-associated antigen 4 blockade and depletion of CD25(+) regulatory T cells in antitumor therapy reveals alternative pathways for suppression of autoreactive cytotoxic T lymphocyte responses. *Journal of Experimental Medicine, 194*, 823-832.
[485] Prudhomme, C.J., Chang, Y. & Li, X. (2002). Immunoinhibitory DNA vaccine protects against autoimmune diabetes through cDNA encoding a selective CTLA-4 (CD152) ligand. *Human Gene Therapy, 13*, 395-406.
[486] Abbas, A.K., Lohr, J., Knoechel, B. & Nagabhushanam, V. (2004) T cell tolerance and autoimmunity. *Autoimmunity Reviews, 3*, 471-475.
[487] Mustelin, T., Wang, T. & Bottini, N. (2005). Protein tyrosine phosphatases and the immune response. *Nature Reviews Immunology, 5*, 43-57.
[488] Roy, G., Mattews, J., Woodford-Thomas, T. & Thomas, M.L. (1995). The function of protein thyrosin phosphatases in immune regulation. *Advances in Protein Phoshatases, 9*, 121-138.
[489] Mustelin, T., Brockdorff, J., Gjorloff-Wingren, A., Tailor, P., Han, S., Wang, X. & Saxena, M. (1998). Lymphocyte activation: the coming of the protein tyrosine phosphatases. *Frontiers in Biosciences, 3*, D1060-D1096.

[490] Hasegawa, K., Martin, F., Huang, G., Tumas, D., Diehl, L. & Chan, A.C. (2004). PEST domain-enriched tyrosine phosphatase (PEP) regulation of effector/memory T cells. *Science, 303*, 685-689.

[491] Gavin, A., Ait-Azzouzene, D., Martensson, A., Duong, B., Verkoczy, L., Skog, J.L., Skog, P. & Nemazee, D. (2004). Peripheral B lymphocyte tolerance. *Keio Jornal of Medicine, 53*, 151-158.

[492] Tsubata, T., Wu, J. & Honjo, T. (1993). B-cell apoptosis induced by antigen receptor crosslinking is blocked by T-cell signal trough CD40. *Nature, 364*, 645-648.

[493] Parry, S.L., Hasbold, J., Holman, M. & Klaus, G.G. (1994). Hypercross-linking surface IgM or IgD receptors on mature B cells induces apoptosis that is reversed by costimulation with IL-4 and anti-CD40. *Journal of Immunology, 152*, 2821-2829.

[494] Mackus, W.J., Lens, S.M., Medema, R.H., Kwakkenbos, M.J., Evers, L.M., Oers, M.H., Lier, R.A. & Eldering., E. (2002). Prevention of B cell antigen receptor-induced apoptosis by ligation of CD40 occurs downstream of cell cycle regulation. *International Immunology, 14*, 973-982.

[495] Mehling, A., Loser, K., Varga, G., Metze, D., Luger, T.A., Schwarz, T., Grabbe, S. & Beissert, S. (2001). Overexpression of CD40 ligand in murine epidermis results in chronic skin inflammation and systemic autoimmunity. *Journal of Experimental Medicine, 194*, 615-628.

[496] Ochi, Y., Inui, T., Kouki, T., Yamashito, K., Hachiya, T. & Kajita, Y. (1998). Thyroid stimulating immunoglobulin (TSI) in Graves' disease. *Endocrine Journal, 45*, 701-718.

[497] Van Kooten, C. (2000). Immune regulation by CD40-CD40-L interactions – 2; Y2K update. *Frontiers in Bioscience, 5,* D880-D893.

[498] Elenich, L.A., Ford, C.S., Collins, J.T. & Dunnick, W.A. (1997). Gamma1 heavy chain transgenes are responsive to IFN-gamma repression and CD40 ligation. *Journal of Immunology, 158*, 4564-5473.

[499] Burdin, N., Van Kooten, C., Galibert, L., Abrams, J.S., Wijdenes, J., Banchereau, J. & Rousset, F. (1995). Endogeneous IL-6 and IL-10 contribute to the differentiation of CD40-activated human B lymphocytes. *Journal of Immunology, 154*, 2553-2544.

[500] Jirapongsananuruk, O., Melamed, I. & Leung, D.Y. (2000). Additive immunosuppressive effects of 1,25-dihydroxyvitamin D3 and corticosteroids on TH1, but not TH2, responses. *Journal of Allergy and Clinical Immunology, 106*, 981-985.

[501] Deluca, H.R. & Cantorna, M.T. (2001). Vitamin D: its role and uses in immunology. *FASEB Journal, 15*, 2579-2585.

[502] Liu, P.Y., Zhang, Y.Y., Lu, Y., Long, J.R., Shen, H., Zhao, L.J., Xu, F.H., Xiao, P., Xiong, D.H., Liu, Y.J., Recker, R.R. & Deng, H.W. (2005). A survey of haplotype variants at several disease candidate genes: the importance of rare variants for complex diseases. *Journal of Medical Genetics, 42*, 221-227.

[503] Yagil, Y. & Yagil, C (2003). Pharmacogenomic considerations for immunosuppressive therapy. *Pharmacogenomics, 4*, 309-319.

[504] Furszyfer, J., Kurland, L.T., McConahey, W.M., Woolner, L.B. & Elveback, L.R. (1972). Epidemiologic aspects of Hashimoto's thyroiditis and Graves' disease in Rochester, Minnesota (1935-1967), with special reference to temporal trends. *Metabolism, 21*, 197-204.

[505] dos Remedios, L.V., Weber, P.M., Feldman, R., Schurr, D.A.& Tsoi, T.G. (1980). Detecting unsuspected thyroid dysfunction by the free thyroxine index. *Archives of Internal Medicine, 140*, 1045-1049.

[506] Jacobson, D.L., Gange, S.J., Rose, N.R. & Graham, N.M. (1997). Epidemiology and estimated population burden of selected autoimmune diseases in the United States. *Clinical Immunology and Immunopathology, 84*, 223-243.

[507] Tunbridge, W.M., Evered, D.C., Hall. R., Appleton, D., Brewis, M., Clark, F., Evans, J.G., Young, E., Bird, T., Smith, P.A. (1977). The spectrum of thyroid disease in a community: the Whickham survey. *Clinical Endocrinology (Oxford), 7*, 481-493.

[508] Berglund, J., Christensen, S.B. & Hallengren, B. (1990). Total and age-specific incidence of Graves' thyrotoxicosis, toxic nodular goitre and solitary toxic adenoma in Malmo 1970-74. *Journal of Internal Medicine* 1990, 227, 137-141.

[509] Haraldsson, A., Gudmundsson, S.T., Larusson, G. Sigurgsson, G. (1985). Thyrotoxicosis in Iceland 1980-1982. An epidemiological survey. *Acta Medica Scandinavica, 217*, 253-258.

[510] Galofre, J.C., Garcia-Mayor, R.V., Fluiters, E., Fernandez –Calvet, L., Rego, A., Paramo, C. & Andrade, M.A. (1994). Incidence of different forms of thyroid dysfunction and its degrees in an iodine sufficient area. *Thyroidology, 6*, 49-54.

[511] Jung, C.H., sung, K.C., Shin, H.S., Rhee, E.J., Lee, W.Y., Kim, B.S., Kang, J.H., Kim H., Kim, S.W., Lee, M.H., Park, J.R. & Kim, S.W. (2003). Thyroid dysfunction and their relation to cardiovascular risk factors such as lipid profile, hsCRP, and waist hip ratio in Korea. *Korean Journal of Internal Medicine, 18*, 146-153.

[512] Maalej, A., Makni, H., Ayadi, F., Bellassoued, M., Jouida, J., Bouguacha, N., Abid, M. & Ayadi, H. (2001). A full genome screening in a large Tunisian family affected with thyroid autoimmune disorders. *Genes and Immunity, 2*, 71-75.

[513] Greenberg, D.A. & Berger, B. (1994). Using lod-score differences to determine mode of inheritance: a simple, robust method even in the presence of heterogeneity and reduced penetrance. *American Journal of Human Genetics, 55*, 834-840.

[514] Abreu, P.C., Greenberg, D.A. & Hodge, S.E. (1999). Direct power comparisons between simple LOD scores and NPL scores for linkage analysis in complex diseases. *American Journal of Human Genetics, 65*, 847-857.

INDEX

A

B

C

D

F

G

H

J

K

L

M

N

O

P

T

U

V

W

X

Y

Z